D0908137

Understanding and Preventing Noncontact ACL Injuries

American Orthopaedic Society for Sports Medicine

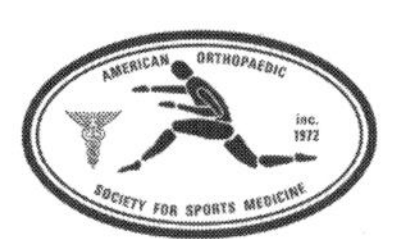

Understanding and Preventing Noncontact ACL Injuries

American Orthopaedic Society for Sports Medicine

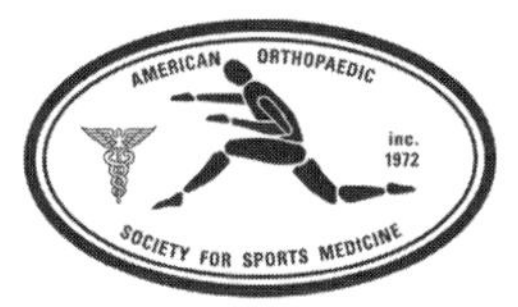

Editors

Timothy E. Hewett
Sandra J. Shultz
and Letha Y. Griffin

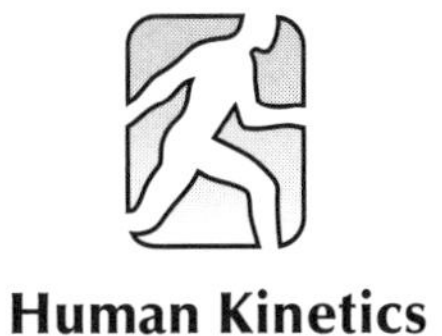

Human Kinetics

Library of Congress Cataloging-in-Publication Data

Understanding and preventing noncontact ACL injuries / American Orthopaedic Society for Sports Medicine ; Timothy E. Hewett, Sandra J. Shultz, Letha Y. Griffin, editors.
p. ; cm.
Includes bibliographical references and index.
ISBN-13: 978-0-7360-6535-1 (hard cover)
ISBN-10: 0-7360-6535-0 (hard cover)
1. Anterior cruciate ligament--Wounds and injuries--Prevention. 2. Sports injuries--Prevention. 3. Knee--Wounds and injuries--Prevention. I. Hewett, Timothy E. II. Shultz, Sandra J., 1961- III. Griffin, Letha Y. IV. American Orthopaedic Society for Sports Medicine.
[DNLM: 1. Anterior Cruciate Ligament--injuries. 2. Athletic Injuries--prevention & control. 3. Knee Injuries--prevention & control. WE 870 U55 2007]
RD561.U53 2007
617.4'7044--dc22

2006038700

ISBN-10: 0-7360-6535-0
ISBN-13: 978-0-7360-6535-1

The Web addresses cited in this text were current as of January 12, 2007, unless otherwise noted.

Acquisitions Editor: Loarn D. Robertson, PhD; **Managing Editor:** Lee Alexander; **Copyeditor:** Joyce Sexton; **Proofreader:** Pam Johnson; **Indexer:** Nancy Ball; **Permission Manager:** Carly Breeding; **Graphic Designer:** Nancy Rasmus; **Graphic Artist:** Denise Lowry; **Photo Manager:** Laura Fitch; **Cover Designer:** Keith Blomberg; **Photographer (cover):** Richard Bergen; **Art Manager:** Kelly Hendren; **Printer:** Edwards Brothers

Printed in the United States of America 10 9 8 7 6 5 4 3 2 1

Human Kinetics
Web site: www.HumanKinetics.com

United States: Human Kinetics, P.O. Box 5076, Champaign, IL 61825-5076
800-747-4457
e-mail: humank@hkusa.com

Canada: Human Kinetics, 475 Devonshire Road Unit 100, Windsor, ON N8Y 2L5
800-465-7301 (in Canada only)
e-mail: orders@hkcanada.com

Europe: Human Kinetics, 107 Bradford Road, Stanningley, Leeds LS28 6AT, United Kingdom
+44 (0) 113 255 5665
e-mail: hk@hkeurope.com

Australia: Human Kinetics, 57A Price Avenue, Lower Mitcham, South Australia 5062
08 8372 0999
e-mail: liaw@hkaustralia.com

New Zealand: Human Kinetics, Division of Sports Distributors NZ Ltd.,
P.O. Box 300 226 Albany, North Shore City, Auckland
0064 9 448 1207
e-mail: info@humankinetics.co.nz

Contents

Contributors xvii
Preface. xix
An Introduction to Understanding and Preventing ACL Injury xxi

Timothy Edwin Hewett, PhD, FACSM

The incidence of anterior cruciate ligament (ACL) injuries in young athletes (<25 years of age) remains high. Despite early recognition, initial appropriate care, adequate surgical stabilization (if needed), and a well-structured rehabilitation program, arthritis of the injured knee frequently develops. Therefore, prevention strategies to decrease its incidence are needed. This book presents the latest research on the causes and prevention of ACL injuries, particularly among female athletes. In particular, we review the effects of programs that have been recently developed to prevent ACL injury and address the following questions: What are the essential components of effective programs? What do the various programs have in common, and can one assume that these shared components are, therefore, the essential components of an ACL prevention program? How do these programs favorably alter neuromuscular risk factors; or, stated in an alternative way, how do they influence biomechanics to decrease risk? What new information on risk factors has come forth that could be used to improve or broaden our present thoughts on prevention strategies or more reliably identify those at increased risk of sustaining an ACL injury?

Summary. xxviii

Part I The Problem of ACL Injuries 1

Part Editor: Letha Y. Griffin, MD, PhD

Chapter 1 Incidence of ACL Injury 5

Stephen W. Marshall, PhD; Darin Padua, PhD, ATC; and Melanie McGrath, MS, ATC

The goal of this chapter is to examine advances in data collection and changes in incidence data regarding noncontact ACL injury. Significant progress has been made in the last five years in developing mechanisms to collect more detailed information on ACL injuries, particularly at the collegiate level. Despite initiation of prevention efforts, the overall risk of ACL injuries in collegiate female soccer and basketball has not declined since 1998, and the risk is still three to four times that of male counterparts in these sports. Anterior cruciate ligament injuries also are a concern in other contact (football) and noncontact (gymnastics) sports; prevention efforts should be focused on these activities as well. Rule modifications implemented at the sport governing board level may be another way to enhance prevention efforts, particularly in contact situations.

Human Movement and ACL Injury . . . 5
What Is Incidence? . . . 6
What Is the Average Incidence of ACL Injury in the General Population? . . . 7
National Ambulatory Care Surveys . . . 7
Summary . . . 9
How Does ACL Injury Incidence Vary by Age and Gender? . . . 9
How Does the Incidence of ACL Injury Vary by Sport and Gender? . . . 12
Literature Review Methods . . . 12
Abstraction of Incidence Data . . . 13
General Results . . . 15
Synthesis and Commentary . . . 26
Conclusions . . . 28
Recommendations for Future Research . . . 29

Chapter 2 Does ACL Reconstruction Prevent Articular Degeneration? . . . 31

The ACL Risk Equation

Paul H. Marks, MD; Kurt P. Droll, MD, MSc, FRCSC; and Michelle Cameron-Donaldson, MD

Osteoarthritis is found more commonly in the knee than in any other weight-bearing joint in the human body. Individuals with ACL insufficiency have been found to have a higher risk for developing osteoarthritis in the knee compared to the general population. Several risk factors have been implicated in the development of osteoarthritis in the ACL-deficient knee, including concomitant meniscal pathology, osteochondral pathology, impaired proprioception, and biomechanical mediators. The chapter reviews the evidence pertaining to these risk factors. In addition, in an effort to aid in the future prognosis of posttraumatic osteoarthritis, we propose that an "ACL risk equation" be developed that would express overall osteoarthritis risk quantitatively. This proposed equation would be a function of all the pertinent risk factors.

Meniscal Pathology . . . 33
Osteochondral Pathology . . . 36
Impaired Proprioception . . . 40
Biochemical Mediators . . . 42
Summary and Future Work . . . 44

Chapter 3 The Costs Associated With ACL Injury . . . 47

Timothy Edwin Hewett, PhD, FACSM;
and Bohdanna T. Zazulak, DPT, MS, OCS

In this chapter, we review the financial and emotion burdens placed on individuals, families, and societies from ACL injuries. We compare these costs with the amount of federal funding that has been expended to research ACL injuries and their prevention. We also present an analysis of the potential savings that would occur if ACL injury prevention programs were instituted on a more extensive basis. It is concluded that greater awareness

at both the governmental and public levels is needed to enhance efforts to reduce the incidence of ACL injury.

Who Pays for ACL Injury Prevention in the High-Risk Female Athlete? 52
Informing the High-Risk Female Athlete 54
Summary 56

Part II ACL Injury Prevention Programs 57

Part Editor: Timothy Edwin Hewett, PhD, FACSM

Chapter 4 Components of Prevention Programs 61

Holly J. Silvers, MPT

Twelve ACL intervention programs that have empirically evaluated outcomes were identified. A component analysis of these programs was performed to identify some of the commonalities among successful ACL intervention protocols. Numerous deficits have been identified in the high-risk female adolescent population. These include faulty landing kinematics (hip and knee extension with valgus perturbation), decreased core stability, decreased hamstring contraction times, decreased hamstring and abductor dynamic control, excessive tibial torsion, and subtalar pronation. The existing programs focus on neuromuscular and proprioceptive interventions in the female athletic population in order to reduce the rate of ACL injury in this population. The commonalities of successful programs are discussed.

Chapter 5 Theories on How Neuromuscular Intervention Programs May Influence ACL Injury Rates 75

The Biomechanical Effects of Plyometric, Balance, Strength, and Feedback Training

Timothy Edwin Hewett, PhD, FACSM; Gregory D. Myer, MS, CSCS; and Kevin R. Ford, MS

A systematic review of the published literature yielded six studies of interventions targeted toward knee or ACL injury prevention in female athletes. Five of the six interventions were reported to reduce injury incidence, four of the six reduced knee injury incidence, and three of the six reduced ACL injury incidence in females. Examination of the similarities and differences among the training regimes gives insight into the development of more effective and efficient interventions. The purpose of this review is to highlight the relative effectiveness of these interventions in altering landing techniques and dynamic balance, as well as the common components of the training. This review focuses on the common components of the various interventions in order to discuss their potential to reduce ACL injury risk and assess their potential for combined use in more effective and efficient intervention protocols.

Single-Component Training 84
Multicomponent Training 87
Effects of a Comprehensive Program Combined With Either Plyometric or Balance Components 89
Conclusions and Future Directions 89

to study the injury in the lab, try to devise prevention strategies, test the prevention strategies, and continually revise the prevention strategies. The prevention programs that have been developed to date target known risk factors, yet several unanswered questions remain. For example, do these training effects generalize to the competitive situation? Do they lead to long-term behavior change? Do they have sufficient power for a reasonable effect size? Do they address potentially important but unexplored variables such as stretching and endurance? Finally, must these programs be completed exactly as prescribed, or can they serve as suggestions for a variety of activities? This chapter explores possible answers to these questions and proposes one central skill that may be the most effective in reducing injury incidence.

ACL-Loading Mechanisms and Risk Factors for Noncontact ACL Injury 109
Current Training Programs 115
Future Training Program Development 117

Chapter 9 Discussion, Summary, and Future Research Goals . . 121

Lars Engebretsen, MD, PhD

This chapter summarizes issues related to successful prevention programs that have recently been evaluated. This includes a discussion of the nature of interventions (cognitive and psychomotor approaches), delivery mechanisms, duration, and follow-up. In addition, we offer suggestions regarding needs for future prevention programs.

Part III Biomechanical and Neuromuscular Mechanisms of ACL Injuries 129

Part Editor: Timothy Edwin Hewett, PhD, FACSM

Chapter 10 Biomechanics Associated With Injury 131

Athlete Interviews and Review of Injury Tapes

Tron Krosshaug, PhD; and Roald Bahr, MD, PhD

A precise description of the biomechanics associated with injury—the injury mechanism—is a key component to understanding the causes of any particular injury type in sport. However, any attempt to describe the injury mechanisms raises a number of issues. A complete understanding of injury causation needs to take into account the multifactorial nature of sport injuries—not only the injury biomechanics, but also the risk factors associated with an increased risk of injury. This chapter reviews studies aimed at assessing multiple variables associated with the specific event in which a noncontact ACL injury occurred, including studies in which athletes have been interviewed about their recollection of these variables and studies in which videotapes of injury events have been analyzed.

Defining “Injury Mechanisms” 131
Describing the Inciting Event 132
Research Approaches to Describe the Injury Mechanisms 134
Literature Search 135
Athlete Interviews 136

Video Analysis . . . 138
Conclusions . . . 140

Chapter 11 Clinical Biomechanical Studies on ACL Injury Risk Factors . . . 141

Laura J. Huston, MS

This chapter reviews clinical studies that have investigated the biomechanics of ACL injury. It is concluded that kinematic and kinetic gender differences exist that may render women more susceptible than men to ACL injury. The most prevalent differences that females exhibited, either when landing from a jump or during a cutting and pivoting maneuver, were reduced hip and knee flexion angles, increased knee valgus, internal rotation of the femur, high quadriceps activity unbalanced by the hamstrings, and inadequate generation of trans-knee muscle stiffness.

Background . . . 141
Kinematic and Kinetic Differences . . . 142
Jump Landings . . . 142
Sidestep and Cutting Maneuvers . . . 147
Muscular Differences . . . 149
Conclusions . . . 153

Chapter 12 Effects of Neuromuscular Training on Lower Extremity Motion Patterns . . . 155

Bing Yu, PhD; and Marlene DeMaio, MD

Understanding the biomechanical changes following training programs is critical in the development of intervention strategies for reducing the risk of sustaining noncontact ACL injuries. Scientifically evaluating the effectiveness of these training programs is difficult. It is helpful to have a good understanding of the effects of various exercises on the biomechanics of the movements in those athletic tasks in which noncontact ACL injuries frequently occur. Such understanding will not only assist clinicians and scientists in deciding which exercises to include in intervention programs, but also provide indirect evidence to support the effectiveness of intervention programs. Biomechanical studies with sophisticated modeling techniques to estimate in vivo ACL loading in athletic tasks are particularly needed to elucidate cause-and-effect relationships between movements and ACL loading and injuries. These types of biomechanical studies will be critical tools for identifying specific motor control–related biomechanical risk factors, as well as for evaluating intervention programs aimed at reducing the risk of noncontact ACL injuries.

Combined Training Programs Including Plyometrics . . . 155

Chapter 13 Sport-Specific Injury Mechanisms Associated With Pivoting, Cutting, and Landing . . . 163

Mary Lloyd Ireland, MD

The typical mechanism of ACL injury in basketball, soccer, and team handball is a rapid but awkward stop and anticipation of lateral move-

of jumping and landing maneuvers required in these activities. Possible reasons for lack of ACL injuries in these populations, such as muscular control, shoe–surface interface, minimal foot fixation, forward center of gravity, landing with flexed knees, and choreographed movements, are examined. Prevention strategies stemming from this examination are discussed.

Muscular Control 191
Shoe–Surface Interface 192
Center of Gravity and Proprioception 192
Choreography 193
Additional Considerations 193
What About Gymnasts? 193
Summary 194

Chapter 17 The Role of Biofeedback in Preventing Noncontact ACL Injuries 195

Julie R. Steele, PhD; and Bridget J. Munro, PhD

A perpetual challenge confronting practitioners implementing ACL prevention programs is the ability to monitor the technique of athletes during training sessions and then to "feed" this information back to athletes in real time so that they can modify their motion to achieve the desired performance. To address this challenge, sophisticated biofeedback devices have been developed to monitor aspects of performance—particularly muscle recruitment patterns and joint motion. Although highly sophisticated, many of the biofeedback devices available typically have rigid components that do not conform to the individual's body shape; thus they interfere with the person's natural motion during performance of a movement and possibly pose a safety hazard. However, recent advances in polymer science now enable the integration of inherently conducting polymers into appropriate host fabrics, creating the opportunity to develop wearable textile sensors that offer novel biomonitoring options for use in ACL injury prevention programs. These fabric sensors, with strain gauge-like properties that have a wide dynamic range, are ideal for biomonitoring applications. They can be worn without interfering with normal human motion and, when connected to appropriate electronic circuitry, can also act as unique systems capable of providing biofeedback to the wearer with respect to joint motion. The chapter provides an overview of biofeedback devices that have been used in landing training programs to reduce the rate of noncontact ACL ruptures.

The Role of Biofeedback in ACL Injury Prevention 195
Biofeedback, Neuromuscular Activity, and ACL Injury Prevention 196
Biofeedback, Knee Joint Motion, and ACL Injury Prevention 201
The Role of Biofeedback in Preventing ACL Reinjury 204
Future Directions for Biofeedback and ACL Injury Prevention 204

Part IV Hormonal and Anatomic Risk Factors and Preventive Bracing for ACL Injuries 207

Part Editor: Sandra J. Shultz, PhD, ATC, CSCS

Chapter 18 Ligament Biology and Its Relationship to Injury Forces 213

James R. Slauterbeck, MD; John R. Hickox, MS; and Daniel M. Hardy, PhD

Recent research indicates that ligament remodeling varies by sex and animal model. It has been demonstrated that tissue remodeling favors strengthening and repair in human males who have a higher ratio of collagen to matrix metalloproteinases (MMPs; MMP3 protein correlates with mRNA). We explore how sex hormones in part regulate collagen synthesis and degradation in humans and the implications for ACL injury.

Relationships Among ACL Injury Factors 214
Effects of Tissue Remodeling 215
Sex, Hormones, and ACL Injury 217

Chapter 19 Hormonal Influences on Ligament Biology 219

Sandra J. Shultz, PhD, ATC, CSCS

Research over the past decade has begun to address the complex relationship between sex hormones and ACL injury through three primary avenues of study. At the microscopic level, sex hormones have been examined for their influence on the structure and metabolism of the ligament through laboratory studies in cell culture as well as animals and human ligament tissues. At a macroscopic level, sex hormones have been investigated for their effects on knee joint laxity and stiffness, with comparisons drawn between males and females as well as within females across different phases of their menstrual cycle. Lastly, epidemiological studies have addressed the relationship between menstrual cycle phase and ACL injury incidence. This chapter critically reviews the evidence in each area of study regarding how sex hormones may play a role in noncontact ACL injury. Further research is needed to determine the effects of sex hormones on ACL biology and function, as well as the changing hormonal profiles in the days immediately preceding ACL injury.

Sex Hormone Profiles: Not All Menstrual Cycles Are Created Equal 219
Sex Hormone Effects on Collagen Structure and Metabolism. 221
Sex Hormones and Knee Joint Laxity and Stiffness 225
Menstrual Cycle and ACL Injury 229
Summary. 233
Birth Control Hormones, Ligament Biology, and ACL Injury 234
Summary. 237

Chapter 20 Anatomical Factors in ACL Injury Risk. 239

Sandra J. Shultz, PhD, ATC, CSCS; Anh-Dung Nguyen, MS Ed, ATC; and Bruce D. Beynnon, PhD

Anatomical characteristics are often cited as one of four risk factor classifications (environmental, anatomic, hormonal, and neuromuscular/biomechanical) that have been proposed to explain the increased risk of ACL injury in females. While much has been learned about gender differences in neuromuscular and biomechanical function in recent years, the influence of lower extremity anatomy on neuromuscular and biomechanical function and ACL risk remains elusive. This chapter reviews what is known about gender differences in lower extremity anatomy and the potential relationships between lower extremity anatomical factors, dynamic knee joint function, and noncontact ACL injury. We present evidence that examining a single anatomical factor without accounting for the presence of other alignment factors may partially explain why it has been difficult to reliably identify relationships between anatomic alignment and ACL injury risk. Postural alignment of the entire lower extremity, from the pelvis to the foot, are considered, as malalignment at one segment or joint may profoundly influence the alignment of other segments or joints and ultimately knee joint function

Notch Size and Width 240
Generalized Joint Laxity 241
Anterior Knee Laxity 243
Anatomical Alignment. 249
Conclusions 257

Chapter 21 Intrinsic and Extrinsic Forces Associated With ACL Injury 259

Can Functional Bracing Reduce the Risk of ACL Injury?

Bruce D. Beynnon, PhD; and James R. Slauterbeck, MD

Three questions are examined in this chapter: What are the intrinsic and extrinsic forces associated with ACL injury? Do the extrinsic forces produced by functional bracing protect the injured ACL or ACL graft? Does functional bracing protect the ACL-deficient knee? After a review of laboratory and video analysis of forces associated with ACL strain and injury, the chapter explores data on the effects of bracing on uninjured, ACL-deficient, and ACL-reconstructed knees. In the past, prophylactic knee braces have not been found to prevent injury in the uninjured. Evidence does suggest that functional knee braces can reduce anterior-posterior laxity of the ACL-deficient knee to within the limits of the normal knee during nonweight-bearing or weight-bearing activities. However, in the ACL-deficient knee, braces cannot reduce the abnormal anterior displacement of the tibia relative to the femur that is produced as the knee transitions from nonweight-bearing to weight-bearing conditions. Field studies

Contributors

Roald Bahr, MD, PhD
Chair, Oslo Sports Trauma Research Center
Professor of Sports Medicine
Chair, Department of Sports Medicine
The Norwegian University of Sport and Physical Education

Bruce D. Beynnon, PhD
Associate Professor
Director of Research
Department of Orthopaedics and Rehabilitation
McClure Musculoskeletal Research Center
University of Vermont

Michelle Cameron-Donaldson, MD
Orthopedic Surgeon
Park Clinic
Livingston Orthopaedic & Rehabilitation Institute

Captain Marlene DeMaio, MD
Bone & Joint/Sports Medicine Institute
Orthopaedics Department
Naval Medical Center Portsmouth

Kurt P. Droll, MD, MSc, FRCSC
Clinical Fellow
Department of Orthopaedics
University of Southern Califormia

Lars Engebretsen, MD, PhD
Oslo Sports Trauma Research Center
The Norwegian University of Sport and Physical Education

Carl F. Ettlinger, MSME
President, Vermont Safety Research

Kevin R. Ford, MS
Research Biomechanist, The Sports Medicine Biodynamics Center
The Human Performance Laboratory
Cincinnati Children's Hospital Medical Center

William E. Garrett, Jr., MD, PhD
Professor of Surgery
Department of Orthopaedics
Duke University Medical Center

Letha Y. Griffin, MD, PhD
Adjunct and Clinical Professor
Department of Kinesiology and Health
Georgia State University
Clinical Staff, Peachtree Orthopaedic Clinic

Daniel M. Hardy, PhD
Assistant Professor
Cell Biology Biochemistry Lab
Texas Tech University

Timothy Edwin Hewett, PhD, FACSM
Director and Associate Professor, The Sports Medicine Biodynamics Center
The Human Performance Laboratory
Cincinnati Children's Hospital Medical Center
University of Cincinnati College of Medicine
Departments of Pediatrics and Orthopaedic Surgery

John R. Hickox, MS
Cell Biology Biochemistry Lab
Texas Tech University

Laura J. Huston, MS
Department of Orthopaedics
Vanderbilt University

Mary Lloyd Ireland, MD
President, Kentucky Sports Medicine Clinic

Robert J. Johnson, MD
McClure Professor of Musculoskeletal Research
Department of Orthopaedics & Rehabilitation
University of Vermont College of Medicine

Tron Krosshaug, PhD
Fellow, Oslo Sports Trauma Research Center
The Norwegian University of Sport and Physical Education

Paul H. Marks, MD
Assistant Professor of Orthopaedic Surgery, University of Toronto
Orthopaedic & Arthritic Institute
Sunnybrook and Women's College Health Sciences Centre

Stephen W. Marshall, PhD
Assistant Professor, Department of Epidemiology
School of Public Health
University of North Carolina

Melanie McGrath, MS, ATC
School of Public Health
University of North Carolina

Bridget J. Munro, PhD
Department of Biomedical Science
University of Wollongong, Australia

Gregory D. Myer, MS, CSCS
Sports Biomechanist, The Sports Medicine Biodynamics Center
The Human Performance Laboratory
Cincinnati Children's Hospital Medical Center

Anh-Dung Nguyen, MS Ed, ATC
Department of Exercise and Sports Science
University of North Carolina at Greensboro

Darin Padua, PhD, ATC
School of Public Health
University of North Carolina

Christine D. Pollard, PhD, PT
Assistant Professor of Research Physical Therapy
Division of Biokinesiology & Physical Therapy at the School of Dentistry
University of Southern California

Christopher M. Powers, PhD, PT
Associate Professor
Director, Program in Biokinesiology
Co-Director, Musculoskeletal Biomechanics Research Lab
Division of Biokinesiology & Physical Therapy, School of Dentistry
Department Radiology & Orthopaedic Surgery, Keck School of Medicine
University of Southern California

Sandra J. Shultz, PhD, ATC, CSCS
Assistant Professor, Co-Director, Applied Neuromechanics Research Laboratory
Department of Exercise and Sports Science
University of North Carolina at Greensboro

Susan M. Sigward, PhD, PT, ATC
Assistant Professor of Research Physical Therapy
Musculoskeletal Biomechanics Research Laboratory
Division of Biokinesiology & Physical Therapy at the School of Dentistry
University of Southern California

Holly J. Silvers, MPT
Director of Research/Physical Therapist
Santa Monica Orthopaedic and Sports Medicine Research Foundation

James R. Slauterbeck, MD
Associate Professor
University of Vermont College of Medicine
Department of Orthopaedics & Rehabilitation

Julie R. Steele, PhD
Department of Biomedical Science
University of Wollongong, Australia

Carol C. Teitz, MD
Professor, Department of Orthopaedics and Sports Medicine
University of Washington

Bing Yu, PhD
Associate Professor
Division of Physical Therapy
Department of Allied Health Sciences
University of North Carolina at Chapel Hill

Bohdanna T. Zazulak, DPT, MS, OCS
Adjunct Faculty/Physical Therapist
Department of Physical Therapy, Quinnipiac University
Department of Rehabilitation Services, Yale Physicians Building
Yale-New Haven Hospital

Preface

It is estimated that each year somewhere between 75,000 and 250,000 individuals in the United States will suffer a new injury to the anterior cruciate ligament (ACL) of the knee. These injuries occur primarily in young, healthy individuals, most commonly as a result of sudden changes in direction or speed during physical activities such as sports. In these situations, the injuries are a product of indirect forces to the knee, as opposed to direct contact with the lower extremity, and are often classified as "noncontact" ACL injuries.

As more girls and young women have become involved in sports such as soccer and basketball in the last three decades, it has become increasingly apparent that females are at much greater risk for noncontact ACL injuries than are males. Studies incorporating injury surveillance methods have consistently shown that the rate of ACL tears by number of exposures is two to eight times greater among females than males. It is estimated that 1.4 million women and girls have torn their ACL over the last decade. The incidence of noncontact ACL injuries in young females has been reported to be as high as one out of 100 high school girls (30,000 each year in the United States) and one out of 10 collegiate women who participate in sports.

In relation to the number of people who sustain an ACL injury, the costs involved with these injuries are equally staggering. The procedure of ACL reconstruction has been listed as the sixth most common surgical procedure performed by orthopedic fellows. If one estimates that 100,000 ACL reconstructions are done each year in the United States (a conservative estimate), at a cost of $17,000 per reconstruction, over 1.5 billion medical dollars are required merely for reconstruction in those with this injury. This cost does not take into account the initial evaluation of those injured, the rehabilitation of those selecting nonoperative care, or the anticipated costs of caring for those who will develop posttraumatic degenerative joint disease 5 to 10 years following their injury.

Not only do noncontact ACL injuries have a severe financial impact on families and on society; they are also associated with significant emotional and physiological consequences to the injured individual. An athlete who tears an ACL is usually forced to miss an entire season of competition. Although current surgical and rehabilitation techniques have accelerated return to play in many athletes, others face a lengthy recovery period of 6 to 12 months. Moreover, 25% of those who suffer an ACL injury do not achieve their previous level of activity after surgery. In addition, osteoarthritis is markedly increased in people who sustain an ACL injury, even following successful ACL reconstruction. Hence, prevention strategies based on understanding of causally related factors are needed.

Unfortunately, the precise mechanisms by which noncontact ACL injuries occur have remained unresolved. It is known that ACL tears tend to occur in situations in which an athlete lands or cuts in an off-balanced, upright position, particularly if there is rotation or inward bend at the knee at the time. It has been speculated that the tear is a product of a large eccentric quadriceps force unopposed by the hamstrings, although the role and source of an intrinsic force remain controversial. Better clarification of the biomechanics of injury-associated maneuvers is needed to help young athletes, particularly young female athletes, avoid the injury. Whether and to what extent environmental factors (e.g., shoe–surface interface), anatomical factors (e.g., size of ACL, notch width), and physiological factors (e.g., hormonal status) influence and contribute to the rate of injury are unknown as well.

It is also imperative that we discover risk factors and mechanisms of injury in order to be able to construct and implement effective prevention programs. The vast majority of active young people do not experience an ACL tear. Consequently, research conducted over the last decade has sought to identify variables that might suggest which individuals are most at risk for ACL injury. The results from these investigations hold promise with respect to the development of targeted, tailored preventive interventions.

The purpose of this book is to provide the most up-to-date research on how noncontact ACL injury occurs, who is most at risk for these injuries, and why female athletes suffer these injuries at a much higher rate than their male counterparts, as well as to discuss the effectiveness of programs designed to reduce one's risk of noncontact ACL injury. We also provide resources for athletic directors, coaches, parents, and athletes who would like to learn more about how to implement a prevention program in their school, sport club, or league.

An Introduction to Understanding and Preventing ACL Injury

Timothy Edwin Hewett, PhD, FACSM

It is estimated that each year, anywhere from 75,000 to over 250,000 individuals in the United States will suffer a new injury to the anterior cruciate ligament (ACL) of the knee. The ACL is a primary ligament holding the knee joint intact and helps to create the hinge joint of the knee (figure I.1). Injuries to this both stabilizing and mobilizing structure of the knee occur primarily in young, healthy individuals, most commonly as a result of sudden changes in direction or speed during physical activities such as sports. In these situations, the injuries are a product of indirect forces to the knee, as opposed to direct contact with the lower extremity, and are often classified as "noncontact" ACL injuries. These noncontact ACL injuries occur at a four- to sixfold higher incidence in female athletes than in male athletes.

The purpose of this book is to provide the most up-to-date research on how noncontact ACL injury occurs, who is most at risk for these injuries, and why female athletes incur these injuries at a much higher rate than their male counterparts, as well as to discuss the effectiveness of programs designed to reduce one's risk of noncontact ACL injury. We also provide resources for athletic directors, coaches, parents, and athletes who would like to learn more about how to implement a prevention program in their school, sport club, or league. Each section of the book includes a summary of "take-home messages" and clinical applications that will relate scientific findings to elements of successful preventive efforts.

The target audience of this book is physicians, scientists, athletic trainers, physical therapists, clinicians, coaches, athletic directors, and athletes and their parents. This book should serve as a valuable reference in the quest to understand ACL injuries in the female athlete, as well as drive you, the reader, toward action in preventing these devastating injuries. We owe this to our young female athletes. I grew up with six sisters; five were older, and at least half of them were better athletes than I was. This upbringing gave me a great

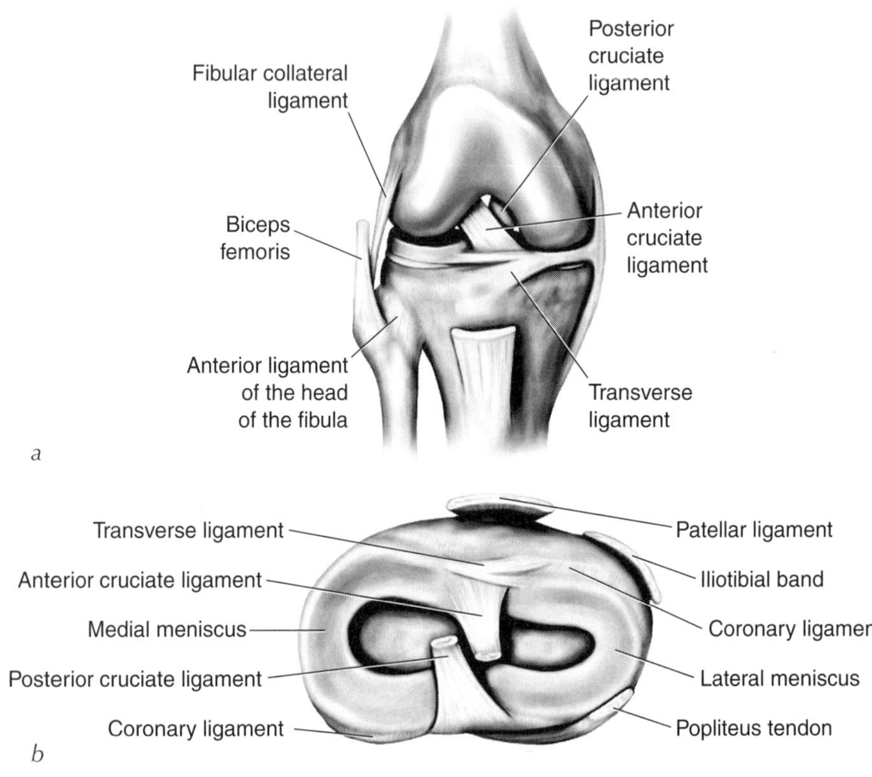

FIGURE I.1 Location of the ACL within the knee: *(a)* anterior view with patella removed and *(b)* superior view.

Reprinted, by permission, from R.S. Behnke, 2006, *Kinetic anatomy,* 2nd ed. (Champaign, IL: Human Kinetics), 194.

appreciation for the talent, power, and toughness of the female athlete. My sister Patti was the fastest kid in our neighborhood in the 1960s. She remained a good athlete in later years, but given the opportunities she might have had under Title IX, she might have accomplished greater goals. My sister Jenny tore her ACL playing basketball. She now lives with debilitating knee arthritis. We have given these girls and women greater opportunities to compete at the levels that boys and men do, but we have not adequately prepared them to compete at those levels. Again, this is something we owe them.

The issues of Title IX, the greater incidence of ACL injuries in females, and the potential contributions of hormonal factors are politically charged and constantly debated. Sometimes a little knowledge can be dangerous; and the idea that a coach, parent, or athletic director, or worse yet a clinician, would limit a young athlete's participation based on which phase of her cycle she is in, is disturbing to those of us in the field. However, as informed clinicians and researchers we should work to set aside the politics and set aside our biases, and examine the relevant data in order to help these young athletes. In the clinical and scientific arenas, there is no room for politics. There is also no room for exaggerations or misconceptions. The sky is not falling on these young athletes.

With the increased media coverage of high-profile female athletes who have suffered ACL injuries, it has been extrapolated that this must in fact be an epidemic in females during athletic participation. This is an important problem, but it is absolutely not an epidemic. An epidemic is defined as "a widespread outbreak of an infectious disease; many people are infected at the same time" or as an outbreak "of disease or anything resembling a disease; attacking or affecting many individuals in a community or a population simultaneously; such as 'an epidemic outbreak of influenza.'" Though ACL injuries occur at a higher incidence in females than males, they constitute an important medical dilemma, but not an epidemic. Young women gain much greater benefits from sport participation than they lose from an approximately 1% chance of an ACL injury.

We should point out that more ACL injuries still occur in men and boys than in women and girls (see chapter 1 for a complete discussion). It is in rate, or incidence, that females far exceed males in ACL rupture. An incidence or rate is the number of injuries per number of exposures (hours of participation in games or practices), whereas prevalence is the absolute number of injuries in a population at a given time. Females have a greater incidence, but not a greater prevalence, of ACL injuries than males. The absolute number remains greater in male athletes.

Title IX Education Amendments of 1972 (Title 20 USC Section 1681) states, "No person in the United States shall, on the basis of sex, be excluded from participation in, be denied the benefits of, or be subjected to discrimination under any education program or activity receiving federal financial assistance" (Shelbourne et al. 1995). This landmark legislation prohibits discrimination in schools on the basis of sex in all curricular and extracurricular activities at educational institutions that receive federal funding. Title IX governs the overall equity of treatment and opportunity in athletics while giving schools the flexibility to choose sports based on student body interest, geographic influence, budget restraints, and gender ratio.

There are three primary areas that may be monitored to determine if an institution is in compliance with Title IX: athletic financial assistance, accommodation of athletic interests/abilities, and interscholastic sport programming. Appraisal of compliance is on a program-wide basis, not on a sport-by-sport basis. Title IX requires schools or other covered educational institutions to offer members of both sexes equal opportunities to play sports, allocate athletic scholarships equitably, and treat male and female athletes equally at all levels.

In the past, ACL injuries often resulted in a premature end to a career in sport, as occurred with Rebecca Lobo, an early star of the WNBA. Rehabilitation following ACL injury and surgical reconstruction has undergone a drastic evolution in the past few decades. Increased knowledge of the ligament remodeling and healing process, as well as of biomechanics in the knee joint after injury and reconstruction, together with physiological and neuromuscular aspects of training, has significantly improved rehabilitation programs. The treatment after rupture of the ACL may be operative or conservative. In both cases, the goal is to reach the best functional level for the athlete without risking new injuries or degenerative changes in the knee.

In the recent past (up to the early 1980s), the recommended treatment to protect the healing knee included 6 to 8 weeks of immobilization, 8 to 12 weeks on crutches, and the avoidance of early isolated quadriceps contractions. Furthermore, a return to sporting activities was not permitted until 9 to 12 months following surgery. In the early 1990s, an accelerated rehabilitation approach to ACL repair was first reported (Shelbourne et al. 1995). The patients who followed this treatment exhibited better strength and range of motion, had fewer patellofemoral complaints, and had an earlier return to sport. In current more accelerated protocols, the patients are allowed to return to light sporting activities such as running at two to three months after surgery and to contact sports, including cutting and jumping, after six months (Kvist 2004). It is our duty as clinicians and researchers to continue clinical research in order to improve our rehabilitation while protecting the healing reconstructed graft as much as possible.

Physicians, physical therapists, athletic trainers, and researchers should play an active role in the multidisciplinary efforts to determine the mechanism and etiology of the gender differences in ACL injuries. Careful and thorough clinical and laboratory investigation will enable us to better understand these knee injuries that are more prevalent in female athletes and help guide us in preventive strategies. Though no definitive etiology for the discrepancy in occurrence of these injuries between the sexes has been established, structural, hormonal, and neuromuscular factors have been proposed (Hewett 2000). These structural and hormonal factors may play a role in ACL injuries, yet no conclusive studies unequivocally demonstrate a difference in ACL injury involving any of these factors. Furthermore, interventions aimed at injury reduction are unlikely to influence less modifiable anatomic and hormonal factors. Therefore, research and clinical efforts are primarily focused on neuromuscular etiologies over which clinicians may have some influence.

Dynamic muscular control of knee joint alignment, specifically differences in muscle recruitment, firing patterns, and strength, may be partially responsible for the gender disparity in incidence of ACL injury (Zazulak et al. 2005). There is evidence that neuromuscular training alters muscle firing patterns, decreases landing forces, improves balance, and reduces ACL injury incidence in female athletes (Hewett et al. 2005c). Current rehabilitation programs focus not only on strengthening exercises, but also on proprioceptive and neuromuscular control drills in order to provide a neurologic stimulus for the athlete to regain the dynamic stability needed for safe participation in athletic competition (figures I.2 and I.3).

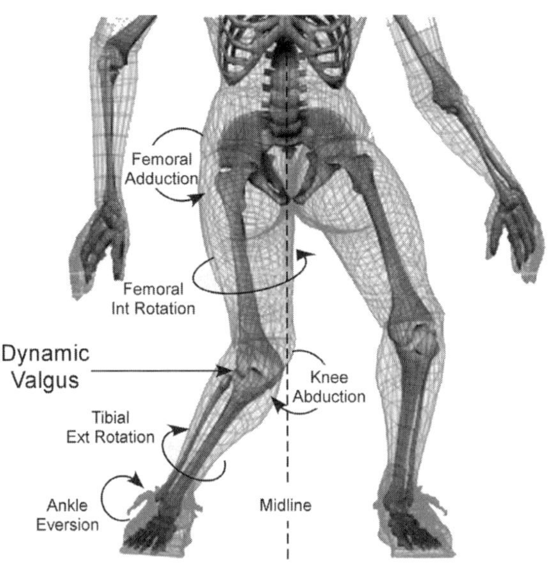

FIGURE I.2 Valgus lower extremity alignment.

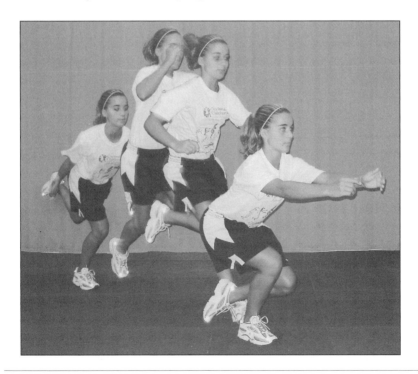

FIGURE I.3 Plyometric-core stability training.

These concepts were central to the recent development of prevention programs to reduce injury rates. Hewett and colleagues recently completed a systematic review of the published studies of interventions targeted toward ACL injury prevention in female athletes (Hewett, Myer, and Ford 2005a). Five of the six studies reviewed demonstrated significant reduction of injuries in general; four of the six showed reduction of knee injuries, and three of the six showed reduction of ACL injury rates specifically (see figure I.4). The common components of the effective interventions emphasized plyometric power, biomechanics and technique, strength, balance, and core stability training. With this evidence in support of the effectiveness of neuromuscular training in knee and ACL injury reduction in female athletes, it is our responsibility as clinicians and health care professionals to implement screening and prevention programs in our communities, as well as to advocate for insurance reimbursement for preventive intervention.

Future approaches could be to use epidemiologic analysis to assess the relative efficacy of these interventions in order to achieve the optimal effect in the most efficient manner possible. Selective combination of neuromuscular training components may provide additive effects, further reducing the risk of ACL injuries in female athletes. Additional research directions include the assessment of relative injury risk using mass neuromuscular screening. The development of screening and intervention protocols may lead to the reduction of ACL injury incidence through identification of the high-risk female athlete displaying neuromuscular control deficits (Hewett et al. 2005b).

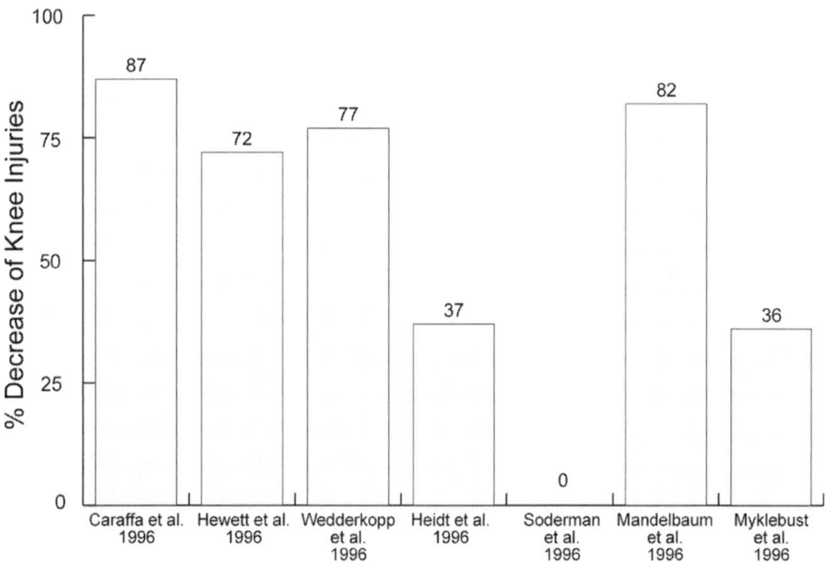

FIGURE I.4 Effects of neuromuscular training on ACL injury.

Regular physical activity is necessary for maintaining normal muscle strength, joint structure, and neuromuscular function. In the range recommended for health, physical activity is not associated with joint damage or development of osteoarthritis and may be beneficial for many people with arthritis. However, sport-related injuries that result from competitive athletics may be associated with the development of osteoarthritis later in life. There is evidence of devastating long-term effects of ACL laxity in young female athletes to the medial tibiofemoral compartment knee joint, as chronic micromotion may lead to cartilage degeneration (Lohmander et al. 2004), greater risk of radiographically diagnosed osteoarthritis (Deacon et al. 1997), and potential long-term disability (see chapter 2) (Ruiz, Kelly, and Nutton 2002). Clinicians and researchers must face this challenge by helping to develop new and improved rehabilitative protocols to minimize the potential of instability, subsequent degenerative osteoarthritis, and disability.

The First World Congress on Sports Injury Prevention was held in June 2005 in Oslo, Norway, with over 550 participants representing 55 different nations. This international multidisciplinary conference of scientists and clinicians marks the importance of this new research field. There is no doubt that long-term epidemiologic studies support a positive relationship between physical activity, physical fitness, and women's health. Several benefits have been identified for individuals who regularly participate in sport and exercise. A lifetime of physical activity and improved fitness decreases the likelihood of developing a number of diseases and conditions like obesity, hypertension, and diabetes; increases longevity; increases bone density; improves mental health; and reduces the overall health care burden in our nation (U.S. Department of Health and Human Services 1996).

Increased sport participation, although beneficial, is also accompanied by increased risk of musculoskeletal injury and subsequent osteoarthritis. To promote sport participation safely in the female population, sports medicine physicians, physical therapists, and athletic trainers must play an active role in the education of athletes and the prevention of injuries. Title IX has allowed the nation's young women more opportunities to play sports and to enjoy the benefits that are derived from athletic participation, including improved health, higher self-esteem, avoidance of risky behaviors, academic success, and preparation for professional success (Freedman et al. 1998). The promotion of safe sport participation is a great public health challenge that we must work quickly to achieve. The stakes are high for these young women at this point in time, yet the potential rewards of athletic involvement are great: the prevention of premature death, illness, and disability; control over health care costs; and the maintenance of a high quality of life. We must preserve this law in order for American girls to grow up strong, healthy, and confident; yet it is important for us to continue research and targeted intervention to provide safer sport participation in the future.

Summary

The gender disparity in noncontact ACL injury risk presents a clinical dilemma. The disparity has also given rise to some common misconceptions about ACL injury risk in girls and women. In summary, it is the responsibility of both clinicians and researchers in the sports medicine field to develop and test strategies for ACL injury prevention in young female athletes. It is imperative that emphasis be placed on the development of preventive interventions to reduce ACL injuries and the morbidity associated with ACL injuries in this population.

Part I

The Problem of ACL Injuries

Letha Y. Griffin, MD, PhD

Chapter 1: Incidence of ACL Injury

Synopsis

The authors begin their discussion and systematic review of the literature on the epidemiology of ACL injuries by distinguishing prevalence from incidence—two basic concepts fundamental to this topic.

Various numbers have been quoted for the incidence of ACL injury and the number of ACL reconstructions done each year. However, consistent epidemiologic data from which to derive these numbers are lacking. Such information would come from large multicenter studies that employ data collection extending across gender and sport lines, as well as across various geographic areas, and that compile the data in not only a global, but also a sport- and sex-specific manner.

The National Ambulatory Care Survey does provide a national representative sample of injuries seen in emergency rooms, hospital-based outpatient centers, and physician offices. These data suggest an estimate of approximately 1 million ACL, PCL, or combined ACL and PCL injuries each year, but this calculation may be in error since the objective criteria used to make the diagnosis of an ACL injury are not clearly defined. Moreover, since one injury can generate several physician visits, the calculations cannot be used to estimate incidence. The actual number of cruciate ligament injuries is most likely much lower, and has been estimated at 200,000 annually in the United States, with the majority of reported injuries occurring in young people.

Key Points

- Incidence quantifies the occurrence of new cases of a given injury in a population. The number can be expressed as an incident rate, which is the rate at which the new injury occurs and is reported as the number of new injuries per athlete-exposures or athlete-hours. Incidence proportion is the number of persons with the injury divided by the size of the population at risk. Prevalence is the proportion of the population that is currently injured at a given point in time.
- The incidence of ACL injury in the general population is largely unknown. Data exist only for Swiss youth, among whom the incidence is less than 1 injury per 100,000 athlete-hours.
- In specialized groups of elite athletes, rates are known and have been reported to be greater than in the general population.
- Within the general population, there are more ACL injuries in men than women, but the incidence rate in certain specific populations appears to be greater in women than in men.
- A great number of ACL injuries occur in the second decade of life.
- Epidemiologic data on ACL injuries are difficult to obtain due to the rarity of ACL injury. Moreover, ACL injury articles are difficult to compare or synthesize since the denominator used to express the incidence of injury varies between number of athletes, athlete-hours of participation, athlete-exposures, and so on. Large-scale multicenter epidemiologic studies are needed to provide reliable data on the incidence of ACL injury within the general population and in specific subsets within the general population.
- When ACL injuries are described, there is no universal agreement on the definition of "contact" and "noncontact." These terms need to be clarified and used similarly by all investigators so that data can be more easily compared and contrasted.

Chapter 2: Does ACL Reconstruction Prevent Articular Degeneration?

Synopsis

The development of osteoarthritis in the ACL-deficient knee is a complex process most likely involving mechanical and endogenous factors as described in this chapter by Dr. Marks.

Mechanical risk factors include injury to the meniscus cartilage, the articular cartilage, and the subchondral bone either at the time of the ACL injury or secondary to chronic ACL laxity. Altered proprioception also likely plays a role as a mechanical risk factor in the development of osteoarthritis, since altered joint sensation can negatively influence protective muscular stabilizing reflexes about the joint. It is unclear whether the altered proprioception is an acute finding that is secondary to alteration of specialized mechanoreceptors such as Golgi tendon organs and Pacinian corpuscles found in the ACL or whether it occurs secondarily to stretching of the capsule in the chronic ACL-deficient knee.

Endogenous factors associated with the development of osteoarthritis in the acute and chronic ACL-deficient knee are still poorly understood. Cartilage failure occurs when an imbalance exists between catabolic and anabolic events within this tissue. This imbalance results in the net loss of proteoglycans and hence loss of the stabilizing matrix. Various cytokines, including interleukin-1-receptor and tumor necrosis factor-alpha, have been implicated in the loss of cartilage matrix homeostasis. As stressed by Dr. Marks, it is probable that no risk factor stands alone, but instead interacts with other factors in the development of osteoarthritis.

Key Points

- Anterior cruciate ligament insufficiency, both acute and chronic, is associated with a high rate of meniscal lesions. Lateral meniscal tears are commonly reported in association with acute ACL injuries, and medial tears are more commonly reported in chronic ACL-injured knees. Fairbank, in 1948, described the association of osteoarthritis with loss of meniscal tissue, and today's evidence still supports this association.
- Bone bruises seen in acute ACL injuries can be divided into geographic lesions (those in a subchondral location within the bone) and reticular lesions (those located in the medullar region of the bone). The latter are not as frequently associated with long-term chondral sequelae as are the geographic lesions.
- Articular cartilage injury is difficult to assess. Trauma can result in physiologic changes that cannot initially be appreciated on gross inspection of the tissue.
- The ACL has Golgi tendon organs and Pacinian corpuscles—that is, mechanoreceptors associated with proprioception.
- There appears to be a relationship between impaired proprioception and osteoarthritis, but this relationship needs further evaluation.
- Cartilage as a tissue is made up of cells, type II collagen, proteoglycans, and water. Net loss of proteoglycans from the extracellular matrix appears to be associated with the development of osteoarthritis.

Chapter 3: The Costs Associated With ACL Injury

Synopsis

Anterior cruciate ligament injuries result in significant financial and emotional cost not only for the injured athlete, but also for the athlete's family and for society as a whole. Therefore, prevention of this injury is critical to decrease pain and suffering and to minimize emotional and financial risk. Only a few controlled, randomized trials examining the effectiveness of prevention programs on injury rates have been reported. Results from these and from several nonrandomized trials are encouraging. Further verification is needed, however.

Prevention programs developed in the last seven years typically consist of one or several of the following components: plyometrics, biomechanics and technique evaluation and feedback, strength, balance, core stability training, and flexibility exercises. The effect of each component or a combination of several components on injury prevention or sport performance is largely unknown at present.

Several research groups are working to develop screening criteria to identify athletes who are at high risk for developing an ACL injury. These athletes may benefit from specialized training over and above what is included in most prevention programs. Funding for screening and intervention programs is often difficult to obtain. The authors of this chapter explore several potential funding sources for screening and prevention programs.

Key Points

- The common components of an effective intervention program for ACL injury include plyometrics, biomechanics and technique evaluation and feedback, strength, balance, core stability training, and flexibility exercises.
- A cost–benefit analysis of potential prevention efforts must consider not only economic aspects of prevention, but also the psychosocial effects of sport injuries.
- Funding for screening and prevention programs is often difficult to obtain.

Chapter 1

Incidence of ACL Injury

Stephen W. Marshall, PhD
Darin Padua, PhD, ATC
Melanie McGrath, MS, ATC

The purpose of this chapter is to review the published data on ACL injury incidence with the goal of addressing four basic questions:

- What is the average incidence of ACL injury in the general population?
- How does ACL injury incidence vary by age and gender?
- How does ACL injury incidence vary by sport and gender?
- What are the limitations in our current epidemiologic knowledge of ACL injury incidence?

To address these questions we undertook a systematic review of the literature. In particular, to address the third question, we attempted to locate all epidemiologic studies published in the peer-reviewed literature within the past decade that have quantified the incidence of ACL injury. For each study, we abstracted data on the number of ACL injuries and the size of the population studied so that we could verify the computations for all incidence estimates and compute confidence intervals.

A major finding that emerged as we undertook this review was that there are few studies addressing the average incidence of ACL injury in the general population, particularly in the United States. We therefore undertook some exploratory data analysis aimed at addressing this gap in the literature, using data from the National Center for Health Statistics.

Human Movement and ACL Injury

Noncontact ACL injury is distinct from many other types of acute injury in that the forces that cause these injuries are generated within the athlete's body. Most other acute injuries involve a transfer of energy from a source external to the athlete (e.g., a collision with another athlete). Before considering the epidemiologic data, we present a brief review of the characteristics of ACL injury.

Boden and colleagues (2000) assembled a general case series of ACL injuries using athlete interviews and videographic review. Boden concluded that around 70% of the injuries were noncontact in nature; that is, there was no external contact to the knee that led directly to injury. All injuries occurred during vigorous athletic tasks, such as planting, cutting, and jumping. Poor alignment of the body, for instance an awkwardly wide stance during landing from a jump, was a characteristic feature. Boden specifically implicated a situation in which one foot is planted and a rapid deceleration occurs. Anterior cruciate ligament injuries in skiers, although quite different in nature from those described by Boden and colleagues, also involve imbalances of body weight and malalignment of body position (Deibert et al. 1998).

What Is Incidence?

Incidence is a basic epidemiologic concept that, although simple, is frequently confused with prevalence. *Incidence* quantifies the occurrence of new cases of a given injury in a population. To measure the incidence of ACL injury, we would ideally identify a group of people who do not currently have an ACL injury, and then prospectively follow them over a defined period of time to identify how many of them sustain an ACL injury. For some research questions, we might want to restrict the study population to those who have no history of ACL injury.

Incidence can be quantified either as an incidence rate or as an incidence proportion. The denominator for incidence rate is person-time at risk (e.g., athlete-exposures or athlete-hours), whereas the denominator for incidence proportion is persons at risk (athletes). The *incidence rate* (also known as incidence density) is the *rate* at which new ACL injuries occur per unit of person-time at risk, that is, the number of new ACL injuries divided by person-time at risk. Person-time at risk is typically measured as either athlete-exposures or athlete-hours (athlete-exposures and athlete-hours are sports medicine adaptations of the epidemiologic concept of person-time at risk). Thus, incidence rates are measured in units of inverse person-time and can range from zero to infinity.

Incidence proportion (also known as cumulative incidence), on the other hand, is the *average risk* of ACL injury, defined as the number of persons who sustain an ACL injury divided by the size of the population at risk, that is, the proportion of the population who sustain an ACL injury over a defined time interval. Unlike rates, risks are proportions, and range from 0 to 1. Note that the numerator and denominator in incidence proportion should both be counts of athletes; thus it is important that the number of injured persons (not the number of injuries) be used as the numerator of incidence proportion. That is, one person who has multiple injuries should be counted only once in the numerator of incidence proportion (whereas all injuries would be counted in the numerator of the incidence rate).

Incidence is often confused with *prevalence*. Prevalence is the proportion of a population that is currently injured at a given point in time. For example, the prevalence of ACL injury could be defined as the proportion of athletes on a team that are unable to play because of a current ACL injury at a given point in the season. Prevalence is always a proportion, not a rate, since no more than 100% can be injured at a given moment in time.

The choice of whether incidence rate, incidence proportion, or prevalence should be used depends on the purpose of the study and the research question being addressed. However, most epidemiologic studies addressing risk factors for incident injury are based (in some way) around the concept of incidence rate.

What Is the Average Incidence of ACL Injury in the General Population?

The best estimate of the average incidence of ACL injury in a country comes from Switzerland. De Loës and colleagues (2000) studied cruciate ligament injury (ACL and posterior cruciate ligament [PCL] combined) in Swiss youth enrolled in a national youth sport program (ages 14-20 years). Approximately 370,000 youth (2/3 of Swiss in this age group) participate in the program. Over a seven-year period, a total of 470 ACL/PCL injuries were reported (annual average of 67 injuries). The incidence rate for females was 0.52 (95% confidence interval [95%CI]: 0.42, 0.61) per 100,000 athlete-hours of exposure to sport. For males, the rate was 0.62 (95%CI: 0.55, 0.68) per 100,000 athlete-hours. The female-to-male rate ratio was 0.84 (95%CI: 0.68, 1.04). Annually, there was approximately 1 ACL or PCL injury per 5000 participants. Males accounted for 76% of the ACL/PCL injuries.

On the basis of these data, it is reasonable to state that the incidence in the general population is low. Note, however, that even if the incidence is low, the burden on the health care system may be high. The high burden of these injuries on the health care system is indicated by de Loës and colleagues' (2000) finding that ACL/PCL injury in the study population had the highest average cost of all knee injuries. As a caveat, we note that de Loës and colleagues (2000) reported incidence estimates that were substantially lower than those from other countries.

National Ambulatory Care Surveys

In an effort to elucidate the absolute incidence of cruciate injuries in the United States, we accessed the 2003 National Ambulatory Care Survey data. These data are collected by the National Center for Health Statistics. This is a large, federally mandated data collection effort. It provides a nationally representative sample of all visits to emergency departments, hospital-based outpatient departments, and all physician offices in the U.S. (federal health facilities are not included). The limitation of this data source is that there is a single code for injury to the cruciate ligaments, which means that injuries to the ACL are grouped with injuries to the PCL (this is an artifact of ICD-9-CM coding, or the International Classification of Disease, version 9, Clinical Modification). However, the incidence of isolated PCL injuries is typically considered to be much lower than the incidence of ACL injury, and so we expect that vast majority of cruciate ligament injuries involve the ACL. For example, Myklebust and colleagues (1997) reported that 94% of all cruciate ligament injuries in Norwegian handball involved the ACL.

Methods Used in National Ambulatory Care Databases

The National Ambulatory Care Survey data come from two separate surveys: the National Ambulatory Medical Care Survey (NAMCS), which is a sample of visits to nonfederally employed office-based physicians who are primarily engaged in direct patient care, and the National Hospital Ambulatory Medical Care Survey (NHAMCS), which is a sample of visits to the emergency departments and outpatient departments of general and short-stay hospitals, exclusive of federal, military, and Veterans Administration hospitals. Both surveys are national probability samples. Both surveys involve comprehensive data checking to ensure that the data are valid and reliable.

In NAMCS, trained interviewers visit the physicians prior to their participation in the survey in order to provide them with survey materials and instruct them on how to complete the forms. Each physician is randomly assigned to a one-week reporting period. During this period, data for a systematic random sample of visits are recorded by the physician or office staff on an encounter form provided for that purpose. In NHAMCS, trained interviewers visit the hospitals prior to their participation in the survey to explain survey procedures, verify eligibility, develop a sampling plan, and train hospital staff in data collection procedures. Hospital staff are instructed to complete forms for a systematic random sample of patient visits during a randomly assigned four-week reporting period. In both surveys, the samples are weighted to facilitate national estimates.

Results From National Health Care Surveys

On the basis of these data, we estimate that in 2003 there were approximately 1 million visits to hospital-based outpatient departments, hospital-based emergency rooms, and physician offices for treatment of injury to a cruciate ligament (95%CI: 220,000 to 1,800,000). This estimate should be treated with extreme caution since it has a very high relative standard error (0.40) and a correspondingly wide 95%CI. More detailed multiyear analyses, which have better precision, are currently in progress but were unavailable at the time of writing.

The number of visits annually in the United States for the care of a cruciate ligament injury—1 million—may seem large, but it is important to place the number in perspective. The total population of the United States in 2003 was approximately 290 million, and the total number of visits to hospital-based outpatient departments, hospital-based emergency rooms, and physician offices for treatment of unintentional injuries was 90 million in 2003. (Information on whether the injury was unintentional or intentional was missing for a large number of records. If the records with missing data for intentional/unintentional were included in the total for unintentional, the total would be 136 million visits.) Nevertheless, the burden of cruciate ligament injury on the health care system is underscored by the fact that possibly as many as 1 out of every 90 physician visits for treatment of unintentional injury pertains to care of an ACL or PCL injury.

This estimate includes all physician visits for cruciate ligament injury and therefore represents the total burden on the physician portion of the health care system. However, one injury will generate many visits, so this is not an estimate of incidence. By limiting the data only to visits for initial care of injury, one could attempt to get a measure of the true incidence of injury. Unfortunately, there are too few such injuries to permit reliable estimates from only one year of data from this source. However, initial exploratory analyses of this data source suggest that there could be around 200,000 cruciate ligament injuries annually in the United States. This suggests that the number of 50,000 to 75,000 ACL reconstructions per annum that is frequently cited may be an underestimate.

Summary

Based on the data from de Loës and colleagues (2000) and preliminary analyses reported here, it is likely that the average incidence of ACL injury in the general population is relatively low. This is probably so because the average person has limited exposure to the athletic tasks that are typically associated with ACL injury. However, the total health care burden of ACL injury appears to be very significant, with approximately 1 million physician visits annually in the United States for treatment of a cruciate ligament injury. The high burden on the health care system is not surprising, given the extensive medical resources consumed in the reconstruction and rehabilitation of ACL injury.

These conclusions are tentative. At this point, we lack good population-based studies that quantify, in an unambiguous manner, both the number of injuries and the population at risk and that therefore would precisely define the average incidence in the population. Addressing this gap in the literature should be a priority for the future research.

How Does ACL Injury Incidence Vary by Age and Gender?

Before we consider the incidence of ACL injury in specific sports, it will be helpful to briefly review some studies presenting case-only data in order to establish the characteristics of ACL injury with regard to age and gender. The age distribution for ACL injuries has been reported by Yu (2002a) and Shea and colleagues (2004). These two sets of age-specific data are shown in figures 1.1 and 1.2.

Yu (2002a) used data from board examinations presented to the American Board of Orthopedic Surgeons. Therefore, these data relate to reconstructions, which are not the same as incident injuries, since an injury that presents with no instability, or in an athlete who does not wish to continue in the sport,

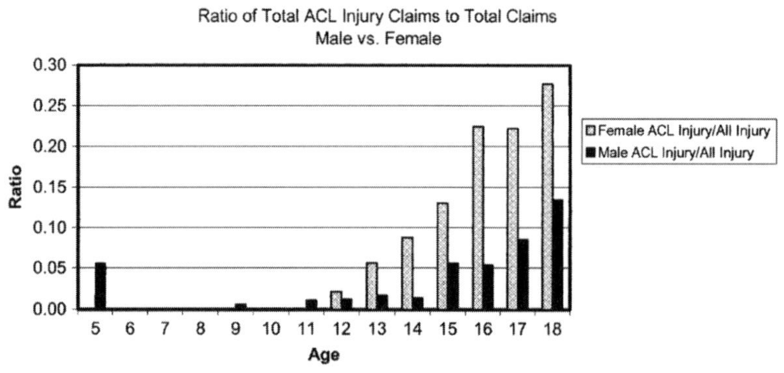

FIGURE 1.1 Incidence of claims for ACL injury in youth soccer, as a percentage of all claims.

Reprinted, by permission, from K.G. Shea et al., 2004, "Anterior cruciate ligament injury in pediatric and adolescent soccer players: An analysis of insurance data," *Journal of Pediatric Orthopedics* 24(6): 623-628.

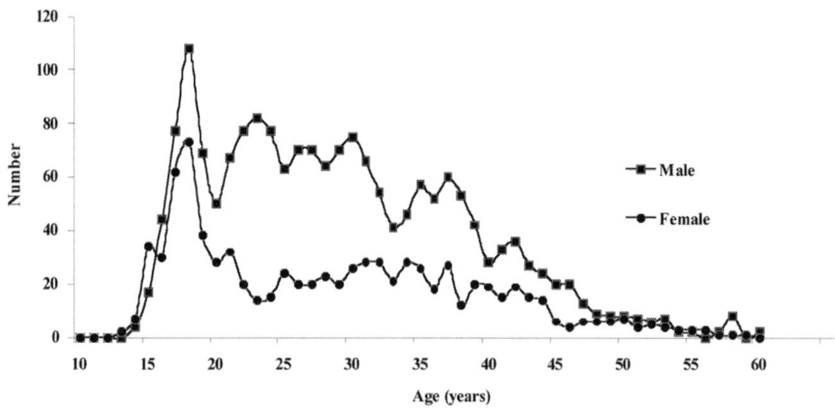

FIGURE 1.2 Number of ACL reconstructions performed by candidates for certification before the American Board of Orthopedic Surgeons in 2000.

Adapted with permission from Yu B, Kirkendall DT, Taft TN, Garrett WE: Lower Extremity Motor Control-Related and Other Risk Factors for Noncontact Anterior Cruciate Ligament Injuries, in Beaty JH, (ed): *Instructional Course Lectures*, volume 51. Rosemont, IL, American Academy of Orthopaedic Surgeons, 2002.

possibly may not be reconstructed. In addition, the biases associated with the case mix for a group of surgeons who are approaching certification should be considered. Nevertheless, the data are informative because they pertain to ACL injury in the general U.S. population.

Shea and colleagues (2004) used insurance data from an insurance agency that covers over 1 million youth soccer players annually in the United States, approximately half of whom are female. However, the insurance agency does not collect details on the age and sex distribution of the covered athletes. To overcome this limitation, Shea's group used the total number of overall injuries (by age and gender) as a surrogate measure of the person-time at risk for the soccer leagues covered by this insurer.

The general age distributions from these two studies are remarkably similar, although the Shea distribution pertains only to youth and adolescents. Both demonstrate a lot of ACL injuries in the 16- to 18-year-old age group. The patterns with regard to gender, however, are very different. According to Yu, males sustain more ACL injuries than females in every age group except age 15. Shea's data, on the other hand, show in youth soccer that females have nearly twice as many ACL injury claims (73 per annum) as males (38 per annum). In every age group, from 12 years through to 18 years, ACL injury claims account for a higher proportion of all injury claims in females than in males (figure 1.1).

This apparent contradiction is, in fact, an established feature of the epidemiology of ACL injury (Garrick and Requa 2001). Males account for the majority of injuries in the general population, but when one conditions on physical activity (by examining specific sports), females are consistently observed to be at higher risk. The fact that males account for more injuries than females in the general population is almost certainly due to their greater exposure to athletic tasks that predispose one to ACL injury, such as cutting and jumping, and to contact sports (such as North American football).

These two case-only studies, although useful, are limited in that they have almost no data about the underlying populations at risk and depend on preexisting administrative databases that were originally assembled for purposes unrelated to learning about ACL injury. It would be extremely useful to have a large case series of well-documented and highly detailed ACL injuries that were prospectively collected in standardized manner. Such a registry would be invaluable in providing more data about injury mechanisms and would be a highly useful tool for researchers. Such a registry does, in fact, already exist for team handball in Norway (Myklebust et al. 1997), and Griffin (In press-b) has called for the expansion of this system to include additional sports and countries.

In summary, comparison of the data from Shea and colleagues (2004) and Yu (2002a) underscores two important points about ACL injury incidence:

- Although males account for the majority of injuries in the general population, within specific sports, females are at higher risk.
- The highest number of injuries occurs in ages 16 to 18 years.

How Does the Incidence of ACL Injury Vary by Sport and Gender?

The most important aspect of quantifying the incidence of ACL injury is perhaps not to establish credible estimates of the average incidence, but rather to determine how the incidence varies with regard to various etiologic factors. These etiologic factors are typically divided into those extrinsic to the athlete (sport, surfacing, footwear) and those that are intrinsic to the athlete (gender, neuromuscular control, hormonal factors, anatomic factors). This section reviews the literature addressing how the incidence of ACL injury varies with regard to sport, or more generally, the type of physical activity. We performed a systematic literature search to identify all papers presenting incidence data for ACL injury that were published in the peer-reviewed literature within the past decade. Even though military training is not a sport, we included studies on the incidence of ACL injury in military training, since it involves athletic tasks commonly associated with ACL injury.

Literature Review Methods

We searched the literature to locate all papers meeting set eligibility criteria. The criteria were English language papers, published in the peer-reviewed literature during approximately the past decade (operationalized as between 1/1/1996 and 10/1/2005), that presented an estimate of the incidence (either incidence rate or incidence proportion) of ACL injury (figure 1.3). To be defined as presenting an incidence estimate, the paper had to quantify both the number of incident ACL injuries and the size of the population at risk; that is, papers that presented a case series of ACL injuries without any information on the underlying population from which the cases arose were ineligible. The methods used to locate the papers included an electronic literature search of the National Library of Medicine's PubMed database. The electronic literature search utilized the search terms listed in figure 1.3. These search criteria yielded a total of 821 papers. The title and abstracts (where electronically available) for these papers were individually reviewed to determine their eligibility.

In addition to the systematic search, an effort was made to manually locate papers meeting the eligibility criteria. The authors were informally aware, through their familiarity with the ACL literature, of a number of other papers that met the eligibility criteria. These were accessed, and their reference lists were reviewed. In addition, the reference lists of several recent review articles (Murphy, Connolly, and Beynnon 2003; Ireland 1999; Hewett 2000; Huston, Greenfield, and Wojtys 2000; Griffin et al. In press-b, 2000; DeMaio and McHale 2003; Traina and Bromberg 1997) were reviewed to identify additional papers that met the eligibility criteria.

Inclusion Criteria Used

English language

Published in the peer-reviewed literature between 1/1/1996 and 10/1/2005

Presents an estimate of the incidence of ACL injury. Must quantify both the number of incident ACL injuries and the size of the population at risk. Could be either incidence rate or incidence proportion.

Search Terms Used in Electronic Search[a]

"Anterior Cruciate Ligament/injuries"[MeSH] or ACL[Text Word]

"wounds and injuries"[MeSH] or injury[Text Word]

"epidemiology"[MeSH/Text Word] or "incidence"[MeSH/Text Word] or "prevalence"[MeSH/Text Word] or "statistics"[MeSH/Text Word]

"humans"[MeSH]

Information Abstracted for Each Paper

First author

Year of publication

Study design

Population (recreational skiers, professional soccer, military cadets, etc.)

Type of sport or activity (basketball, soccer, military training, etc.)

Number of ACL injuries

Denominator (number)

Denominator type (athlete-exposures, athlete-hours, athletes, games, teams)

Rate or risk as reported by authors

Rate ratio or risk ratio for women versus men as reported by authors

Percentage noncontact injuries

[a]MeSH = Major Subject Heading (National Library of Medicine)

FIGURE 1.3 Methodological details of literature review.

Abstraction of Incidence Data

A total of 39 papers were located that met the eligibility criteria. Of the 39 papers, 24 were found by both the electronic and manual search, 7 were located only by the electronic search, and 8 were located only by the manual search. In addition to the 39 papers reviewed here, we identified three studies (Shelbourne,

Davis, and Klootwyk 1998; Carson 2004; Micheli et al. 1999) that almost met the eligibility criteria but that we elected to exclude from review. Shelbourne and colleagues 1998 was excluded because it was limited to a group of injured subjects, Carson 2004 because it did not reliably enumerate the population at risk, and Micheli and colleagues 1999 because it did not include all injuries in the population at risk.

All 39 papers were reviewed, and all data on ACL incidence were abstracted and entered into a database. The type of information abstracted for each study is shown in figure 1.3. Specifically, we abstracted the number of ACL injuries, the denominator reported by the authors, and the incidence estimate (risk or rate) reported by the authors. We recomputed all incidence estimates (risk or rate) to verify the authors' calculations. In some cases minor differences were found, possibly due to rounding error in the author's original computations or the author's handling of missing data in the datasets. Where minor differences existed, we reported the rates and rate ratios that we computed rather than the authors' original estimates. We also computed 95%CI for all estimates so that the precision of the estimate could be considered. Many of the incidence estimates in these studies were based on a relatively small number of ACL injuries. A few authors reported confidence intervals in the original studies (e.g., Olsen et al. 2003; Myklebust 2003), but most did not. If the number of injuries is less than five, the 95%CI itself becomes unstable, and we did not include 95%CI in the tables in these cases.

We computed a female-to-male rate ratio for all studies that included both male and female injuries. In forming our conclusions, however, we gave more weight to the studies with at least five male and five female ACL injuries, because we consider those rate ratios to be estimated with better precision than in studies with fewer than five male or five female injuries.

Studies were classified into four main groups based on the type of denominator used to compute the measure of incidence. Group 1 comprised studies using athlete-exposures as the denominator. For these studies, the measure of incidence was the rate per 1000 athlete-exposures. Group 2 comprised studies using athlete-hours as the denominator. For these studies, the measure of incidence was the rate per 1000 athlete-hours (data from studies that presented rate per 10,000 athlete-hours were rescaled). Group 3 comprised studies using athletes as the denominator. Technically, these studies estimate average risk, not rate. The measure of incidence typically reported by these authors was incidence proportion over one season (note that many authors mistakenly report this as a rate rather than as an average risk). One study reported recalled lifetime incidence of ACL injury (Stevenson et al. 1998). Group 4 comprised studies that did not use individual athletes in the denominator, but rather used teams, games, or team-games (Orchard and Powell 2003; Meyers and Barnhill 2004; Orchard et al., 1999, 2001). There was no easy way for us to utilize these studies to make inferences about individual-level risk or rate, so they were excluded from further consideration.

We also classified the studies according to the sport or activity for which they presented incidence, and tabulated the major groups of sports (tables 1.1 to 1.5). Because we focused on sport and gender, we did not tabulate studies that did not present incidence data broken out by sex or did not explicitly state the gender of the study population. These included Caraffa and colleagues 1996, Deibert and colleagues 1998, and Oates and colleagues 1999. If the study was an intervention trial (Hewett et al. 1999; Heidt et al. 2000; Mandelbaum et al. 2005), we tabulated the incidence in the control group under the assumption that this was the best estimate of background incidence of ACL injury in the study population. If the study addressed a phased intervention (Pope 2002; Myklebust et al. 2003), we tabulated the incidence in the preintervention phase.

General Results

As already stated, we computed a female-to-male rate ratio (or risk ratio) and 95%CI based on the authors' published data. We found that in studies that had at least five ACL injuries in males and at least five ACL injuries in females, females had an injury rate that was 1.5 to 4.6 times higher than in males. Studies have sometimes reported rate ratios that are above 5. For example, Gwinn and colleagues (2000) reported an ACL injury rate for females in military training that was up to 10-fold greater than the rate for males at the U.S. Naval Academy (95%CI: 3, 32). However, we found that all estimates of the female-to-male rate ratios above 5 were based on relatively small numbers of injuries (e.g., the 10-fold estimate in Gwinn's study was based on five female and six male injuries) and consequently should be viewed as preliminary, subject to the conduct of larger studies.

Most studies focused on specific sports or populations. Only de Loës and colleagues (2000) were able to adopt a comprehensive population-based approach and compared the incidence of ACL injury across multiple sports. De Loës and colleagues found that females had a higher rate of ACL injury than males in 11 of the 12 sports studied, and in 6 sports, the female-to-male rate ratio was 2.0 or higher. Only 11 of the 39 studies (Agel, Arendt, and Breshadsky 2005; Arendt, Agel, and Dick 1999; Faude et al. 2005; Giza et al. 2005; Hewett et al. 1999; Lambson et al. 1996; Myklebust et al. 1998; Myklebust 2003; Oliphant and Drawbert 1996; Orchard et al. 1999, 2001) classified the injuries as contact or noncontact and reported the proportion of injuries that were noncontact. The overall proportion of injuries that were noncontact was at least 50% wherever it was documented, and sometimes ranged up to 100%. One study (Uhorchak et al. 2003) was restricted to noncontact injuries.

It was often problematic to synthesize data across multiple studies because of the many different measures of incidence used by authors. In order to facilitate meaningful comparisons, the studies in tables 1.1 through 1.5 are grouped by the type of incidence measure used by the authors (rate per athlete-exposures,

TABLE 1.1 Incidence of ACL Injury in Soccer

				FEMALES			MALES			FEMALE VS. MALE
Study	Design/ Methodology	Population	Setting	No. of ACL injuries	Rate or risk (95%CI)	Percent noncontact	No. of ACL injuries	Rate or risk (95%CI)	Percent noncontact	Rate or risk ratio (95%CI)
STUDIES USING ATHLETE-EXPOSURES AS THE DENOMINATOR. *Measure of incidence: rate per 1000 athlete-exposures*										
Agel, Arendt, and Breshadsky 2005	Injury surveillance	Collegiate, USA	NCAA, 1990-2002	394	0.31 (0.28, 0.34)	58%	192	0.11 (0.09, 0.13)	50%	2.8 (2.3, 3.3)
Arendt, Agel, and Dick 1999	Injury surveillance	Collegiate, USA	NCAA, 1994-98	158	0.33 (0.29, 0.38)	--	77	0.12 (0.09, 0.15)	--	2.7 (2.1, 3.6)
Gwinn et al. 2000	Prospective injury registration	Collegiate, USA	US Naval Academy	5	0.8 (0.1, 1.4)	--	1	0.1 --	--	6.7 (1.5, 31)
Gwinn et al. 2000	Prospective injury registration	Intramural college, USA	US Naval Academy	2	2.7 --	--	10	0.4 (0.2, 0.6)	--	9.5 (1.1, 81)
Harmon and Dick 1998	Injury surveillance	Collegiate, USA	NCAA, 1989-96	88	0.33 (0.26, 0.39)	--	53	0.12 (0.09, 0.16)	--	2.7 (1.9, 3.7)
Hewett et al. 1999	Controls in intervention study	High school, USA	Vicinity of Cincinnati, Ohio	2	0.2 --	100%	1	0.1 --	100%	1.9 (0.2, 21)
Mandelbaum et al. 2005	Controls in intervention study	Youth soccer league	Southern California	67	0.49 (0.37, 0.60)	--	--	--	--	--

STUDIES USING ATHLETE-HOURS AS THE DENOMINATOR. *Measure of incidence: rate per 1000 athlete-hours*										
Bjordal et al. 1997	Retrospective injury review	Recreational league, Norway	Club games in Hordaland	43	0.10 (0.07, 0.13)	--	133	0.06 (0.05, 0.07)	--	1.8 (1.2, 2.5)
de Loës, Dahlstedt, and Thomee 2000[a]	Prospective injury and exposure registration	Recreational and elite youth, Switzerland	National League	9	0.019 (0.006, 0.031)	--	225	0.009 (0.008, 0.010)	--	2.1 (1.1, 4.1)
Faude et al. 2005	Prospective cohort	Pro league, Germany	Elite games	11	2.2 (0.9, 3.4)	64%	--	--	--	--
Faude et al. 2005	Prospective cohort	Pro league, Germany	Elite practices	0	0 --	--	--	--	--	--
Giza et al. 2005	Prospective injury registration	Pro league, USA	Elite games	5	0.9 (0.1, 1.7)	75%[b]	--	--	--	--
Giza et al. 2005	Prospective injury registration	Pro league, USA	Elite practices	3	0.04 --	--	--	--	--	--
STUDIES USING ATHLETES AS THE DENOMINATOR. *Measure of incidence: average risk (incidence proportion) over one season*										
Heidt et al. 2000	Controls in intervention study	High school, USA	Cincinnati, Ohio	8	3.1% (1.0, 5.2)	--	--	--	--	--

[a]Includes PCLs.

[b]Percentage noncontact for games and practices combined.

-- = no data available.

TABLE 1.2 Incidence of ACL Injury in Basketball

				FEMALES			MALES			FEMALE VS. MALE
Study	Design/ Methodology	Population	Setting	No. of ACL injuries	Rate or risk (95%CI)	Percent noncontact	No. of ACL injuries	Rate or risk (95%CI)	Percent noncontact	Rate or risk ratio (95%CI)
STUDIES USING ATHLETE-EXPOSURES AS THE DENOMINATOR. *Measure of incidence: rate per 1000 athlete-exposures*										
Agel, Arendt, and Breshadsky 2005	Injury surveillance	Collegiate, USA	NCAA, 1990-2002	514	0.27 (0.25, 0.30)	75%	168	0.08 (0.07, 0.09)	70%	3.6 (3.0, 4.2)
Arendt, Agel, and Dick 1999	Injury surveillance	Collegiate, USA	NCAA, 1994-98	194	0.29 (0.25, 0.33)	--	75	0.10 (0.08, 0.12)	80%	2.9 (2.2, 3.8)
Gwinn et al. 2000	Prospective injury registration	Collegiate, USA	US Naval Academy	5	0.5 (0.1, 0.9)	--	1	0.1 --	--	5.4 (0.6, 46)
Gwinn et al. 2000	Prospective injury registration	Intramural college, USA	US Naval Academy	0	--	--	5	0.2 (0.1, 0.3)	--	--
Harmon and Dick 1998	Injury surveillance	Collegiate, USA	NCAA, 1989-96	85	0.29 (0.23, 0.35)	--	22	0.06 (0.04, 0.09)	--	4.6 (2.9, 7.4)
Hewett et al. 1999	Controls in intervention study	High school, USA	Vicinity of Cincinnati, Ohio	3	0.3 --	100%	0	0	--	--
Lombardo, Sethi, and Starkey 2005	Prospective injury registration	Pro league, USA	NBA games	--	--	--	14	0.2 (0.1, 0.3)	100%	--

Meeuwisse, Sellmer, and Hagel 2003	Prospective injury and exposure registration	Collegiate, Canada	Canada West, CIAA	4	0.1 --	--	--	--	--	--
STUDIES USING ATHLETE-HOURS AS THE DENOMINATOR. *Measure of incidence: rate per 1000 athlete-hours*										
de Loës, Dahlstedt, and Thomee 2000[a]	Prospective injury and exposure registration	Recreational and elite youth, Switzerland	National League	14	0.011 (0.005, 0.016)	--	13	0.007 (0.003, 0.011)	--	1.6 (0.7, 2.2)
Gomez, DeLee, and Farney 1996	Prospective injury and exposure registration	High school, USA	Texas	16	0.15 (0.08, 0.22)	--	--	--	--	--
Lombardo, Sethi, and Starkey 2005	Prospective injury registration	Pro league, USA	NBA games	--	--	--	14	0.49 (0.24, 0.75)	100%	--
Messina, Farney, and DeLee 1999	Prospective injury and exposure registration	High school, USA	Texas	11	0.09 (0.03, 0.15)	--	4	--	--	3.8 (1.2, 12)
STUDIES USING ATHLETES AS THE DENOMINATOR. *Measure of incidence: average risk (incidence proportion) over one season*										
Lombardo, Sethi, and Starkey 2005	Prospective injury registration	Pro league, USA	NBA games	--	--	--	14	4.6% (2.2%, 7.0%)	100%	--
Oliphant and Drawbert 1996	Retrospective injury registration	Collegiate, USA	Wisconsin	26	4.8% (2.9, 6.6)	81%	13	2.1% (1.0, 3.2)	69%	2.8 (1.2, 4.4)

[a]Includes PCLs.

-- = no data available.

TABLE 1.3 Incidence of ACL Injury in Team Handball

				FEMALES			MALES			FEMALE VS. MALE
Study	Design/ Methodology	Population	Setting	No. of ACL injuries	Rate or risk (95%CI)	Percent noncontact	No. of ACL injuries	Rate or risk (95%CI)	Percent noncontact	Rate or risk ratio (95%CI)
STUDIES USING ATHLETE-HOURS AS THE DENOMINATOR. *Measure of incidence: rate per 1000 athlete-hours*										
de Loës, Dahlstedt, and Thomee 2000	Prospective injury and exposure registration	Recreational and elite youth, Switzerland	National League	30	0.012 (0.001, 0.034)	--	58	0.005 (0.003, 0.007)	--	1.4 (0.9, 2.2)
Myklebust et al. 1998	Prospective cohort	Norway	Elite and recre-ational clubs	21	0.31 (0.19, 0.42)	89%[a]	3	0.06 --	--	5.2 (1.5, 17)
Myklebust et al. 2003	Year 1 in a phased intervention	Norway	Elite and recreational clubs	29	0.14 (0.09, 0.19)	62%	--	--	--	--
Olsen et al. 2003	Secondary data	Norway	Elite and recreational clubs	44	0.77 (0.54, 1.00)	--	9	0.24 (0.08, 0.40)	--	3.2 (1.6, 6.5)
STUDIES USING ATHLETES AS THE DENOMINATOR. *Measure of incidence: average risk (incidence proportion) over one season*										
Myklebust et al. 1997	Prospective injury registra-tion	Norway	Elite and recreational clubs	54	1.6% (1.2, 2.0)	--	33	1.0% (0.6, 1.3)	--	1.6 (1.1, 2.5)

[a]Females and males combined; most injuries (21/24) were to females.

-- = no data available.

TABLE 1.4 Incidence of ACL Injury in Skiing

Study	Design/ Methodology	Population	Setting	FEMALES No. of ACL injuries	FEMALES Rate or risk (95%CI)	FEMALES Percent noncontact	MALES No. of ACL injuries	MALES Rate or risk (95%CI)	MALES Percent noncontact	FEMALE VS. MALE Rate or risk ratio (95%CI)
STUDIES USING ATHLETE-HOURS AS THE DENOMINATOR. *Measure of incidence: rate per 1000 athlete-hours*										
de Loës, Dahlstedt, and Thomee 2000[a]	Prospective injury and exposure registration	Recreational and elite youth, Switzerland	National League	19	0.007 (0.004, 0.010)	--	19	0.005 (0.003, 0.008)	--	1.4 (0.7, 2.6)
Viola et al. 1999	Retrospective review	Ski instructors and patrollers, USA	Vail, Colorado	10	0.044 (0.017, 0.071)	--	21	0.042 (0.024, 0.060)	--	1.0 (0.5, 2.2)
STUDIES USING ATHLETES AS THE DENOMINATOR. *Measure of incidence: average risk (incidence proportion) over one season*										
Beynnon 2003	Prospective cohort	Competitive skiers, USA	Northeast USA	9	10.3% (4.0, 16.7)	--	7	5.1% (1.4, 8.8)	--	2.0 (0.8, 5.4)
Stevenson et al. 1998[b]	Retrospective questionnaire	Ski racers, USA	Colleges and clubs in New England	36	22%[b] (16, 30)	--	18	7%[b] (4, 11)	--	3.1 (1.7, 5.4)

[a]Includes PCLs.

[b]Incidence of any ACL injury during lifetime (retrospective recall).

TABLE 1.5 Incidence of ACL Injury in Collision Sports

					FEMALES			MALES			FEMALE VS. MALE
Sport	**Study**	**Design/ Methodology**	**Population**	**Setting**	**No. of ACL injuries**	**Rate or risk (95%CI)**	**Percent noncontact**	**No. of ACL injuries**	**Rate or risk (95%CI)**	**Percent noncontact**	**Rate or risk ratio (95%CI)**
STUDIES USING ATHLETE-EXPOSURES AS THE DENOMINATOR. *Measure of incidence: rate per 1000 athlete-exposures*											
Australian rules football	Orchard et al. 2001	Prospective injury and exposure registration	Australian football league	Elite games	--	--	--	83	0.82 (0.64, 1.00)	76%	--
Rugby	Gwinn et al. 2000	Prospective injury registration	Intramural college, USA	US Naval Academy	3	0.4	--	4	0.2	--	2.0 (0.5, 9.0)
Rugby	Levy et al. 1997	Retrospective questionnaire	Intramural college, USA	College clubs	21	0.36 (0.20, 0.51)	--	--	--	--	--
STUDIES USING ATHLETE-HOURS AS THE DENOMINATOR. *Measure of incidence: rate per 1000 athlete-hours*											
Ice hockey	de Loës, Dahlstedt, and Thomee 2000[a]	Prospective injury and exposure registration	Recreational and elite youth, Switzerland	National League	1	0.012	--	25	0.005 (0.003, 0.007)	--	2.2 (0.3, 16)
STUDIES USING ATHLETES AS THE DENOMINATOR. *Measure of incidence: average risk (incidence proportion) over one season*											
North American football	Lambson, Barnhill, and Higgins 1996	Prospective injury and exposure registration	High school, USA	Texas	42	1.3% (0.9, 1.8)	55%	--	--	--	--

[a]Includes PCLs.

rate per athlete-hours, or risk per athlete per season). Note that although Agel and colleagues 2005, Arendt and colleagues 1999, and Harmon and Dick 1998 are listed in the tables as separate studies, all three studies used a common data source, the National Collegiate Athletic Association's (NCAA) Injury Surveillance System.

Soccer

Most of the soccer studies (six) reported incidence using athlete-exposures as the rate denominator (table 1.1). For these studies, the reported female rate of ACL injury in collegiate, high school, and youth soccer was generally between 0.3 and 0.8 injuries per 1000 athlete-exposures. One study reported a much higher rate (Gwinn et al. 2000), but had very few female injuries. The reported rate of male ACL injury was around 0.1 per 1000 athlete-exposures, ranging up to 0.4 in U.S. Naval Academy intramural soccer.

Four studies reported incidence using athlete-hours as the denominator. A very wide range of incidence was reported in these studies, from 0.02 in the national youth Swiss league to 2 per 1000 athlete-hours in games in the German professional league. This enormous variation—a 100-fold range of magnitude—is likely due to a number of factors, one of which is the increased intensity of competition in professional sports. However, methodologic factors likely also play a critical role. In particular, Bjordal and colleagues (1997) and de Loës and colleagues (2000) reported an overall injury rate, whereas Giza and colleagues (2005) and Faude and colleagues (2005) reported separate rates for games and practices. Giza and Faude did not include sufficient information for us to compute an overall rate (games and practices combined) from their data.

The female-to-male rate ratio ranged from 1.8 to 2.8 in studies that included at least five male and five female ACL injuries. Gwinn and colleagues (2000) reported female-to-male rate ratios well above 2.8 (6.7 for collegiate and 9.5 for intramural soccer), but these were based on smaller numbers. For intramural and collegiate combined, the rate ratio for Gwinn and colleagues was 3.3 (95%CI: 1.3, 8.6).

Basketball

As with soccer, most studies (seven) reported incidence using athlete-exposures as the rate denominator (table 1.2). The rate of female ACL injury ranged from 0.1 to 0.5 per 1000 athlete-exposures, whereas the rate in males ranged from 0.06 to 0.2. In both soccer and basketball, some of the highest rates of ACL injury were in the professional levels of the sport. Lombardo and colleagues (2005), using data from professional men's basketball, reported incidence using three different types of denominator (rate per athlete-exposures, rate per athlete-minutes, and average risk per athlete), so we included all three incidence estimates in the table (the rate per athlete-minutes was rescaled to athlete-hours).

As with soccer, the studies that used athlete-hours as the denominator showed a much greater range of incidence estimates than the studies using athlete-exposures as the denominator. The range was eightfold (from 0.01 to 0.09); however, no study to date has addressed professional women's basketball. If professional women's basketball were included, the range in incidence would be greater.

The percentage of injuries that were noncontact in collegiate basketball was around 70% to 80% (Agel, Arendt, and Breshadsky 2005; Arendt, Agel, and Dick 1999; Oliphant and Drawbert 1996), higher than the 50% to 60% observed in collegiate soccer (Agel, Arendt, and Breshadsky 2005). The female-to-male rate ratio ranged from 1.6 to 4.6 in studies that included at least five male and five female ACL injuries. The one study that reported a female-to-male rate ratio above 4.6 (5.4 for Gwinn et al. 2000) was based on only five female injuries and one male injury. Generally, the rate ratios in basketball tended to be higher than the rate ratios in soccer.

In general, the rate of ACL injury was lower in basketball than in soccer, but a higher proportion of the injuries were classified as noncontact in basketball. This suggests that the rate of noncontact ACL injuries may be similar in the two sports, but that the rate of contact ACL injuries may be higher in soccer than in basketball. This conclusion must be viewed as tentative, especially because there is no standardized definition of what constitutes a "noncontact" injury. However, this interpretation is consistent with the observation that rate ratios in basketball tended to be higher than the rate ratios in soccer.

Handball

Data on ACL injury in team handball (table 1.3) were available from five studies in two countries, Norway (four studies) and Switzerland (one study). The rates were much higher in the Norwegian studies, but this is likely a methodologic artifact rather than a real difference between the two countries. Olsen and colleagues (2003) compared the incidence of ACL injury on two different types of flooring, using the data from three previous studies (Myklebust et al. 1997, 1998; Myklebust 2003). We used Olsen's aggregate total rate (both types of surfacing pooled). The incidence rate was approximately similar to the rates reported for soccer and basketball. The female-to-male rate ratio ranged from 1.6 to 3.2 in studies with at least five male and five female ACL injuries.

Skiing

The data on the incidence of ACL injury in skiing were difficult to interpret (table 1.4). Two studies using athlete-hours as the denominator indicated a lower rate of ACL injury in skiing than in soccer, basketball, and handball (de Loës, Dahlstedt, and Thomee 2000; Viola et al. 1999). They also gave relatively modest female-to-male rate ratios (1.4 and 1.0). However, skiing studies that used athletes as the denominator showed higher average risks of ACL injury than in any other sport and higher female-to-male rate ratios (2.0 and 3.1). More research is needed to clarify these apparent inconsistencies.

Collision Sports

We classified sports with full-body contact and high transfer of kinetic energies as collision sports (table 1.5). A priori, we expected that studies of collision sports would show a lower proportion of noncontact injuries, but this was not the case. Lambson, Barnhill, and Higgins (1996) and Orchard and colleagues (2001) reported that 55% and 76% of injuries were noncontact, respectively, and this was similar to the range of estimates for the other sports reviewed. Furthermore, the injury incidence reported and the female-to-male rate ratios were similar to those for the other sports reviewed (although all the female-to-male rate ratios for collision sports involved small numbers).

Military Training

Military training is not a sport, but it is a vigorous physical activity involving running and jumping. Pope (2002) and Gwinn's (2000), Uhorchak's (2003), Belmont's (1999), and Lauder's (2000) groups have reported data on the incidence of ACL injury in military personnel. Unfortunately, methodologic complexities preclude us from forming any firm conclusion from these studies. The measures of incidence used and the type of training performed vary greatly among these studies. In addition, Belmont and Lauder did not distinguish between ACL injuries in sport and ACL injuries in training. Obstacle courses were noted as a significant source of ACL injuries; these were the entire focus of Pope (2002) and accounted for 64% (7/11) and 33% (1/3) of ACL injuries related to military training at the U.S. Naval Academy and U.S. Military Academy, respectively (Gwinn et al. 2000; Uhorchak et al. 2003).

Other Sports

We also identified ACL injury incidence estimates for three other sports: floorball, gymnastics, and volleyball. Incidences in these sports tended to be lower than those reported for soccer and basketball. Snellman and colleagues (2001) reported that the average risk in Finnish floorball (a sport similar to ice hockey, but with less body contact) was 2.4% per season (95%CI: 0.6, 4.1). De Loës and colleagues (2000) reported incidence rates of 0.006 and 0.001 per 1000 athlete-hours for females and males in Swiss youth gymnastics, respectively. De Loës and colleagues (2000) also reported an ACL injury rate of 0.004 and 0.002 per 1000 athlete-hours in females and males in volleyball. Arendt and colleagues (1999) reported that the ACL injury rate was 0.11 per 1000 athlete-exposures in NCAA (female) collegiate volleyball.

It was surprising to us that only two studies in the past decade had provided ACL injury incidence data for volleyball, and only one study had dealt with gymnastics. Also, we did not locate any studies giving incidence estimates for lacrosse (one of the fastest-growing sports in the United States) or professional or amateur dance. However, our search was confined to the past 10 years of peer-reviewed literature.

Synthesis and Commentary

The number of females participating in high school and collegiate athletes is steadily increasing (NCAA 2004; National Federation of State High School Associations [NFHS] 2005). Over the course of the past two decades (from the 1983-1984 school year to the 2003-2004 school year), the number of females participating in NCAA sports rose by 92%, whereas the number of male participants grew by only 15% (NCAA 2004). At the high school level, the growth in participation over the same time period was 64% for girls and 33% for boys (NFHS 2005). As the number of females participating in competitive and recreational physical activity increases, the number of female ACL injuries can also be expected to increase. Thus, addressing the cause and prevention of ACL injury is one of the major challenges currently facing sports medicine.

Our knowledge of ACL injury has advanced significantly in the past 10 years. However, the basic conclusions of this review remain similar to those of a review published five years ago (Garrick and Requa 2001). The majority of injuries appear to be noncontact (or do not involve direct contact to the knee). Men account for most of the injuries, but this is likely due to their higher exposure to "high-risk" athletic tasks and their greater involvement in contact sports. Studies examining specific sporting subpopulations that had reasonable precision for gender comparisons have consistently shown that females have an injury rate 1.5 to 4.6 times higher than males. Rates for females up to 10-fold greater than those in males have been reported (e.g., Gwinn et al. 2000, for military training); however, these are based on smaller numbers of injuries and should be viewed as preliminary, subject to the conduct of larger studies.

Only one study (de Loës, Dahlstedt, and Thomee 2000) dealt with the background incidence in a large segment of the general population. The reason is that most studies have concentrated on specific high-risk athletic subpopulations, probably in order to maximize the number of injuries observed in the study. Apart from military training, no study has ever quantified the incidence of ACL injury outside of organized sport. Although the rate of ACL injury is highest in the setting of organized sport, there are likely a significant number of ACL injuries that occur outside of formal sport settings, such as pickup basketball at home.

Only in Switzerland does registration of ACL injury in a large segment of the general population exist. This lack of information on the incidence of ACL injury in the population as a whole is a major gap in our knowledge of the epidemiology of ACL injury. There is a need to develop multicenter registries of ACL injuries so that a large case series can be assembled and studied. Ideally, researchers should collectively develop a template set of standardized injury report forms so that data could be pooled between studies.

Another gap in our knowledge relates to the classification of ACL injuries as contact or noncontact. We were surprised how few studies (11 of the 39) reported the percentage of injuries that were noncontact in nature. Given that the intrinsic forces are assumed to play a criterion role in the causation of many ACL injuries, we had expected that more researchers would define the proportion of their injuries that were classified as noncontact. However, the lack of an agreed-upon definition of "noncontact" in the literature may limit researchers' ability to classify their injuries as contact or noncontact. We urge that researchers develop some standard definition and guidelines for classifying ACL injuries according to the degree of contact. At the Atlanta, Georgia, meeting that led to the development of this book, a classification scheme for ACL injuries based on direct contact with the knee, contact with parts of the body other than the knee (indirect contact), and noncontact was proposed. In the interest of stimulating discussion in this area, this proposed schema is reproduced (with some elaboration) in figure 1.4.

Most of the 39 studies we reviewed were of high quality, and some investigators have been careful to ensure that all ACL injuries conform to some standard criteria (such as arthroscopic examination). However, comparisons between the studies are extremely problematic because of methodologic differences in the way in which the incidence is reported. Some studies report incidence

Type I: Direct Contact

External force was directly applied to injured knee and was probably the proximate cause of injury.

- Example: Injured knee was forcefully struck by another player.
- Example: Athlete tripped and fell, striking injured knee on goalpost with significant force.

Type II: Indirect Contact

External force was applied to athlete but not directly to the injured knee. The force was involved in the injury process but was probably not the proximate cause.

- Example: Injured athlete was struck and knocked off balance by an opponent in an area distal to the knee (i.e., the torso or thigh). Athlete's resultant movement led to the injury without direct contact to the knee.

Type III: Noncontact

Forces applied to the knee at the time of injury resulted from the athlete's own movements and did not involve contact with another athlete or object.

- Example: Athlete landed from a jump and attempted to cut to one side.

FIGURE 1.4 Proposed classification scheme for ACL injuries by type of contact.
Reprinted, by permission, of the attendees of the Atlanta meeting.

rates per player-hours at risk; some studies use rates per athlete-exposure; and others have used risk measures based on the athlete, the team, or the game. This confusion of methodology is very frustrating for researchers attempting to synthesize data across multiple studies. We suggest that authors be encouraged to report their denominator data in detail so that incidence can be recomputed by readers of the paper and compared across studies. Synthesis of data across studies is far easier if authors devote a table to fully presenting the denominator data (e.g., Myklebust et al. 1998; Lombardo et al. 2005). In many (if not all) of the studies that used athlete-hours as the denominator, the authors could readily have additionally reported (in a table) their denominator in terms of athlete-exposures. If they had done this (as in Lombardo et al. 2005), we would have been able to recompute their incidence rates based on athlete-hours to incidence rates based on athlete-exposures. This would have meant that data from *almost all* studies could have been compared.

Conclusions

We set out in this chapter to address four questions. Question 1 was "What is the average incidence of ACL injury in the general population?" We conclude that this is currently unknown except for youth in one country (Switzerland), where the incidence is less than 1 injury per 100,000 athlete-hours of sport exposure. In specific athlete subgroups, the rate rises dramatically, up to 1 per 1000 athlete-hours for females in professional soccer games (Faude et al. 2005; Giza et al. 2005). Thus, the rate may be 10 times to 100 times higher in elite athletes than in recreational athletes.

Question 2 was "How does ACL injury incidence vary by age and gender?" On a population basis, there are more injuries in males than in females. However, this is likely an artifact of males' higher exposure to the type of activities that generate ACL injury. Most injuries appear to occur in the 16- to 18-year-old age group.

Question 3 was "How does ACL injury incidence vary by sport and gender?" For the sports detailed in tables 1.1 through 1.5, the incidence of ACL injury has been consistently higher in females than in males. The reported ACL injury rates in females in these sports are 1.5 to 4.6 times higher than those in males. Female-to-male rate ratios above 4.6 have been reported; however, they are based on small numbers of injuries and should be viewed as preliminary, subject to confirmation by larger studies. Surprisingly, the incidence of ACL injury seems relatively similar among the sports reviewed here. However, comparisons between different studies are problematic because of methodologic differences in the manner in which researchers collect and report denominator data, and because of the relatively small number of injuries observed in most studies.

Question 4 was "What are the limitations in our current epidemiologic knowledge of ACL injury incidence?" One major limitation is that the general incidence in the United States and most other countries is unknown. In addition, although it is clear that many of the injuries do not involve direct contact to the injured knee, the proportion of noncontact injuries is frequently unreported, perhaps because there is no clear consensus on how to define "noncontact" (or lack of direct contact).

Recommendations for Future Research

On the basis of this review, we recommend the following:

1. Research should be conducted on the average incidence of ACL injury in the general population. The incidence of ACL injury needs to be quantified in settings other than organized sport. Researchers should publish their denominator data in detail, perhaps using a table, so that information on number of players per team, number of games and practices, number of athlete-exposures, and length of follow-up can be readily abstracted from papers.

2. Consideration should be given to establishing multicenter ACL injury registries so that a large prospective case series of ACL injuries can be established and systematically built up over time from the individual studies being conducted. Researchers should collectively work to standardize the type of data collected on ACL injuries, as well as the way the data are coded.

3. Researchers should develop guidelines for the classification of ACL injuries as contact versus noncontact (or direct contact, indirect contact, and noncontact), so that data on the proportion of ACL injuries that do not result from direct contact can be meaningfully compared across studies. These data should be collected and reported in all epidemiologic studies of ACL injury.

Chapter 2

Does ACL Reconstruction Prevent Articular Degeneration?

The ACL Risk Equation

Paul H. Marks, MD
Kurt P. Droll, MD, MSc, FRCSC
Michelle Cameron-Donaldson, MD

Osteoarthritis is found more commonly in the knee than in any other weight-bearing joint in the human body. Individuals with ACL insufficiency have been found to have a slightly higher risk for developing osteoarthritis in the knee compared to the general population. Several risk factors have been implicated in the development of osteoarthritis in the ACL-deficient knee, including concomitant meniscal pathology, osteochondral pathology, impaired proprioception, and biochemical mediators. This chapter reviews the evidence pertaining to those risk factors. In addition, in an effort to aid in the future prognosis of posttraumatic osteoarthritis, we propose that an "ACL risk equation" be developed that would express the overall osteoarthritis risk quantitatively and would include all of the pertinent risk factors.

Osteoarthritis (OA) is one of the most common diseases in the world, and it has been estimated that 10% of the general population of North America has this disorder (Cunningham and Kelsey 1984). Osteoarthritis, also known as degenerative joint disease, is found more commonly in the knee than in any other weight-bearing joint in the human body (Slemenda 1992). The principal pathologic features of this disease include progressive focal degradation of the articular cartilage lesion and at the joint margins (i.e., osteophytes) (Brandt

1985). These structural changes in the knee can manifest clinically as joint pain, stiffness, crepitations, loss of motion, and enlargement. Consequently, OA in the knee joint may significantly impair lower extremity function, thus making it extremely disabling and limiting physical functioning such as traveling up or down stairs or engaging in "heavy chores" (Davis et al. 1991). From an economic perspective, it has been postulated that the annual cost of OA in the United States is $82 billion (Centers for Disease Control 2003). Since the knee is the most common site, it is without a doubt responsible for a large proportion of this financial burden. As a result, OA of the knee joint is a major public health problem worldwide.

Even though OA of the knee is relatively prevalent in the population, the etiology and prognostic factors for this disease are poorly understood. Several studies, however, have implicated ACL insufficiency as a precursor for degenerative change in the knee (Sherman et al. 1998; Giove et al. 1983; Pattee et al. 1989; Hawkins, Misamore, and Merrit 1986). These studies showed that individuals with chronic ACL deficiency are at a significantly higher risk for developing OA than the general population. Anterior cruciate ligament insufficiency is a relatively common condition. Neilson and Yde (1991) reported an ACL injury rate of 0.3 per 1000 inhabitants in Denmark during a one-year period among a community of 256,000 inhabitants (i.e., 76 ACL injuries). Another population-based study from San Diego Kaiser Health Plan evaluated knee injuries over a three-year period from among 280,000 inhabitants. The rate of ACL injury was reported to be 0.34 per 1000 individuals (Miyasaka et al. 1991).

As expected, rupture of the ACL is a more common event in athletes. A large proportion of ACL ruptures occur during participation in sporting activities, principally those that involve deceleration, twisting, cutting, and jumping movements. In a study of ski injuries, Feagin and associates (Feagin et al. 1987) reported 72 ACL injuries per 100,000 skier days and estimated over 100,000 ACL injuries in the United States per year from skiing alone. In addition, a football injury study showed 42 ACL injuries per 1000 players, which extrapolated to a 16% chance of ACL injury in a four-year collegiate career and a 100-fold increased risk for ACL injury compared with that for the general population (Hewson, Mendini, and Wang 1986). As reported in the Kaiser study, sport activities such as football, baseball, soccer, basketball, and skiing accounted for approximately 78% of the ACL injuries sustained during participation in sports (Miyasaka et al. 1991). Consequently, many individuals rupture their ACL each year, which results in an increased likelihood of becoming disabled with OA in the future.

The natural history of the ACL-deficient knee has yet to be completely elucidated. Therefore, much debate exists regarding the relationship between OA and the ACL-deficient knee. In addition to pain and swelling (Noyes et al. 1983), previous studies have documented that ACL rupture often leads to joint instability (Hawkins, Misamore, and Merrit 1986; Feagin and Curl 1976). These data have provided the impetus for many researchers to postulate that repetitive anterior tibial subluxation episodes under weight-bearing conditions can cause intra-articular damage to structures such as the articular cartilage, menisci, joint capsule, and ligamentous restraints. This results in additive trauma and progressive deterioration of the joint and in turn OA (Johnson et al. 1992). Many researchers, such as Lynch and Henning (1994), are convinced of this casual relationship and support the belief that degenerative arthritis in the ACL-deficient knee is inevitable. However, controversy surrounds the topic because several studies do not directly support this theory. Ferretti and colleagues (1991) and more recently Daniel and associates (1994) reported that individuals who underwent ligament reconstruction acutely have an overall higher likelihood of developing arthrosis in the affected knee. This suggests that the etiology of the osteoarthritic changes seen after ACL rupture is multifactorial and not solely due to biomechanical disturbances. Therefore the purpose of this chapter is to outline several risk factors that have been implicated as playing a role in the development of OA in the ACL-deficient knee, such as concomitant meniscal pathology, osteochondral pathology, impaired proprioception, and biochemical mediators in the knee joint.

Meniscal Pathology

Structure and Function of Normal Meniscus

The menisci are crescent-shaped wedges of fibrocartilage located between the condyles of the femur and tibia. These structures are composed of primarily type I collagen (accounts for 90% of total collagen within meniscus) and other components that are found in much smaller quantities such as noncollagenous protein, proteoglycans, and interstitial fluid (McDevitt and Webber 1989). The vascular supply of the menisci originates predominantly from the inferior and superior lateral and medial geniculate arteries. The degree of peripheral vascular penetration, however, has been found to be only 10% to 30% of the outer width of the adult meniscus (Arnoczky and Warren 1982). Therefore the majority of the meniscus is avascular, which profoundly influences its ability to heal from injury. Several studies have shown that the menisci have a characteristic pattern of collagen fiber orientation. The majority of collagen fibers are aligned in a circumferential fashion, yet there are some that are oriented radially, particularly at the meniscal surfaces (Bullough et al. 1970; Ahmed and Burke 1983). The biomechanical functions of the meniscus stem from the physical properties of this matrix.

The menisci were for many years believed to be simply vestigial structures. However, a large body of evidence from the last few decades has suggested that the meniscus serves a variety of significant functions. Biomechanical studies have established that the meniscus has an important role as a load-bearing structure, for it has been reported that 50% to 85% of the compressive load of the knee joint is transmitted through the meniscus (Ahmed and Burke 1983). In addition, the viscoelastic properties of menisci allow them to function as shock absorbers in dampening the load generated during weight-bearing activity (Johnson and Pope 1978). As a result, intact menisci transmit load and absorb energy, thus protecting the articular surfaces from compressive stress. In the kinematics of a normal knee (see figure 2.1), there is both sliding and rolling motion of the femur on the tibia. This is accomplished as a rounded femoral condyle is articulated with a relatively flattened tibial plateau. Consequently, only a small region of the femur is in direct contact with the tibia. The menisci decrease joint incongruity by filling in the space between the tibia and the femur (Simon, Freidenberg, and Richardson 1973). In increasing joint congruity, the menisci are able to assist in joint stability by deepening the articular surfaces of the tibial plateau (Smillie 1971). This is particularly relevant in the ACL-deficient knee, for Levy and associates (1982) showed that the posterior horn of the medial meniscus acts as a posterior wedge and thus serves as a secondary restraint to anterior tibial translation. Furthermore, during joint motion the menisci contribute to joint lubrication by spreading synovial fluid over the articular surfaces, and during weight bearing serve to compress nutrients in the articular cartilage (Renstrom and Johnson 1990).

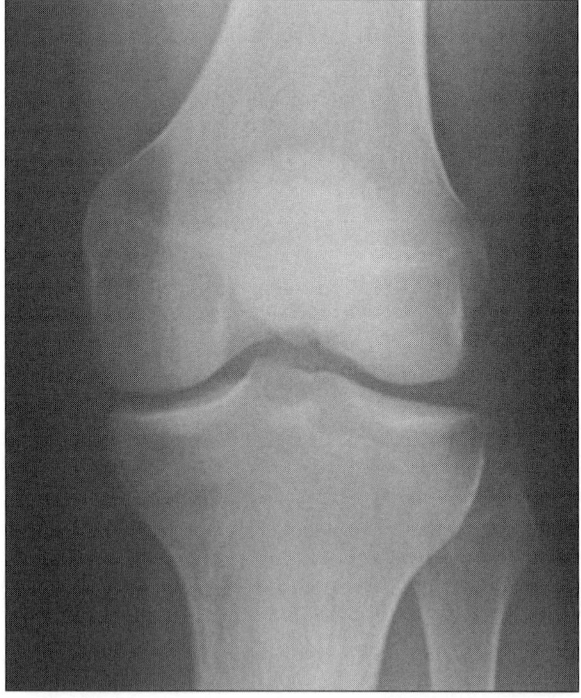

FIGURE 2.1 Radiograph of normal knee.

Prevalence and Pattern of Meniscal Injury in ACL-Deficient Knees

Anterior cruciate ligament insufficiency is associated with a high rate of concomitant meniscal lesions. In acute ACL deficiency, the incidence of meniscal tears has been reported to range from 41% to 77% (DeHaven 1980; Noyes et al. 1980; Woods and Chapman 1984; Indelicato and Bittar 1985; Hirshman, Daniel, and Miyasaka 1990; Shelbourne and Nitz 1991; Paletta et al. 1992). In contrast, the reported rate of meniscal injury in the intact ACL knee is 15% to 25% (Noyes et al. 1980; DeHaven 1980). In the chronic ACL-deficient knee, the incidence of meniscal damage is reported to be even higher, with rates ranging from 73% to 98% (Indelicato and Bittar 1985; Warren and Marshall 1978; McDaniel and Dameron 1980; Noyes et al. 1983; Fowler and Regan 1987). Woods and Chapman (1984) compared a group of patients with chronic injuries to a group with acute injuries and reported that the incidence of meniscal tears almost doubled (88% vs. 45%, respectively). Therefore, some meniscal injuries occur at the time of ACL injury, while others may result from recurrent giving-way episodes long after the ACL was disrupted.

While the type of injury is obviously influenced by mechanism of injury, lateral meniscal tears are more common in acute ACL ruptures (Fowler and Regan 1987; Cooper, Arnoczky, and Warren 1990), and medial tears predominate in chronic insufficiency (Woods and Chapman 1984; Indelicato and Bittar 1985), indicating continued injury to the medial meniscus over time due to knee instability. In the chronic setting, MacIntosh has called the ACL the "watchdog" of the medial meniscus (personal communication). In both the acute and chronic ACL deficiency situations, the peripheral posterior horns of the meniscus are at greatest risk of tearing and account for more than half of the meniscal injuries identified (Thompson and Fu 1993). However, differences in the type of meniscal tear are evident depending on whether it is located in the medial or lateral meniscus. A peripheral longitudinal tear is the most common medial meniscal lesion, while the lateral meniscus is more at risk for radial tear (Cerabona et al. 1998). The type of meniscal tear and its association with OA are discussed later.

Meniscal Pathology and Osteoarthritis of the ACL-Deficient Knee

The role of meniscal lesions in the pathogenesis of OA in the knee continues to be the focus of considerable discussion. Loss or damage of this structure has been associated with an accelerated development of OA (McDaniel and Dameron 1980; Fairbank 1948; Satku, Kumar, and Ngoi 1986). Fairbank, in his classic paper from 1948, described postmeniscectomy (i.e., removal of meniscus) roentgenographic changes that included joint space narrowing, osteophyte development, and flattening of the femoral articular surface. He reported that these changes were present in 50% to 66% of the knees studied after meniscectomy and in only 5% of the contralateral knees. Consequently, Fairbank was one of the first to postulate that loss of the load-bearing role of the meniscus leads to degenerative changes.

The importance of an intact meniscus in the prevention of OA in an ACL-deficient knee has been well documented. Sherman and associates (1998) reported a significantly higher incidence of degenerative change in ACL-insufficient knees with prior meniscectomy compared to those without meniscectomy. This is in agreement with the findings of several authors (Lynch and Henning 1994; Noyes et al. 1983; Sommerlath 1989). Furthermore, individuals who had both menisci removed were reported to have a higher frequency of OA than individuals with unilateral meniscectomy or meniscal repair (Sommerlath 1989). In addition, Sommerlath and Gillquist (1987) found, in a seven-year follow-up of subjects with intact ligaments, that degenerative arthritis occurred more frequently in patients with total meniscectomy than in those with only partial meniscectomy.

Meniscectomy has been shown to profoundly affect the manner in which load bearing occurs in the knee joint. As a result of partial or total meniscectomy, the contact area between the tibia and femur is decreased approximately 30% (Kurosawa, Fukubayashi, and Nakajima 1980). The reduced contact area increases the stresses of compression and shear across the articular cartilage, likely resulting in degenerative change (DeHaven 1990).

The progression of articular degeneration in the knee can also be influenced simply by one's having a meniscal injury, without a history of meniscal surgery. Satku and associates (1986) reported that all ACL-deficient subjects with clinical evidence of meniscal injury but no meniscectomy had degenerative change in the knee. However, not all meniscal tears are associated with damage of the articular cartilage. Unstable tears, such as bucket handle, longitudinal tears with broken handles, and complex tears, have been shown to correlate with an increased incidence of OA (Lynch and Henning 1994; Lewandrowski, Muller, and Schollmeier 1997).

Nevertheless, it has been demonstrated that damaged menisci still distribute some load and that knees with damaged menisci are less likely to have OA complications than those knees treated with partial or total meniscectomy (Casscells 1978; Lynch, Henning, and Glick 1983). Consequently, the risk of degeneration appears to be influenced by the degree of meniscal pathology, and thus the primary goal of management is to preserve the meniscus if at all possible.

Osteochondral Pathology

Prevalence and Patterns of Osteochondral Pathology in ACL-Deficient Knees

The increasing utilization of magnetic resonance imaging (MRI) and arthroscopy in the management of musculoskeletal trauma has allowed investigators to reliably identify lesions of articular cartilage and bone within the knee joint (Vellet et al. 1991; Engebretsen, Arendt, and Fritts 1993; Lahm et al. 1998).

These lesions were previously not visualized on routine roentgenograms. An acute rupture of the ACL has been shown to be associated with damage to both these structures in the knee (Bray and Dandy 1989; Indelicato 1983).

The reported incidence of chondral injury in the acutely ruptured ACL knee ranges from 18% to 46% (Daniel et al. 1994; Lynch, Henning, and Glick 1983; Bray and Dandy 1989; Indelicato 1983; Hardacker, Garret, and Basset 1990; Spindler et al. 1993). These studies commonly defined articular cartilage injuries as any chondromalacia, fractures, impaction, creases, or fissures upon observation; an example can be seen in figures 2.2 and 2.3. Furthermore, the medial compartment has been reported to be more at risk of sustaining damage than the lateral compartment (Daniel et al. 1994; Hirshman, Daniel, and Miyasaka 1990). However, the two studies that analyzed the location of the chondral injury did so three months after the injury. Therefore it is possible that these studies did not accurately document articular damage at time of injury but rather subsequent damage due to altered pathomechanics (i.e., giving-out episodes) of the ACL-deficient knee.

In 1989, Mink and Deutsch coined the term "bone bruise" to describe the posttraumatic subcortical regions of altered signal intensity in the femur or tibia (or both) on T_1- and T_2-weighted MRI images. The lesions on T_1-weighted

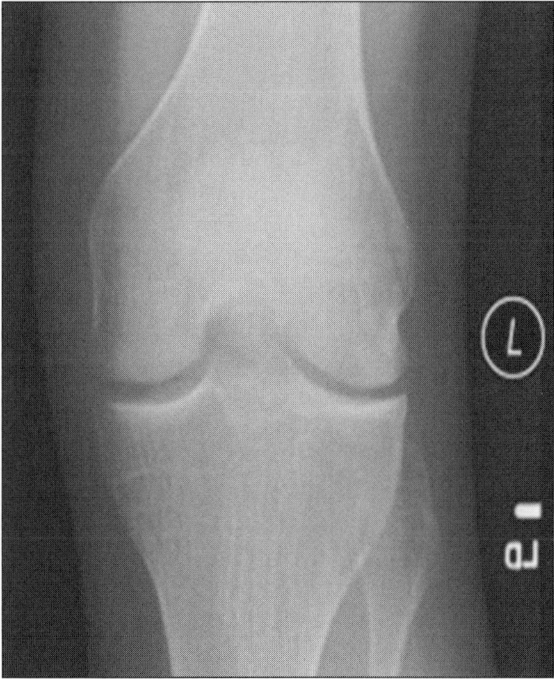

FIGURE 2.2 Radiograph of moderate osteoarthritis.

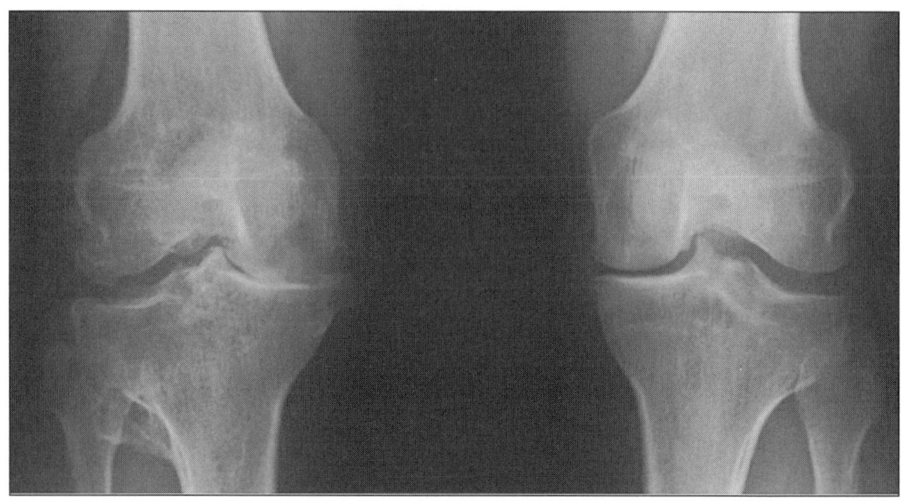

FIGURE 2.3 Radiograph of severe osteoarthritis.

images are characterized by decreased signal intensity, while on T_2-weighted images there is a corresponding increase in signal intensity. These "bone bruises" were subsequently classified by Vellet and colleagues (1991) according to their architectural appearance, their spatial relationship with cortical bone, and their short-term osteochondral sequelae. There is general agreement that the pathogenesis of these identifiable lesions on MRI results from microtrabecular fracture. This bone injury and its sequelae, that is, hemorrhage, edema, and inflammation, are responsible for the abnormal signals seen on imaging (Mink and Deutsch 1989).

The reported incidence of bone bruises with acute ACL rupture is even higher than that observed for articular cartilage injury. Several studies have revealed that approximately 80% of patients with a complete tear of their ACL have concomitant bone bruises (Vellet et al. 1991; Spindler et al. 1993; Speer et al. 1992; Rosen, Jackson, and Berger 1991). Bone bruises are evident in many sites within the knee joint; however, approximately 80% occur in the lateral compartment (Spindler et al. 1993; Graf et al. 1993). The sulcus terminalis of the lateral femoral condyle and the posterior tibial plateau are the most common areas involved. The high frequency of bone bruises in the lateral compartment of the acute ACL-deficient knee suggests that the mechanism of injury includes anterior subluxation, increased internal rotation of the tibia, and valgus stress. This would position the lateral femoral condyle over the posterior edge of the lateral tibial plateau. With subsequent valgus stress, impaction of these structures occurs, resulting in localized osseous contusions (Speer et al. 1992). In addition, bone scintigraphy has confirmed the location and presence of bone bruises in acute ligamentous knee injuries (Marks et al. 1992).

Osteochondral Pathology and Osteoarthritis of the ACL-Deficient Knee

Direct chondral injuries such as those identified by arthroscopy have been shown to initiate the process of OA (Arnoczky et al. 1991). It has been postulated that this occurs due to the limited ability of articular cartilage to repair itself. The impaired ability to heal stems from the lack of blood supply and also from the inability of articular cartilage chondrocytes to form adequate new tissue (Martin 1994). The severity of chondral injury appears to play a role in the progression of OA, as demonstrated by animal model studies. Injuries graded as "superficial" may cause death of cells surrounding the injury; however, they do not necessarily lead to OA unless there is accompanying joint incongruity (Arnoczky et al. 1991). Deep penetrating injuries, on the other hand, heal inadequately, because the defect fills in with cartilaginous tissue that is not articular cartilage but rather a mixture of hyaline and fibrocartilage. This new tissue does not remain intact over time and thus contributes to the further development of cartilage degeneration (Mankin 1982). With regard to the ACL-deficient knee, repeated episodes of anterior subluxation can exacerbate existing articular cartilage damage (Mankin 1982). Thus, the chondral lesion accompanying the acute rupture of the ACL may provide a focus for deterioration of the articular cartilage.

The natural history of bone bruises and their pathodegenerative implications within the knee joint remain largely unknown. Bone bruises represent a blunt injury to the overlying articular cartilage, subchondral bone, and inner marrow. Because of their relatively high occurrence in acute ACL injuries, they have generated a renewed interest in the etiology of posttraumatic knee OA. A number of animal model studies have addressed this possible relationship. Mankin (1982) reported that a single, supraphysiological blow to the surface of canine knee articular cartilage exceeding a critical threshold serves as a precursor for OA. Whether the trauma experienced at the time of ACL trauma is significant enough to exceed this threshold remains unknown. Donohue and associates (1983) noted that blunt trauma to adult canine articular cartilage produced changes in its histological, biochemical, and ultrastructural characteristics without articular surface disruption. In addition, they showed that it may be weeks or months before surface abnormalities become apparent. Consequently, the articular cartilage could be damaged yet appear normal on arthroscopic evaluation immediately following injury, and degenerative change may not become visibly apparent until much time later. This is consistent with clinical results reported by Graf and associates (1993) and Mink and Deutsch (1989), both of whom found no correlation between the location of bone bruises on MRI and articular cartilage damage in acute ACL-deficient knees.

There is a lack of data concerning this topic from human studies in the literature; however, Vellet and associates (1991) prospectively studied bone bruises and acute ACL tears. They reported that bone bruises localized in the medullary area (i.e., reticular) resolved completely within three months.

Lesions characterized by their contiguity with the adjacent cortical bone (i.e., reticular) resolved completely within three months, but lesions characterized by their contiguity with the adjacent cortical bone (i.e., geographic) had evidence of osteochondral sequelae at follow-up 6 to 12 months later. These changes included subcortical sclerosis, cartilage thinning, cartilage loss, and cortical impaction.

Coen and associates (1996) have recently reported a phenomenon they have termed "dimpling," which refers to softening of articular cartilage overlying an occult osseous injury. The cartilage transiently indents after gentle placement of a probe. The long-term sequelae of dimpling are unknown. However, dimpling may prove to be an early prognostic indicator of OA. Researchers have postulated that the mechanism for posttraumatic OA from a bone bruise is one in which the subchondral bone heals via callus formation, resulting in a stiffer construct than the previous normal bone. The decreased compliance of the new subchondral bone would require the articular cartilage to absorb more of the compressive forces and thus possibly lead to degenerative change (Rosen, Jackson, and Berger 1991). The evidence published to date, though minimal, nevertheless indicates that blunt trauma to the articular cartilage, even when not visible on initial inspection, may have profound effects on future cartilage integrity.

Impaired Proprioception

Proprioception in the Normal Knee

Recently, it has become apparent that most intra-articular and periarticular knee joint structures, in addition to their mechanical function, also play an important role in knee proprioception (Kennedy, Alexander, and Hayes 1982; Zimney 1988). Proprioception is considered a specialized variation of the sensory modality of touch and encompasses the sensations of joint movement (i.e., kinesthesia) and position (i.e., joint position sense) (Lephart et al. 1992). Proprioception in the knee has been shown to be provided by mechanoreceptors localized in the muscle, tendon, skin, capsule, and ligaments (Kennedy, Alexander, and Hayes 1982; Zimney 1988). Recent neuroanatomical studies have demonstrated that specialized mechanoreceptors respond to mechanical deformation (e.g., tension) of the tissue and serve to translate the stimulus into specific neuronal signal(s) (Schutte et al.1987). These mechanoreceptors have been found to be more active at the extreme ranges of motion and also responsible for initiating reflex contraction about the knee joint; both these properties may serve a protective or stabilizing role (Kennedy, Alexander, and Hayes 1982; Solomonow et al. 1987). Consequently, the ACL provides important neurologic feedback to the central nervous system that directly mediates joint position sense and protective muscular stabilization reflexes about the joint (Lephart et al. 1995; Solomonow et al. 1987). Therefore, a lack of afferent input from these mechanoreceptors may contribute to the progressive functional decline of the knee joint.

Impaired Proprioception and Osteoarthritis in the ACL-Deficient Knee

A significant deterioration in the proprioception of the knee joint occurs with an ACL rupture compared to that in the noninjured contralateral knee joint or in an age-matched control group, as well documented by several investigators (Barrack, Skinner, and Buckley 1989; MacDonald et al. 1996; Corrigan, Cashmen, and Brady 1992; Beard et al. 1993; Barrett, Cobb, and Bentley 1991). As mentioned previously, complete ACL insufficiency, and thus loss of this ligament's mechanical function, creates an unstable knee. Loss of ACL proprioceptive function, as originally proposed by Kennedy and associates (1982), is thought to contribute to this increasing instability over time through loss of the dynamic stabilizing reflexes. If this were the case, then proprioceptive loss would be expected to be present acutely as well as chronically. If loss of the ACL simply resulted in loss of passive restraint, which leads over time to mechanical stretching of capsular structures and thus to a possible change in response of capsular receptors, loss of proprioceptive ability would be expected chronically but not acutely. Barrack and associates (1989) and MacDonald and associates (1996) showed no difference in proprioception deficits between knees with acute and chronic injuries, thus suggesting that proprioceptive loss can be a cause of increased joint laxity and not just the result of it.

Appropriately coordinated and timed muscle coactivation normally attenuates load across the articular cartilage. Muscle activity is a critical determinant of the mechanical stiffness of the joint, which relates to its ability to resist disturbances and to maintain articular congruence (Johansson, Sjolander, and Sojka 1991). Afferent signals from mechanoreceptors in the ACL have been shown to initiate joint-protective muscular reflexes. Joint instability that occurs when muscular reflex stabilization of the knee is lacking is associated with a diminished sensory feedback mechanism, which causes a latent motor response of the hamstring muscles. Beard and associates (1993) reported in 1993 that reflex hamstring contraction latency is significantly slower in ACL-deficient knees than in the contralateral noninjured knee. Furthermore, they claimed that the greater the latency, the greater the instability. These data suggested that the loss of proprioceptive input from the ruptured ACL—evident as the longer response time required for the ACL-hamstring reflex to become active—contributes significantly to the functional instability of the knee. This corroborates Kennedy's original theory.

The relationship between impaired proprioception and OA has been minimally evaluated. Barrett and associates (1991) reported that joint position sense was impaired in a cohort of patients with osteoarthritic knees; however, this was not a longitudinal study, so it is difficult to conclude that the loss of position sense is a cause or a consequence of OA (or both). Many osteoarthritic patients have an abnormal wide-based gait, but this may not necessarily be related to the pain experienced. Instead it may be due to the loss of proprioception. Some authors have proposed that the abnormal gait results from an effort to maximize proprioceptive input (Barrett, Cobb, and Bentley 1991; Stauffer, Chao, and Gyory 1997, Berchuk et al. 1990). A similar effect observed in the ACL-deficient knee is designed to prevent excessive anterior displacement of the tibia, and is reported to result from abnormal proprioception (Barrett, Cobb, and Bentley 1991; Stauffer, Chao, and Gyory 1997). After an ACL rupture, proprioception must arise from other intact structures within the knee joint. However, the ACL-deficient knee has been shown to move in a nonphysical axis (resulting in alterations in gait and movement) (Berchuk et al. 1990). Thus the remaining proprioceptive output is nonphysiologically disorganized. Consequently, patients feel the knee to be unstable because cortical interpretation and analysis of knee position are disturbed. Therefore, the lack of proprioceptive feedback resulting from a rupture of the ACL leads to poor spatial and temporal coordination of muscle activity and limb position. This is characterized clinically by joint instability and an abnormal gait. This in turn causes an increased, repetitive, poorly distributed load across the joint surface, which leads to progressive degenerative change in the knee (Barrett 1991; Sharma and Pai 1997). Longitudinal studies are required to fully elucidate the relationship between impaired proprioception and OA in ACL-deficient knees.

Biochemical Mediators

Biochemistry of Articular Cartilage

Articular cartilage is a highly differentiated tissue consisting of four major components: chondrocytes, type II collagen, proteoglycan, and water. The three latter components form the extracellular matrix (ECM) of the cartilage, whose conformation provides the property of resilience. As a result, the articular cartilage located in the knee joint is able to resist load-bearing forces (Maroudas et al. 1986). Chondrocytes, although few in number, play a key role in matrix homeostasis. Matrix integrity is maintained through the regulation of degradative and synthetic events. This regulation is mediated by biological agents known as cytokines. Cytokines are polypeptides released by living cells, which act as local intercellular messengers to regulate host cell function (Nathan and Sporn 1991). Specifically, catabolic cytokines act on chondrocytes and synovial cells to induce production of matrix-degrading enzymes, such as metalloproteases. This is normally balanced by anabolic cytokines, which act on chondrocytes to induce production of cartilage matrix (Westacott and Sharif 1996). Alterations in the concentrations of any of the components responsible for this homeostasis may shift the equilibrium in favor of either overproduction of matrix proteins or net degradation.

Biochemical Mediators of Osteoarthritis in an ACL-Deficient Knee

The reported frequency of posttraumatic OA following ACL injury has been rather variable. This has led researchers to postulate that endogenous factors, in addition to mechanical factors, contribute to the development of knee OA. Osteoarthritis is characterized by slow changes in matrix metabolism. Initially there is an increase in water content of cartilage, implying a failure in the elastic restraint of the collagen network. Shortly afterward, an increased turnover of proteoglycans occurs, followed by an eventual net loss of proteoglycans from the ECM as catabolic events dominate over anabolic events (Heinegard and Oldberg 1989; Mankin and Brandt 1992). Therefore, an imbalance between the anabolic and catabolic events occurs in OA, resulting in the loss of cartilage matrix. The role of cytokines in this process has received particular attention because of their function, as already described, in regulating articular cartilage matrix homeostasis. The intra-articular cytokines most commonly implicated in the pathogenesis of OA have been interleukin (IL)-1, 6, and 8; interleukin-1-receptor antagonist protein (IL-1RA); tumor necrosis factor-alpha (TNF-α); and granulocyte macrophage-colony stimulating factor (GM-CSF).

Interleukin-1 exists in two isoforms, alpha (α) and beta (β); and they both have the biological ability to suppress the synthesis of type II collagen, which is a major constituent of articular cartilage matrix (Arner and Pratta 1989). Furthermore, IL-1 promotes the resorption of the cartilage matrix by inducing the production of specific matrix-degrading enzymes known as metalloproteases (Pelletier et al. 1991). Interleukin-1 also stimulates chondrocytes and synoviocytes to produce IL-6, which is believed to act as a cofactor for the inhibition of proteoglycan synthesis by IL-1 (Neitfeld et al. 1990). The cytokine IL-1RA has been shown to antagonize the activity of both isoforms of IL-1 (Seckinger, Williamson, and Balavoine 1987). This occurs because IL-1RA is a specific antagonist that competitively inhibits binding of IL-1 to its receptors. Interleukin-1RA is further characterized as having no intrinsic agonist activity (Carter, Beibert, and Dunn 1990). Consequently, IL-1RA can neutralize the catabolic effects of IL-1α and IL-1β.

The actions of TNF-α are very similar to those observed with IL-1. Tumor necrosis factor-alpha is a macrophage-derived cytokine that also promotes the degradation of cartilage and that suppresses the synthesis of cartilage proteoglycans (Saklatuala 1989). Like IL-1, TNF-α stimulates the secretion of IL-6 from chondrocytes. Furthermore, increased synthesis of IL-1 and metalloprotease has been shown to promote intra-articular inflammation, which results in the production of more IL-1 and TNF-α (Pelletier et al. 1991). Therefore, these latter cytokines induce cartilage degradation indirectly via their inflammatory properties.

Only recently have researchers investigated the role of intra-articular cytokines in the pathogenesis of posttraumatic OA. Several researchers have reported that IL-1α levels do not change in acute or chronic ACL-deficient knees compared to uninjured knees (Cameron et al. 1994; Marks, Cameron, and Regan 1998). However, levels of IL-1β have been shown to increase after an acute ACL injury; and they remain elevated, approximately fourfold when compared to levels in uninjured knees, in the chronic setting (Marks, Cameron, and Regan 1998). The level of chondroprotective IL-1RA is also increased acutely; however, only a slight increase, if any, is observed in chronic knees (Cameron et al. 1994; Marks, Cameron, and Regan 1998). This suggests the loss of an important chondroprotective cytokine in subjects with chronic ACL deficiency. The chronic absence of IL-1RA may allow IL-1 to act unabated and thus inflict more damage on the articular cartilage. Increased expression of IL-1 receptors on OA chondrocytes suggests that only small amounts of IL-1α or -1β, such as those levels seen normally, are needed to trigger catabolic enzyme production in OA joints (Roos et al. 1995).

The levels of TNF-α have been reported to increase acutely; and while their levels fall over several weeks, they still remain elevated compared to uninjured knee values (Cameron et al. 1994; Marks, Cameron, and Regan 1998). This suggests that TNF-α may play a role in chronic cartilage loss after ACL rupture. High levels of IL-6 and -8 have been noted in the acute phase of ACL injury but have been shown to fall back to the normal range by three months after injury. Conversely, the concentration of GM-CSF assists in propagating chronic chondral destruction. Recent work by Marks, Cameron, and Regan (1998) demonstrated increased expression of IL-1β and TNF-α with increasing grades of chondrosis in a chronic ACL-deficient knee. Furthermore, they showed decreasing IL-1RA levels with increasing grades of chondrosis. This suggests that certain cytokine profiles are associated with greater risk for developing posttraumatic OA in the ACL-deficient knee.

Summary and Future Work

The etiology of degenerative change in the knee following rupture of the ACL remains uncertain. The development of OA in the ACL-deficient knee is a complex process, with many factors likely contributing to its initiation, perpetuation, or both. This chapter has focused on the role of biomechanical, neuroanatomical, and biochemical factors in the development of knee OA. Along with instability of the knee, the degree of meniscal pathology has been well established as having a profound influence on modifying OA risk. Meniscectomy, partial or total, appears to present the greater OA risk, more so than damaged or repaired menisci. The magnitude of risk is illustrated by the fact that if a meniscectomy is performed, the development of OA is independent of the stabilization achieved with the ACL reconstruction (Ferretti et al. 1991). Consequently, preservation of the meniscus should be a primary goal of management. Occult osseous lesions or bone bruises represent traumatic injuries to bone. They occur in more than 80% of individuals with complete ruptures of the ACL, and have been shown to have degenerative osteochondral sequelae. Therefore, MRI-detected bone bruises are an important variable to consider. In addition, an ACL-insufficient knee has been shown to have deficits in proprioceptive function. This results in alterations in gait, with resulting modifications in weight-bearing loads in the knee joint, which may lead to degenerative changes. The role of cytokines in promoting cartilage degradation has recently received attention. Individuals with relatively high concentrations of chondrodestructive cytokines, such as IL-1β and TNF-α, and correspondingly low levels of chondroprotective cytokines such as IL-1RA, are at increased risk for developing posttraumatic OA in the ACL-deficient knee.

It is important to understand that all the risk factors discussed here do not act in isolation, but rather interact with each other to produce the degenerative changes. Moreover, other endogenous factors such as increasing age (Roos et al. 1995), obesity (Lynch and Henning 1994), abnormal alignment of the knee joint (Coventry 1973), genetic predisposition (Ala-Kokko et al. 1990), and high levels of activity (Lynch and Henning 1994), although not profiled in this chapter, have also been implicated as risk factors for knee OA. Therefore, many factors may contribute to OA, and orthopedic surgeons need to be aware of all the possible risks in order to determine the proper prognosis for OA after ACL rupture. Consequently, in an effort to aid in the future prognosis of posttraumatic OA, we propose the development of an "ACL risk equation" that would express overall OA risk quantitatively. This proposed equation would be a function of all the pertinent risk factors. To properly generate the ACL risk equation, a multiple-variable analysis of the degree of interaction among these risk factors (which ultimately produce posttraumatic OA) is necessary. The ability to determine an individual's level of OA risk would aid the surgeon in tailoring pre- and postoperative management. Finally, novel therapeutic strategies such as gene therapy may be subsequently developed in order to counteract or neutralize the relevant factors and thus protect the ACL-insufficient knee from degenerative changes.

Chapter 3

The Costs Associated With ACL Injury

Timothy Edwin Hewett, PhD, FACSM
Bohdanna T. Zazulak, DPT, MS, OCS

Since its passage 30 years ago, Title IX has led to greater opportunities for girls and women to play sports, receive scholarships, and obtain other important benefits resulting from athletic participation. As a result, there has been a large increase in female sport participation (figure 3.1). In 1972, 1 in 27, or fewer than 300,000 girls nationwide, participated in high school varsity sports. By 2002, the proportion of female participants rose to 1 in 2.5, the number approaching 3 million girls nationwide. Title IX has also made a tremendous difference in female athletic participation at the collegiate level. Prior to Title IX, 2% of college athletes were female, but by 2001 this had increased to 43% of college athletes—a change from 32,000 to over 150,000 (National Coalition for Women and Girls in Education 2002). The passage of Title IX in 1972 has increased female participation in sport by almost 500% at the college level and more than 1000% at the high school level (National Coalition for Women and Girls in Education 2002).

The NCAA Injury Surveillance System (1998-2002) showed that ACL injury rates for females were two to three times higher than those of males in soccer and five to eight times greater in basketball (National Collegiate Athletic Association 2002). More than two-thirds of ACL injuries are sustained in noncontact situations, with the majority occurring during landing from a jump (Boden et al. 2000; Griffin et al. 2000; McNair, Marshall, and Matheson 1990). This elevated risk of ACL injury, coupled with the aforementioned dramatic increase in participation in jumping and cutting sports (i.e., basketball, volleyball, and soccer), has led to a dramatic rise in ACL injuries in female athletes. Many of these injuries require surgical and rehabilitative intervention, with the financial burden of ACL injuries in females approaching $650 million annually for the

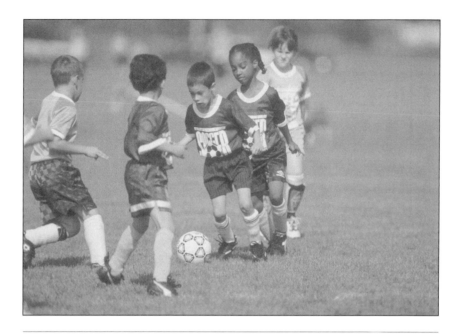

FIGURE 3.1 Since the inception of Title IX there has been a large increase in female sport participation, including coed sports at a young age.
© Human Kinetics

combined secondary and collegiate levels (Myer, Ford, and Hewett 2004b). Conversely, probably less than $10 million of federal funds has been awarded to research ACL injuries and their prevention over the same period. Most funding has been awarded in just the last couple of years. If it were possible to eradicate the approximate 5-to-1 gender disparity in ACL injury rates in gender-matched pivoting and cutting sports, the financial burden of the female ACL dilemma could drop by 80%. If ACL injury costs are estimated at $650 million, this amount could theoretically be reduced to $130 million annually.

A cost–benefit analysis of potential prevention efforts should consider not only the economic aspects of prevention but also its impact on the psychosocial effects of sport participation for female athletes (figure 3.2). We should be prepared to deal with the potential psychological and emotional sequelae surrounding the gender disparity in ACL injury incidence. These may include the deleterious effects of entire lost seasons of sport participation or scholarship funding (or both) and the long-term effects of lowered academic performance; the pressures from parents and coaches on the medical provider's judgment of the patient's readiness to return to play; and increases in the incidence of factors such as teenage pregnancy, illicit drug use, and smoking that occur more often in nonparticipants (Freedman et al. 1998; Miller et al. 1999; Naylor, Gardner, and Zaichowsky 2001). These social and psychological factors can also influ-

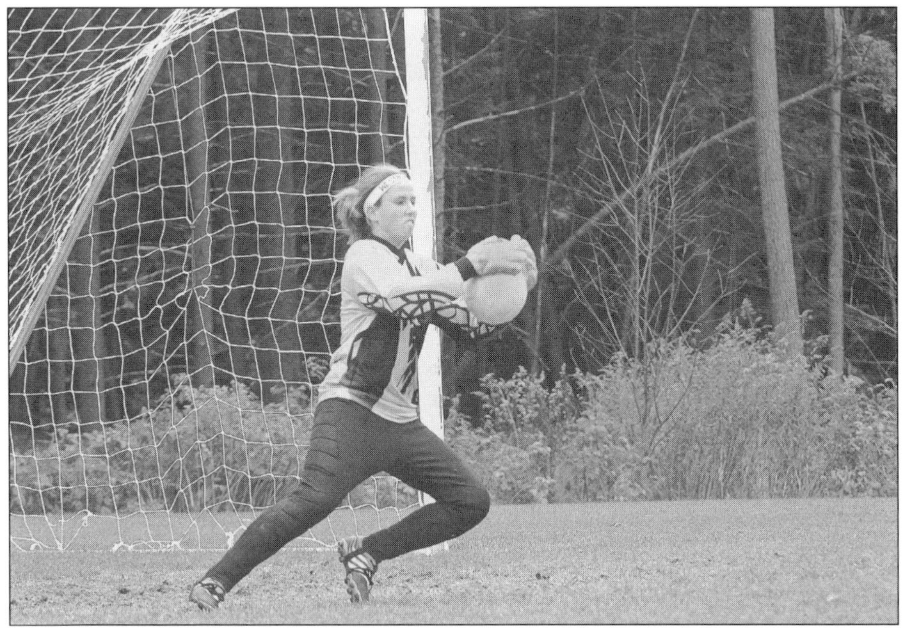

FIGURE 3.2 A cost–benefit analysis of potential prevention efforts should consider not only the economic aspects of prevention but also its impact on the psychosocial effects of sport participation for female athletes.
© Richard Bergen

ence the athlete's ability to return to participation and should be considered throughout the course of treatment and rehabilitation. Despite the potential negative side effects of sport participation, the rise in sport participation for young women is associated with considerable favorable outcomes for both mental and physical health. The U.S. Surgeon General reported that regular physical activity relieves symptoms of depression and anxiety and may improve mood and reduce the risk of developing depression (U.S. Department of Health and Human Services 1996). In general, sport participation improves health-related quality of life in female athletes by enhancing psychological well-being and by improving physical function (U.S. Department of Health and Human Services 1996) (figure 3.3).

There is evidence that neuromuscular training alters muscle firing patterns as it decreases landing forces, improves balance, and reduces ACL injury incidence in female athletes (Hewett et al. 2005c). Hewett, Myer, and Ford (2005d) recently completed a systematic review of the published studies of interventions targeted at ACL injury prevention in female athletes. Five of the six studies in the review demonstrated a significant reduction of injuries in general; four of six showed a reduction of knee injuries; and three of six showed a reduction of ACL injury

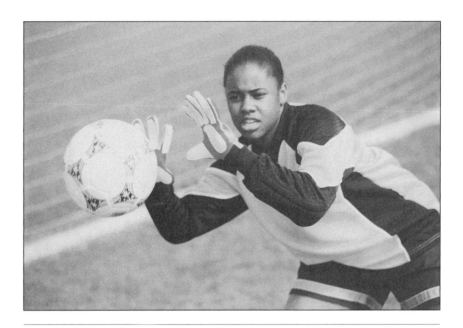

FIGURE 3.3 There are numerous psychosocial effects of sport participation for female athletes.

rates specifically. The common components of the effective interventions were plyometrics, biomechanics and technique evaluation with feedback, strength, balance, and core stability training. With strong evidence in support of the effectiveness of neuromuscular training on knee and ACL injury reduction in female athletes, health care providers and researchers should implement screening and prevention programs in their communities and advocate for insurance reimbursement for preventive intervention (figure 3.4).

Though preventive intervention may reduce ACL injury incidence in female athletes, the rate of ACL injury, regardless of mechanism of injury, continues to be significantly higher for female athletes than for male athletes (Agel, Arendt, and Bershadsky 2005). Despite the significant attention paid to the discrepancy between ACL injury rates in men and women, these differences remain prevalent; this may indicate a problem with a lack of widespread implementation of these programs. One of the most important factors that limit the use of preventive services is the insufficient health insurance coverage for these services. Until recently, most public and private health insurance plans have excluded coverage of preventive care options, especially in fields related to "quality of life" like sports medicine. The remainder of the current review examines sources of funding for preventive services in the past, present, and potentially the future, including employer-based coverage, federal sources, and private insurance organizations.

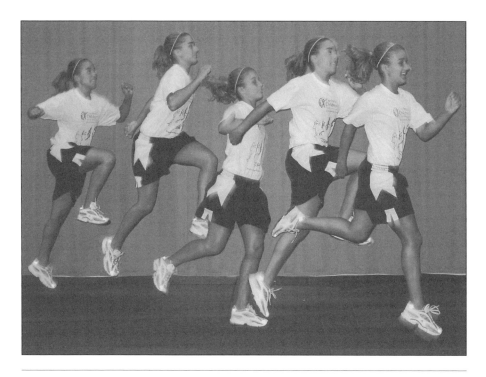

FIGURE 3.4 Neuromuscular training programs appear to reduce the incidence of ACL injury.

Workers' compensation may be the leader on the frontier of reimbursement for injury prevention. Workers' compensation programs are state regulated and covered by third-party insurers based on federal standards (Kissick 1994). Workers' compensation insurance covers employees when they become sick or injured or are killed on the job. This insurance generally provides coverage for any necessary medical treatment related to the injury or illness and compensation for lost wages. Benefits include medical expenses, lost wages, vocational rehabilitation, and death benefits.

Injury prevention in the workplace now includes the prevention of occupational overuse injuries, manual handling injuries, psychological hazards, and other injuries and illnesses that affect the worker's ability to perform assigned duties. These types of preventive interventions include ergonomic assessments for work areas, education for supervisors, local athletic programs, and skills training in proper posture and body mechanics for work groups. Numerous studies support the effectiveness of these types of consultative workplace risk assessments and preventive interventions in the reduction of the rate and severity of workplace injury (Carrivick, Lee, and Yau 2002; Coleman and Hansen 1994; McGrail, Tsai, and Bernacki 1995; Wood 1987). Federal legislation has been instrumental in the development of many of the injury prevention strategies in these state-run programs and will continue to be significant due to increased awareness of the importance of these services. Potential further federal legislation (e.g., amendment to Title IX) could lead to greater use of prevention strategies for female athletes.

Who Pays for ACL Injury Prevention in the High-Risk Female Athlete?

Despite the recognition of the importance of prevention, the federal government's approach to this sport injury dilemma is divided among numerous federal organizations: the Centers for Disease Control and Prevention, the National Center for Injury Prevention and Control, and the Department of Health and Human Services. Working independently, it is challenging for these federal agencies to collectively support scientific research and collection of data. The fragmented approach to the amelioration of this problem contributes to the inadequate nationwide recognition of the gender disparity in ACL injury rates. It would seem prudent to form a unified, proactive federally funded program targeted toward safety in sport in order to guide the provision of a coordinated infrastructure with the sole purpose of injury prevention. Establishment of such a national group with authority and equal representation would expedite the widespread implementation of ACL injury prevention programs for the at-risk female athlete.

Funding by sport organizations, university athletics departments, and school districts is another potential option. The Fédération Internationale de Football Association (FIFA) has developed, through an international network and its own funding sources, the nine-step F-MARC program to prevent injuries in football (soccer). Other international programs include injury prevention in skiing. Switzerland's social insurance system has launched a program designed to minimize risk of skiing accidents (Ramseier and Odermatt 1993). The Institute for Preventative Sports Medicine is an organization in the United States devoted to the development of preventive sports medicine practice. Funds for research and operation of the institute are obtained entirely through tax-deductible contributions from individuals, foundations, and corporations and with grants from public and private agencies.

Private health coverage has been slow to follow the public sector's lead in funding prevention initiatives. In the United States, private insurance is provided primarily by two different types of entities: state-licensed health insuring organizations and self-funded employee health benefit plans. State-licensed health insuring organizations are regulated under state law, although federal law includes additional standards and in some cases supersedes state authority. There are three primary types of state-licensed health insuring organizations: commercial health insurers, government-sponsored plans, and health maintenance organizations. Preventive ACL intervention is generally not covered by most private insurance programs. With health care reform, private health organizations have begun to recognize the cost benefits of prevention, particularly in covering specific clinical preventive services such as well-child visits, prenatal care, immunizations, family planning, and cancer screening. The prevention benefits least likely to be included in health care reform are coverage for counseling services, community-based health promotion, wellness programs, and injury prevention.

Despite the inadequacies in the current approach, change is imminent as more and more insurance companies are recognizing the importance of these types of preventive services and the potential liability of an absence of support for these intervention strategies. For example, if a patient is identified as high risk for ACL injury and the primary physician refers the patient for preventive training, private insurers may be pressured to change their current practice of flatly denying claims for preventive interventions and begin to cover these important, validated interventions. There are isolated examples of private insurer sponsorship for community ACL injury prevention training. However, this action does not translate into specific reimbursement for an enrollee for prevention training. Health maintenance organizations are chartered to maintain health and not just contain the cost of injury treatment. The recognition that injury prevention should be a mandate for managed care organizations may lead to a growing trend toward coverage for prevention and health promotion services.

Self-pay is another method for funding these potential prevention strategies and interventions. Secondary to athletic department-funded programs (both collegiate and secondary), self-pay is the most common form of payment for ACL injury prevention programs. The biggest potential problem with this method is the inequity in the delivery of these preventive services. To construct an equitable system for increasing access to preventive services, it may be necessary to consider improvements in both public and private coverage of these services, in order that high risk athletes may be screened, identified and given access to effective preventative interventions.

Insurance companies should both be pressured and have incentives to reimburse for these interventions. Researchers and clinicians must demonstrate the potential long-term cost savings of these preventive strategies. In the meantime, it is important for the lay public, and perhaps even more importantly researchers and health care professionals, to maintain persistent pressure on insurance companies, organized athletic groups, sport organizations, and other for-profit and nonprofit organizations to promote preventive interventions. Without effective leadership and promotion by researchers and clinicians, these important programs will not be adequately instituted. Without these preventive interventions, ACL injuries will continue to inequitably affect young female athletes and continue to stress overextended health care systems.

This is the era of both evidence-based medicine and easy accessibility of medical information to the lay public. Thus, for successful prevention, specific scientifically based strategies should be employed and the important findings quickly made available to both the insurance companies and the athletic community. Like any medical intervention, preventive practice relies on good scientific data. Well-designed, clinically relevant research programs should continue to be developed in order to study the effectiveness of various prevention programs in both the short and long term. In order for ACL injury prevention programs to be recognized as potentially important for the long-term health and well-being of young female athletes, as well as for health care cost containment, sound scientific research findings must be brought to the public forum through academic lectures and the lay media. The public's awareness of preventive measures may be increased if this scientific evidence is shared with state and federal government representatives. Enlisting government representatives as advocates for ACL injury prevention, as well as use of the media, will increase the awareness of coaches, athletic trainers, parents, athletes, and the general public.

Informing the High-Risk Female Athlete

Neuromuscular training programs appear to reduce the incidence of ACL injury (figure 3.5) (Hewett, Myer, and Ford 2005d). Though preventive intervention programs may reduce ACL injury incidence in female athletes, the rate of ACL injury continues to be significantly higher for female athletes than for male athletes (Agel, Arendt, and Bershadsky 2005). Despite the significant attention paid to the disparity between ACL injury rates in men and women, these differences remain prevalent, perhaps indicating a lack of sufficient implementation of these scientifically validated programs. Greater awareness in both the private and public sectors may be required in order to enhance efforts to promote these programs and to result in more widespread availability and use of these interventions by the female athlete. The current sources of information available to the female athlete regarding ACL injury prevention include direct personal communication (with coaches, physicians, physical therapists, and athletic trainers), the news media, and the World Wide Web. Here we discuss the usefulness of each of these sources of information in assisting athletes to recognize the efficacy of neuromuscular training programs and the options for coverage of knee injury preventive measures in the high-risk female athlete. We also outline future directions for helping female athletes recognize the benefit and cost implications of coverage for potential preventive needs.

The news media has greatly contributed to public awareness of the disparity between the sexes in ACL injury incidence. One of the first high-profile examples of the news media's influence in nationwide recognition of the ACL problem was the 1995 feature by Frank DeFord in *Sports Illustrated* on the loss of three of the University of Tennessee women's basketball team's starting players. More recent examples of female ACL injuries that received significant news media attention include those of Rebecca Lobo of the New York Liberty professional women's basketball team in 1999 and Shea Ralph, the starting point guard on the University of Connecticut women's basketball team, who suffered this devastating injury on three separate occasions, one during the NCAA Championship playoffs.

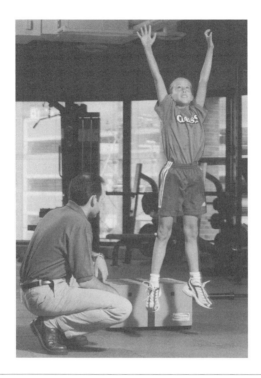

FIGURE 3.5 Screening programs appear to reduce the incidence of ACL injury.
Reprinted, by permission, from G.D. Meyer, K.R. Ford, and T.E. Hewett, 2004, "Rationale and clinical techniques for anterior cruciate ligament injury prevention among female athletes" *Journal of Athletic Training* 39(4): 352-364.

The identification of successful intervention strategies for the reduction of ACL injury incidence in female athletes has spurred additional media coverage. A paper presented at the 1998 American Orthopaedic Society of Sports Medicine meeting demonstrated that neuromuscular training could significantly reduce the risk of ACL injury in female athletes to a level equal to that for males (Hewett et al. 1999). This important finding launched significant subsequent media coverage from several avenues regarding the gender disparity in ACL injury, including *Good Morning America, Wide World of Sports,* ESPN, several other television programs, and many radio interviews, as well as the *New York Times* and hundreds of newspaper and magazine articles. Although the media has been successful in achieving widespread public recognition of this serious problem, little has been presented concerning the relative efficacy of interventions aimed at ACL injury reduction for the at-risk female athlete, or private and public insurance coverage for such prevention programs.

A recent study examined how adolescent girls access the Internet, with the aim of determining its viability as a source of health information for this population at high risk for ACL (Borzekowski and Rickert 2000). As anticipated, this group proved to be technologically savvy. The authors reported that private high school girls spent significantly more time online than urban public school girls; however, the urban girls did utilize the Web frequently to retrieve health information. The study demonstrates that adolescent girls do use the Internet, especially for health information, and shows the significance of this resource for the provision of valuable information to the female athlete regarding ACL injury prevention. However, limited information is available on the Web regarding ACL injury prevention, and even less is available regarding the options for insurance coverage for these important preventive services.

The utility of prevention training is slowly disseminated by word of mouth from physical therapists, athletic trainers, coaches, and athletic directors to school administrators, parents, and athletes. However, little information passes by word of mouth regarding insurance reimbursement for prevention training. This situation may be improved through involvement and education of hospital administrators, patient advocates, and both public and private insurers as well as physical therapists, athletic trainers, coaches, and athletic directors regarding the efficacy and insurability of these programs. ACL injury risk increases significantly at puberty (on average 10-12 years of age in American females), and the number of ACL reconstructive surgeries peaks at age 16 in females. The institution of preventive interventions near the time of puberty could close this gap and reduce four to five years of increased risk exposure in the high-risk athlete. The cost of these injuries currently reaches in excess of $650 million annually in high school and collegiate varsity sports alone. Potentially large savings would occur within the health care system if ACL injury prevention programs were instituted on a more timely and extensive basis.

Summary

In this chapter we discussed the financial burdens placed on individuals, families, and society due to the gender disparity in noncontact ACL injury risk. We compared these costs with the relatively sparse federal funding expended to research ACL injuries and their prevention. In addition, we presented an analysis of the potential savings that might occur if ACL injury prevention programs were instituted on a more extensive basis. It may be concluded that greater awareness at many levels, including the government, the general public, and insurance organizations (both public and private), is necessary to enhance efforts to reduce the incidence of ACL injury, especially in female athletes. In summary, it is the responsibility of the health care provider within the field of sports medicine to implement strategies for sport injury prevention, specifically for the prevention of noncontact ACL injuries. It is imperative that emphasis be placed on the development of preventive interventions to reduce ACL injuries and the associated subsequent osteoarthritis, joint replacements, and long-term disabilities, as well as the other financial, psychological, and emotional costs accompanying these devastating injuries in young female athletes.

Part II

ACL Injury Prevention Programs

Timothy Edwin Hewett, PhD, FACSM

Examination of the similarities and differences among training regimes gives insight into the development of more effective and efficient interventions. The purpose of this section of the book is to highlight the relative effectiveness of these interventions in reducing ACL injury rates and to evaluate the training components among the training studies (see the following figures). Also discussed are the level of rigor of these interventions, the costs and the difficulty of implementation, compliance with these interventions, and performance benefits. This section of the book summarizes conclusions based on evidence from the common components of the various interventions in order to discuss their potential to reduce ACL injury risk and assess their potential for combined use in more effective and efficient intervention protocols.

Neuromuscular training programs may assist in the reduction of ACL injuries in female athletes if the common effective components as reported in these chapters include the following:

1. Plyometrics and balance and strengthening exercises are incorporated into a comprehensive training protocol.
2. The training sessions are performed more than one time per week.
3. The duration of the training program is a minimum of six weeks.

The clinical significance of these findings is that prevention and intervention programs should be designed using the most effective components. The

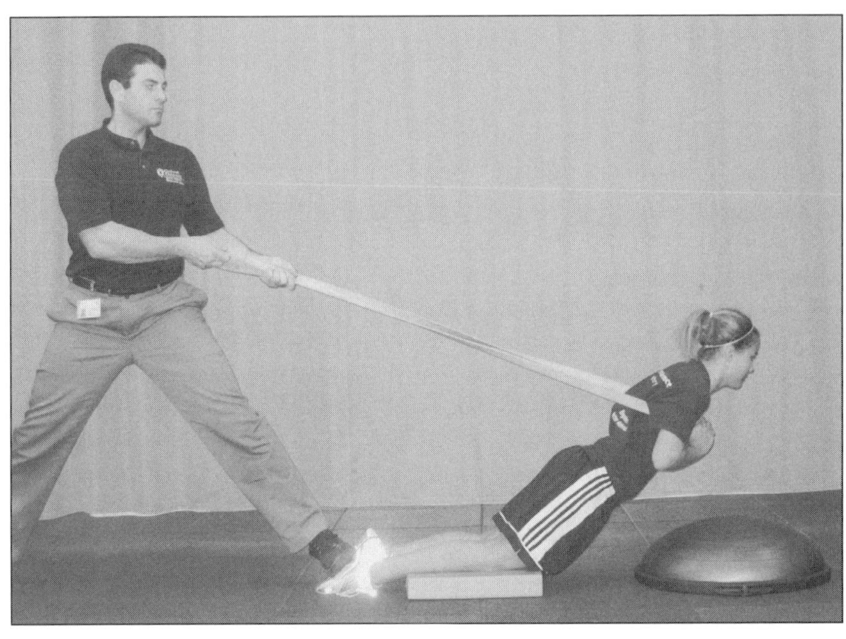

Hamstrings strength training using a modified (with band) Russian hamstrings curl.

Plyometric training with feedback.

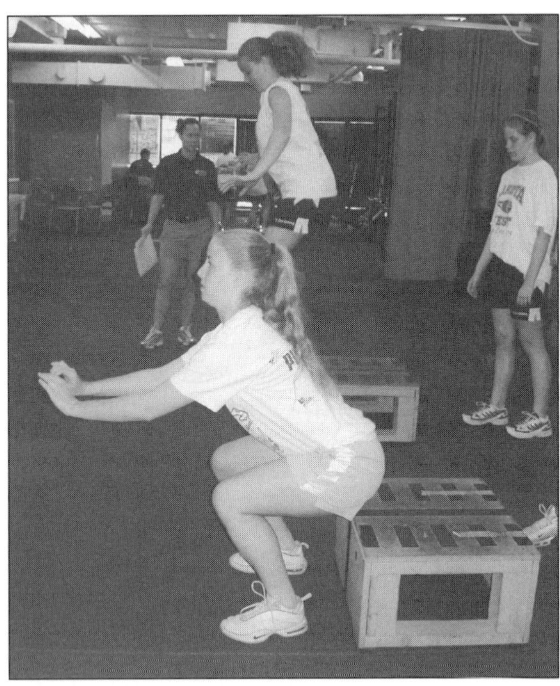

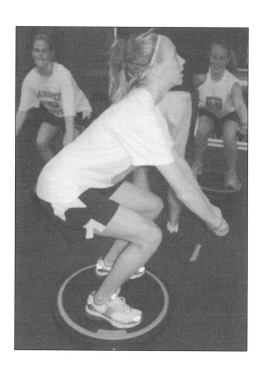

Balance training.

studies that were effective at reducing ACL injury risk all incorporated into the intervention high-intensity plyometric movements that progressed beyond footwork and agility. The studies that were ineffective did not. The studies that incorporated high-intensity plyometrics reduced ACL risk, while the studies that did not incorporate high-intensity plyometrics did not reduce ACL injury risk. The plyometric component of these interventions, which trains the muscles, connective tissue, and nervous system to effectively carry out the stretch–shortening cycle and focuses on proper technique and body mechanics, appears to reduce ACL injuries.

Chapter 4

Components of Prevention Programs

Holly J. Silvers, MPT

The occurrence of ACL injuries has reached record proportions, particularly within the female athlete population (Bjordal et al. 1997; Caraffa et al. 1996; Engstrom, Johansson, and Tomkvist 1991; Griffin et al. 2000; Heidt et al. 2000; Mandelbaum et al. 2005). The medical community has been entrusted to understand the epidemiology, etiology, and mechanisms of such injuries in order to develop effective injury prevention strategies. A multidisciplinary meeting was held in Hunt Valley, Maryland, in 1999 to delineate specific risk factors that were thought to be directly correlated to the increased incidence of ACL injuries in the female athlete (Griffin et al. 2000). The risk factors that were identified included anatomy, hormones, environment, and biomechanics. This meeting had many positive outcomes, including the generation of increased interest in research and development with respect to ACL injury prevention protocols. This meeting was revisited during the Hunt Valley II meeting held in Atlanta in January 2005. The topics of the 1999 meeting were addressed, as well as the new research findings that had been published since that initial meeting.

Twelve injury prevention programs that were empirically evaluated with regard to epidemiology and outcome measures were identified and are discussed in this chapter. These programs were analyzed with regard to the following criteria: sport specificity, frequency and duration of the intervention, whether or not the study design included randomized controlled trials, equipment needs, type of strength training, flexibility components, sport-specific agilities, plyometric training, proprioceptive components, strengths and relative weaknesses of the specific intervention program, and functional outcome measures (table 4.1).

Caraffa and colleagues (1996) conducted a nonrandomized prospective study with 600 semiprofessional and amateur soccer players in Umbria and Marche in Italy. Twenty teams (10 amateur and 10 semiprofessional: group A) underwent

TABLE 4.1 ACL Injury Prevention Studies

Author	Sport	Duration	Randomized	Equipment	Strength	Flexibility
Caraffa et al. 1996	Soccer semi-professional and amateur males; N = 600 on 40 teams (20 intervention, 20 control)	3-season intervention (preseason)	Prospective, nonrandomized	Rectangular, oblique, circular, and BAPS boards (20 min from level I to V) over 3 to 6 days a week with self-determined advancement to next level = 30 preseason days	PNF exercises	No
Ettlinger et al. 1995	Alpine skiing; N = 4000 ski personnel in 20 ski areas	1-year intervention (1993-94) with two previous years of historic controls (1991-93)	Prospective, nonrandomized	Educational video clips of skiers sustaining ACL injuries and those that avoided injury in very similar falls; injury prevention education utilized (mechanism of injury, avoidance of high-risk behavior, fall technique)	No	No
Gilchrist et al. 2004a (abstract only)	Soccer U-18 to U-22; 561 Div I NCAA females (61 universities)	1-year intervention	Yes	Educational video, cones, soccer ball	Glut med, abd, ext, HS, core training	Yes
Henning et al. 1990	BB females	8-year intervention	Prospective, nonrandomized	No	No	No
Mandelbaum et al. 2005	Soccer U-14 to U-18; N = 1041 (year 1) and 844 (year 2) females	2-year intervention	Prospective, nonrandomized	Educational video, 2 in. cones, soccer ball	HS, core training	Yes

Agility	Plyometric	Proprioception	Strengths	Weaknesses	Outcome
No	No	Balance board activities: multi-level I-V on four boards	Mechanoreceptor/Proprio training	Additional equipment (BAPS board); not cost-effective in a large-scale cohort	87% decr. in NC ACL injury: 1.15/team/season in control group compared to 0.15/team/season in intervention group ($p < 0.001$)
No	No	No	Fall analysis and accident and injury analysis; cost-effective intervention and highly feasible with large skiing populations	Nonrandomized; not all potential participants trained; historic controls; exact diagnosis of serious knee sprains not always available; exact exposure to risk cannot be precisely determined	Severe knee sprains reduced by 62% among trained skiers (patrollers and instructors) compared to unperturbed group, who had no improvement during study period
Deceleration, sport specific	Hip and knee position, landing technique, multiplanar	Strength on field perturbation on grass	Instructional video; Web site; compliance monitored (random site visits)	Randomized, 1-year intervention, begun at day 1 of season	Overall 72% reduction in ACL injury; 100% reduction in practice contact and NC ACLs; 100% reduction in contact and NC ACLs in last 6 weeks of season
Yes	Landing technique (knee and hip flexion)	Rounded cut, deceleration patterns (3-step shuffle)	Changing cutting, deceleration, and landing techniques (encouraging knee and hip flexion)	Nonrandomized; not published (abstract only)	89% decr. in NC ACL injury in female basketball athletes
Soccer specific with deceleration techniques	Hip and knee, landing technique, multiplanar	On-field program: strength, plyo, agilities on grass	Instructional video; Web site; compliance monitored (random site visits)	Nonrandomized; inherent selection (motivational) bias	Injury rates: year 1—88% reduction in NC ACL injury; year 2—74% reduction in NC ACL injury

(continued)

TABLE 4.1 *(continued)*

Author	Sport	Duration	Randomized	Equipment	Strength	Flexibility
Myklebust et al. 2003	European team handball; N = 900 female Div I-III	3-year intervention, five-phase program	Prospective, nonrandomized	Educational videotape, poster, wobble board, balance foam mats	No	Yes
Pfeiffer et al. 2004	Soccer, VB, BB HS females; N = 577 intervention, N = 862 control	2-year prospective intervention over a 9-week treatment, 15 min, two times a week	Prospective, nonrandomized	No	Yes	No
Soderman et al. 2000	Soccer females; N = 121 (control N = 100); only 62 intervention and 78 control completed study	1-season intervention (April-Oct), 10-15 min	Prospective, randomized	Balance board, 10-15 min training program in addition to regular training	No	No
Hewett et al. 1999	BB, VB, soccer; N = 1263: male (N = 434), female (N = 366 trained and 463 untrained)	6-week preseason intervention, 1-year monitoring, 60-90 min/day for 3 days a week	Prospective, nonrandomized	Plyometric jump box, and balance	Yes	Yes
Heidt et al. 2000	Soccer; 300 females	7-week preseason intervention, 1-year monitoring, 3 days a week (one plyo and two treadmill)	Prospective, nonrandomized	Treadmill, sports cord, plyometric box jump	Yes	Yes

Agility	Plyometric	Proprioception	Strengths	Weaknesses	Outcome
Planting, cutting, NM balance control activities	Landing technique (knee and hip flexion)	Balance activity on foam mats and boards	Compliance monitored by PT; instructional video and poster	Nonrandomized; insufficient power	In elite division, risk of injury reduced among those who completed the program (OR: 0.06 [0.01-0.54]) compared with control; overall 53.8% and 61.5% reduction of ACL injury
No	Landing technique	No	Compliance monitored; sig. reduction in GRF and RFD in intervention	No decr. in injury in intervention group; performed posttraining; fatigue phenomenon; only 9 weeks in duration	6 NC ACL injuries: 3 intervention and 3 control = no effect
No	No	Balance	Randomized clinical trial; sig. more injuries in control vs. intervention	37% dropout rate; not all subjects received same amount of training; unknown if training other than balance board was the same; numbers of ACL injuries very small	The training did not reduce the risk of primary traumatic injuries to the lower extremities; four of five ACL injuries occurred in the intervention group
No	Yes	Yes	Videotape, decr. peak landing forces, decr. valgus/varus perturbation, incr. vert. leap, incr. hamstring strength and decr. time to hamstring contraction	Nonrandomized; low VB enrollment; motivational bias; 1-on-1 program in sport facility; not feasible to implement across large cohort	14 ACLs reported: female injury rates 0.43 untrained vs. 0.12 trained vs. male control 0.9 over 6-week program; untrained group 3.6-4.8 higher injury rates of ACL injury
Yes	Yes	Yes	Incr. strength, lower overall injury rates	Not stat. sig.; 7 weeks insufficient time for NM reeducation to occur at mechanoreceptor level	61.2% injuries in knee/ankle; 2.4% injury rate in intervention vs. 3.1% in control

(continued)

TABLE 4.1 ***(continued)***

Author	Sport	Duration	Randomized	Equipment	Strength	Flexibility
Olsen et al. 2005b	European team handball (123 teams); N = 1837 players: 1586 female, 251 male	15-20 min training, 8 months (one handball season), 15 consecutive sessions and once a week thereafter	Randomized, controlled cluster trial	Wobble board (Norpro), balance foam mats (Airex)	Squats and power (bounding)	Yes
Wedderkopp et al. 2003	European team handball; 236 females (17-18 years), 20 teams	10-month intervention (one season)	Randomized, controlled cluster trial	Balance board (proprioceptive) in four levels	Yes	No

NM = neuromuscular; PNF = proprioceptive neuromuscular facilitation; NC = non-contact; GRF = ground reaction force;

proprioceptive preseason training in addition to their regular training session. The control group (group B) consisted of 20 teams (10 amateur and 10 semiprofessional) and continued training in their usual fashion. The intervention (group A) was a five-phase progressive balance training program consisting of four balance boards: rectangular, round, combination rectangular and round), and a BAPS board (Camp Jackson, MI). The intervention took place during the preseason. The duration and frequency were 20 min per day on two to six days per week, which equated to 30 exposures. The groups were followed for three years. Group A reported 10 ACL injuries over three seasons (0.15 ACL injuries per team/season) compared to group B (control), which reported 70 ACL injuries (1.15 ACL injuries per team/season) ($p < 0.001$). These injuries were confirmed through magnetic resonance imaging and arthroscopy. Contact and noncontact ACL injuries were not differentiated during the reporting process. This program was limited to balance training and proprioceptive neuromuscular facilitation (PNF) strengthening. No component of flexibility, agility, or plyometric training was utilized in this protocol.

Ettlinger and colleagues (1995) conducted a nonrandomized prospective study using an ACL awareness training videotape depicting 10 recorded ACL injuries that were sustained by alpine skiers of various levels. This videotape

gility	Plyometric	Proprioception	Strengths	Weaknesses	Outcome
lanting, utting, NM ontrol	Knee over toe, proper landing technique	Balance activity on single/double leg, mats and boards	Randomized; compliance monitored; reduction of injury; structured warm-up	Uncertain what parameter of program effective; male and female; cannot extrapolate to other sports	129 acute knee and ankle injuries overall; 81 in control (0.9 overall, 0.3 trained, 5.3 matched) vs. 48 in intervention (0.5 overall, 0.2 trained, 2.5 matched); 80% reduction of ACL injuries
lo	Yes	Balance training with ankle discs	Randomized clinical trial	Specific injury types not given; description of ankle disc training not given; "warm-up" exercises also provided to trained group but not specified; compliance with all exercises not mentioned	Ankle injuries sig. greater in control group (2.4 vs. 0.2); unspecified knee injuries not sig. less in trained group (6.9 vs. 0.6); 5 knee sprains and 1 knee "luxation" in control group vs. 1 knee sprain in trained group

D = rate of force development; PT = patient; VB = volleyball; BB = basketball; HS = high school.

utilized guided discovery, which allowed the viewer (alpine ski instructor or patroller) to visualize carefully selected stimuli (ACL injuries) and to make suppositions of high risk positions based on their exposure to the viewing of these injuries. This information, in contrast to didactic learning, would be incorporated into the viewers' skiing in order to allow them to avoid high-risk behavior, prevent high-risk situations, and act readily and effectively to reduce the risk of ACL injury. During the 1993-1994 ski season, 4000 on-slope ski personnel in 20 ski areas completed training and reporting requirements. The training kit included a 19 min video, a supplemental leader guide, a flip chart for quick review of the video images, and a workbook. An awareness training session included proper body positioning and information on the phantom foot ACL injury mechanism, and strategies to avoid high-risk positions and effective reaction strategies were discussed.

The data collected indicated 31 serious ACL sprains sustained by area employees over the course of the first two seasons (historic control) and 16 (10 trained and 6 untrained) for the intervention season. After the data were normalized, the expected number of ACL injuries was calculated to be 26.6, whereas the actual number reported for trained individuals was 10. This translates into an overall 62% reduction ($p < 0.005$) of overall ACL sprains for the ski patrol staff. This study was limited to injury prevention from an awareness perspective. There was no physical biomechanical intervention. The strengths of this specific research study demonstrate the value of injury prevention awareness, education, and visual aids in effectively reducing the number of significant ACL injuries experienced by the alpine skiing population. This type of prevention effort could potentially be bolstered if it were combined with a biomechanical intervention to address the neuromuscular deficits leading to the phantom foot or the boot-induced types of ACL injury mechanisms commonly seen in ACL injuries in skiers.

Henning implemented a prevention study in two Division I basketball programs over the course of eight years (Griffin 2000). He proposed that the increased rate of ACL injury is due to the quad–cruciate interaction: As the knee extends, the quadriceps exerts a significant anterior translational force on the tibia that imparts a sheer force on the ACL. In contrast, as the knee moves into flexion, the anterior translational force on the tibia is decreased, thereby decreasing the torque on the ACL. In order to decrease the risk of ACL injury, Henning proposed that the athletes cut, land, and decelerate with knee and hip flexion. In addition, he proposed a rounded cut maneuver instead of utilization of a sharp or more acute angle during the cut cycle. He also proposed that a one-step stop deceleration pattern be avoided and that a three-step quick stop be instituted instead. This intervention program was geared toward changing player technique—stressing knee flexion upon landing, accelerated rounded turns, and deceleration with a multistep stop. Henning noted an 89% reduction in the rate of occurrence of ACL injuries in his intervention group. Sadly, Dr. Henning's death in 1991 prevented the publication of this research. However, this work served as the crucial foundation for the numerous prevention programs that ensued. Henning's program incorporated biomechanical components, addressing landing in genu valgum or excessive hip and knee extension, multistep deceleration to dissipate forces over three steps instead of one, and avoiding acute cutting angles. This protocol was completed on the basketball court without any additional equipment requirements.

Mandelbaum and colleagues developed the Prevent Injury and Enhance Performance (PEP) program for female soccer players (Mandelbaum et al. 2005). The PEP program focused on biomechanical risk factors, stressed avoidance of high-risk behaviors, and addressed the deficits most commonly demonstrated by adolescent female athletes. The program consisted of an educational videotape/DVD that demonstrated proper and improper biomechanical technique for each prescribed therapeutic exercise. This prospective nonrandomized study involved competitive female club soccer players between the ages of 14 and 18 over the course of two years. During the first year of the study (2000), 1041 female club soccer players (52 teams) performed the PEP program, and 1902 players (95 teams) served as the age- and skill-matched controls. There were two ACL tears (0.2 ACL injuries/AE [AE= athlete exposures]) in enrolled subjects versus 32 ACL tears (1.7 ACL injuries/AE) in the control group—an

88% decrease in ACL ligament injury. In year 2 (2001) of the study, four ACL tears were reported in the intervention group, with an incidence rate of 0.47 injuries/AE. Thirty-five ACL tears were reported in the control group, with an incidence rate of 1.8 injuries/AE. This corresponds to an overall 74% reduction in ACL tears in the intervention group compared to an age- and skill-matched control group in year 2.

The limitations of this study include nonrandomization of the subjects, no consistent direct oversight of the intervention, and completion of compliance measurements in a small subset of intervention teams. The strengths of the PEP program include the fact that it is an on-field warm-up program that requires only traditional soccer equipment (cones and soccer ball). It is completed two to three times a week over the course of the 12-week soccer season and is 20 min in duration. It includes progressive strength, flexibility, agility, and plyometric and proprioceptive activities to address the deficits most commonly demonstrated in the female population. Deceleration patterns are addressed; the multistep deceleration pattern and proper landing technique are emphasized, as are knee and hip flexion during landing on the ball of the foot and avoiding genu valgum through use of the abductors and lateral hip musculature

Mandelbaum and colleagues' study was followed by a randomized controlled trial using the PEP program in Division I NCAA women's soccer teams in the 2002 fall season (Gilchrist et al. 2004b). Sixty-one teams with 1429 athletes completed the study; 854 athletes participated on 35 control teams, and 575 athletes participated on 26 intervention teams. No significant differences were noted between intervention and control athletes with regard to age, height, weight, or history of past ACL injuries. After one season of the PEP program, there were seven ACL injuries in the intervention athletes (IA) (rate of 0.14) versus 18 in control athletes (CA) (rate of 0.25) ($p = 0.15$). No ACL injuries were reported in IA during practices versus six in CA (0.10) ($p = 0.01$). During game situations, the difference was nonsignificant (IA 7 vs. CA 12; $p = 0.76$). Noncontact ACL injuries occurred at over three times the rate in CA ($n = 10$; 0.14) as in IA ($n = 2$; 0.04) ($p = 0.06$). Control athletes with a prior history of ACL injury suffered a reoccurrence five times more frequently than the IA group (0.10 vs. 0.02; $p = 0.06$); this difference reached significance when limited to noncontact ACL injuries during the season (0.06 vs. 0.00; $p < 0.05$). There was a significant difference in the rate of ACL injuries in the second half of the season (weeks 6-11; IA 0.00 vs. CA 0.18) ($p < 0.05$). This would support the concept that it takes approximately six to eight weeks for a biomechanical intervention program to impart a neuromuscular effect.

Anterior cruciate ligament injuries in European team handball have also been problematic. Myklebust and colleagues conducted a nonrandomized prospective study utilizing 900 Division I-III competitive handball players over a three-year period in Norway (Myklebust et al. 2003). Sixty teams (942 players in the 1998-1999 season) served as the control athletes (CA), and 58 teams (855 players in 1999-2000) and 52 teams (850 players in the 2000-2001 season) served as the intervention athletes (IA). A five-phase 15 min program served as the neuromuscular intervention. The program focused on landing technique and cutting and planting technique. Special equipment included an instructional videotape, a poster delineating the tasks to be completed, six balance mats, and six balance boards. A physical therapist was designated to each team to assess compliance during the second intervention season (2000-2001).

There were 29 ACL injuries during the control season, 23 injuries during the first intervention season (OR [odds ratio]: 0.87; CI, 0.50-1.52; p = 0.62), and 17 injuries during the second intervention season (OR: 0.64; CI, 0.35-1.18; p = 0.15). When the data were stratified to the elite division, 13 ACL injuries were reported during the control season, six injuries during the first intervention season (OR: 0.51; CI, 0.19-1.35; p = 0.17), and five injuries in the second intervention season (OR: 0.37; CI, 0.13-1.05; p = 0.06). For the entire cohort, there was no difference in injury rates during the second intervention season between those who complied and those who did not comply (OR: 0.52; CI, 0.15-1.82; p = 0.31). In the elite division, the risk of injury was reduced among those who completed the ACL injury prevention program (OR: 0.06; CI, 0.01-0.54; p = 0.01) compared with those who did not. This study demonstrated an overall 61.5% and 53.8% reduction in ACL injury, respectively, between the two intervention seasons. The intervention included elements of plyometric activities, proprioception, and agilities. It did not include any elements of strength. Limitations of the study include nonrandomization of the subjects, insufficient power, and control data that were collected during an earlier season. Strengths of the study include measures of compliance by a medical clinician (physical therapist) and the use of an educational videotape and poster. These findings may indicate that the inclusion of a neuromuscular balance-based training program may impart some protective benefit to the ACL.

Pfeiffer and Shea and colleagues (2004) developed the Knee Ligament Injury Prevention (KLIP) program for female soccer, volleyball, and basketball high school-aged athletes. This two-year nonrandomized prospective study incorporated strength and plyometric activities in a 15 min intervention program with a frequency of two times a week. Forty-three schools participated in the first season (17 BB: N = 191; 11 soccer: N = 189; 15 VB: N = 197), and 69 schools served as the control group (28 BB: N = 319; 14 soccer: N = 244; 27 VB: N = 299). The study design included a training session for the coaches of each sport and the athletic trainers. There were weekly compliance checks for athlete participation for both games and practices. Three arthroscopically confirmed ACL injuries were reported in the intervention athletes compared to four in the control group. Average weekly exposure (games and practices) and numbers of participants were used to calculate the odds ratio (KLIP to control: 2.38 OR; ACL tear for KLIP: 0.20 OR) (Pfeiffer et al. 2004). The strengths of the KLIP program include the study design, which used a thorough and consistent measure of compliance and a significant number of participating athletes. The KLIP program included elements of strengthening and plyometrics and did not address flexibility, balance, or agilities. This program was conducted two times a week over nine weeks (18 exposures). Due to the abridged duration of this intervention program, there may not have been sufficient exposure to the injury prevention elements to have an effect. In addition, since neuromuscular reeducation typically takes six to eight weeks to demonstrate an effect, it would be interesting to see if the KLIP program would be beneficial if initiated in the preseason. Furthermore, this program was conducted posttraining; therefore the element of neuromuscular fatigue may have eradicated any preventive benefit the KLIP program could potentially impart.

Soderman and colleagues (2000) conducted a balance board training program in female soccer players participating on 13 teams in the Swedish second and third divisions. Seven teams (N = 121, 62 completed) served as the intervention group, and six teams (N = 100, 78 completed) served as the age- and skill-matched control group throughout one outdoor season. The intervention consisted of a 10 to 15 min balance board training program in addition to regularly scheduled games and practices. Injuries were assessed with regard to number, incidence, type, and location. Four ACL injuries were reported in the intervention group as opposed to one in the control group. The balance board program included elements of balance and did not include strength, plyometrics, flexibility, or agility. Strengths of this study include the fact that it was randomized and was continued over the course of a six-month season (April-October). The limitations include the fact there was a 37% dropout during the study and the insufficient power of the study design. In addition, the study failed to include elements of compliance and supervision. Use of equipment such as a balance board on a wide-scale basis may have inherent cost-effectiveness and feasibility limitations.

In another study, Hewett and colleagues (1999) researched the effect of neuromuscular training on the incidence of knee injury in high school-aged female athletes. Forty-three (N = 1263 athletes) soccer, volleyball, and basketball teams from 12 area high schools participated in the six-week preseason intervention program. The program incorporated flexibility, strengthening (through weight training), and plyometric activities. Fifteen female teams (N = 366) elected to utilize the program; 15 additional female teams (N = 463) served as the same-sex untrained control, and 13 male sport teams (N = 434) served as the male control group. The program was 60 to 90 min in length and was performed three days a week on alternate days for at least four weeks. There were three phases to the program: the technique phase, the fundamental phase, and the performance phase. Exercises in the first two phases were increased in duration, and 1 to 2 min of recovery time was permitted between the plyometric exercises. The flexibility portion took place before plyometric training, which was then followed by weight training.

Hewett and colleagues (1999) found that the incidence of ACL injuries (N = 14) was 0.43/AE in the untrained group, 0.12/AE in the trained group, and 0.09/AE in the male control group. Nine of the serious knee injuries (N = 14) were noncontact injuries. The incidence of noncontact ACL injuries was 0.35/AE in the untrained group, 0.0/AE in the trained group, and 0.05/AE in the male control group. Stratification of the data according to sport showed that no ACL injuries were reported in volleyball players. For soccer, five ACL injuries were reported in the untrained athletes (0.56/AE), zero in the trained athletes (0.0/AE), and one in the male control group (0.12/AE). For basketball, eight ACL injuries were reported—five in the untrained athletes (0.48/AE), two in the trained athletes (0.42/AE), and one in the male control group (0.08/AE). The strengths of this program include the relative ease of implementation and its general effectiveness in reducing the overall rate of ACL injury. The limitations include the study design, which was nonrandomized, and discrepancy in the number of athletes in each sport and in the respective training groups. In addition, the number of ACL injuries reported throughout this prospective study was low in comparison to historic controls (Engstrom, Johansson, and Tomkvist 1991; Feagin et al. 1987; Griffin et al. 2000; Heidt et al. 2000; Hertling 1996; Huston, Greenfield, and Wojtys 2000; Kirkendall and Garrett 2000; Lloyd 2001; Silvers and Mandelbaum 2001). The notion of continuing this type of neuromuscular conditioning program throughout the entirety of a season, using the concept of periodization, might be considered so that one could see its effect on overall injury rates over the course of a season. Further research efforts may elucidate whether or not there is a regression in the neuromuscular gains made by trained athletes throughout a preseason training program if the program is not continued throughout the entire season.

Heidt and colleagues (2000) used the Frappier Acceleration Program as a seven-week preseason training program to address injuries in the female soccer population (14 to 18 years of age). Three hundred female soccer players participated in the intervention over the course of one year (one high school season and one club/select season). A subset of 42 athletes participated in the Frappier Acceleration Program. This consisted of sport-specific aerobic conditioning, plyometrics, sports cord resistance drills, strength training, and flexibility that was individually customized by sport, player position, and specific deficits. The plyometric progression was as follows: unidirectional, bidirectional, multidirectional, and vertical challenge (2 in. [5 cm] increments utilizing foam obstacles). Seven injuries were reported in the trained athletes (14%, P = 0.0085) compared to 91 injuries in the 258 untrained athletes (37%). Nine ACL tears were reported: one in the trained group (2.4%) compared to eight in the untrained group (3.1%). This difference was not statistically significant (Heidt et al. 2000).

This study incorporated elements of strength, flexibility, plyometrics, and agilities. The program required the training to be completed in a facility, secondary to the equipment needs (treadmill, plyometric box). Similar to Hewett's program, this program was designed as a preseason protocol and did not offer an in-season continuation of the prescribed activities. In addition, the cohort of trained individuals was quite small (N = 42) and not sufficiently powered to offer statistical significance.

Olsen and colleagues (2005) conducted a study that examined whether or not exercises can be used to prevent lower limb injury in youth athletics. European team handball clubs (N = 120; 61 intervention teams, 59 teams in the control group) participated in an eight-month 15 to 20 min intervention program that consisted of four sets of exercise, increasing in difficulty. Each club was instructed on how to perform the program and was issued a training handbook, five wobble boards (Norpro), and five balance mats (Airex). The program focused on proper biomechanics during landing, core stability, and interrater feedback between team members. The intervention teams consisted of 16- to 17-year-old males and females who completed 15 consecutive training sessions at the start of the season, followed by one training session per week. The training consisted of warm-up exercises (jogging, backward running, forward running, sideways running, and speed work), technique (plant, cut, and jump shot landing), balance (passing, squats, bouncing, perturbation), and strength and power (squats, bounding, jumps, hamstrings).

Sixty-six (6.9%) lower limb injuries were reported in the intervention group compared to 115 (13.1%) in the control group (0.51: 95%CI, $P < 0.001$). Three ACL injuries were reported in the intervention group compared to 14 in the control group (0.20; 95%CI, $P < 0.01$), which was equivalent to an 80% reduction. The compliance reached 87% among the youth clubs. This may be attributed to increased media attention to ACL injury or motivational influence from coaches, parents, or peers. This study elucidates the need to begin the implementation of injury prevention programs in a younger cohort in order to integrate proper biomechanics and neuromuscular control at an earlier age. If these programs are implemented prior to the high-risk age range, the incidence of ACL injury may be decreased even further. Future clinical research, focusing on the 8- to 12-year-old cohort and following them longitudinally through pubescence, will shed light on this prospect.

Wedderkopp and colleagues (2003) compared two intervention programs in female European handball athletes. European team handball is a highly popular sport in Denmark, with over 130,000 players registered with the national Danish Handball Association. Sixteen handball teams (N = 163, aged 14-16) participated in the study and were randomized into one of two groups, one using an ankle disc and one not. Eight teams (N = 77) were randomized to the intervention group while eight teams (N = 86) were relegated to the control group. This systematic four-step program included functional strengthening and balance training (ankle disc). The study was conducted over the course of one season (August to April). The group using the ankle disc incurred six injuries compared to 16 injuries in the control group. The incidence of traumatic injury in the intervention group was 2.4 injuries/1000 match hours (95%CI, 0.7; 6.2) and 0.2 injuries/1000 practice hours (95%CI, 0.02; 0.7). The incidence of traumatic injury in the control group (without the ankle disc) was 6.9 injuries/1000 match hours (95%CI, 3.3; 12.7) and 0.6 injuries/1000 practice hours (95%CI, 0.2; 1.3). Furthermore, the intervention group had significantly fewer major and moderate injuries. This research study suggests that the inclusion of a proprioceptive balance device, such as an ankle device, may significantly reduce the number of significant injuries in the female handball population.

Several of the prevention programs were performed as a preseason or in-season intervention prior to training. Therefore, fatigue did not interfere with neuromuscular motor control and performance of the prescribed activities (Irmischer et al. 2004). In contrast, a critical review of Pfeiffer and colleagues' (2004) paper reveals that there was no effect of this intervention with regard to reduction of ACL injury. Interestingly, the KLIP program was the only injury prevention program that was implemented posttraining, in direct contrast to the 11 other injury prevention training programs that were designed to be instituted prior to training. Johnston and colleagues (1998) studied the effect of fatigue during single-leg balance activities. Twenty healthy subjects were statically and dynamically balance tested (unilaterally and bilaterally). The subjects were then fatigued to less than 50% of their initial force on an isokinetic dynamometer. Further analysis of the pre- and postfatigue balance testing indicated significant decreases in motor control performance on the three static tests in all subjects ($p < 0.001$). These studies demonstrate the critical need for further randomized clinical trials on the relevance of fatigue, the timing of utilization of a neuromuscular injury prevention program, and the role of fatigue with regard to injury.

Chapter 5

Theories on How Neuromuscular Intervention Programs May Influence ACL Injury Rates

The Biomechanical Effects of Plyometric, Balance, Strength, and Feedback Training

Timothy Edwin Hewett, PhD, FACSM
Gregory D. Myer, MS, CSCS
Kevin R. Ford, MS

A major theory to account for higher knee and noncontact ACL injury incidence in female athletes is the absence of neuromuscular control of the knee joint, due to training deficiencies, developmental differences, or perhaps hormonal influences. This chapter focuses on the neuromuscular theory, in which adaptation to training readily occurs, and where intervention and prevention are likely to have the greatest impact. There is good evidence that neuromuscular control issues play an important role in the gender disparity in ACL injury risk. If specific training can increase neuromuscular control of the joint and decrease knee and ACL injury risk, it is likely that the mechanisms underlying the increased risk are neuromuscular (figure 5.1).

Several prospective studies have demonstrated that neuromuscular training for female athletes has the potential to decrease knee injuries in general and

ACL injuries in particular (Heidt et al. 2000; Hewett et al. 1999; Mandelbaum et al. 2005; Myklebust et al. 2003; Soderman et al. 2000; Wedderkopp et al. 1999) (see figure 5.2). Intensive short-term neuromuscular training may induce a "neuromuscular spurt" that may otherwise be absent in adolescent females (Hewett et al. 1996; Hewett, Myer, and Ford 2004; Myer et al. 2004; Myer, Ford, and Hewett 2004; Quatman et al. 2006). Even if neuromuscular training and strength differences account for only a portion of the increased incidence of noncontact ACL injury in female athletes, lowering these high figures by even a percentage could have a significant effect on the number of these injuries. Such training, if effectively implemented on a widespread basis, could help to significantly decrease the number of female athletes injured each year.

A recent systematic review of the literature (Hewett, Myer, and Ford 2005a) yielded six studies of interventions targeted toward knee or ACL injury prevention in female athletes (Heidt et al. 2000; Hewett et al. 1999; Mandelbaum et al. 2005; Myklebust et al. 2003; Soderman et al. 2000; Wedderkopp et al. 1999) (figure 5.2). Five of the six interventions reduced injury incidence, four of the six

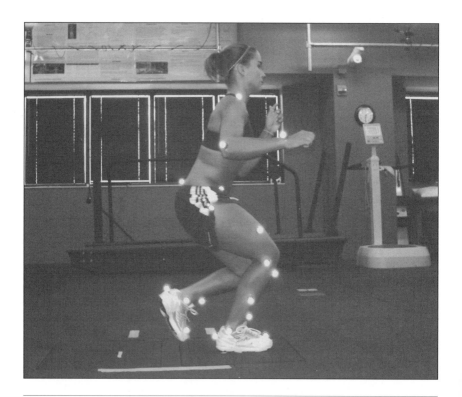

FIGURE 5.1 If specific training can increase neuromuscular control of the joint and decrease knee and ACL injury risk, it is likely that the mechanisms underlying the increased risk are neuromuscular in nature.

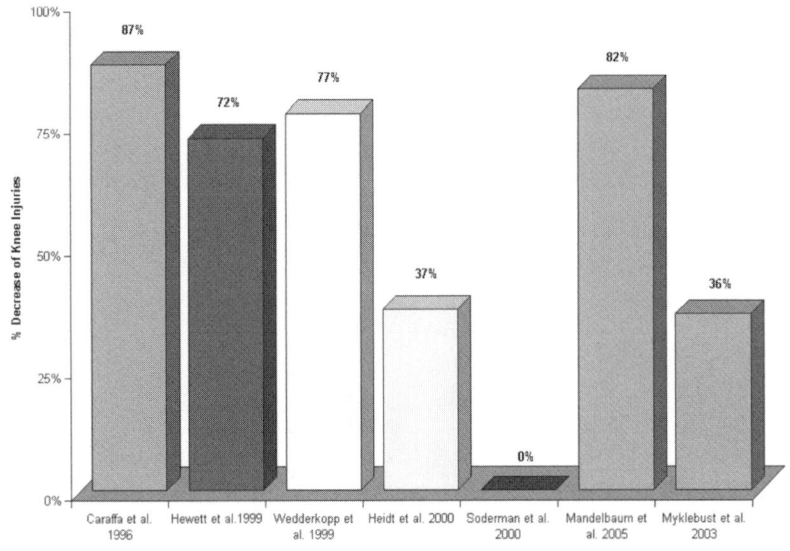

FIGURE 5.2 A recent systematic review of the literature by Hewett, Myer, and Ford (2005a) yielded six studies of interventions targeted toward knee or ACL injury prevention in female athletes.

Data adapted from Heidt, Sweeterman, et al. 2000; Hewett, Lindenfeld, et al. 1999; Mandelbaum, Silvers, et al. 2005; Myklebust, Engebretsen, et al. 2003; Soderman, Werner, et al. 2000; Wedderkopp, Kaltof, et al. 1999.

reduced knee injury incidence, and three of the six reduced ACL injury incidence in females. Examination of the similarities and differences between the training regimes helps afford insight into the development of more effective and efficient interventions. The purpose of this chapter is to evaluate the biomechanical effects of (1) plyometrics (figures 5.3-5.7), (2) balance (figure 5.8), (3) biofeedback (figures 5.9 & 5.10), and (4) resistance (strength) (figure 5.11) training components of neuromuscular training programs, in isolation and in combination, with respect to their relative effectiveness in reducing ACL injury. The chapter focuses on the common components of the various interventions in order to discuss their potential to reduce ACL injury risk and assess their potential for combined use in more effective and efficient intervention protocols.

Assessment of the relative efficacy of these four common components of neuromuscular training programs (plyometrics, balance, biomechanical feedback, and strength training interventions, alone and in combination) is important in order to optimize the potential positive effects on ACL injury prevention. The comprehensive interventions currently utilized in ACL injury prevention programs often involve large time commitments that may deter coaches from including them in preseason conditioning programs (Holm et al. 2004; Myer et al. 2004; Wedderkopp et al. 1999). In addition, the increased volume of training, especially plyometric training, may place undue stress on

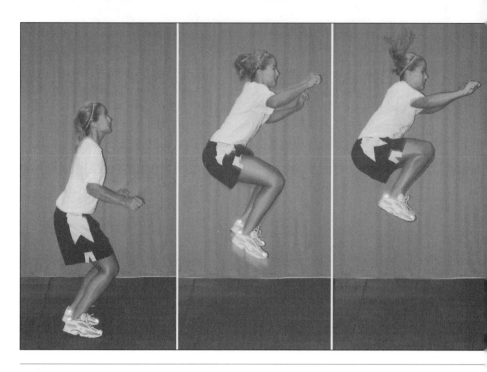

FIGURE 5.3 Plyometrics: tuck jump.

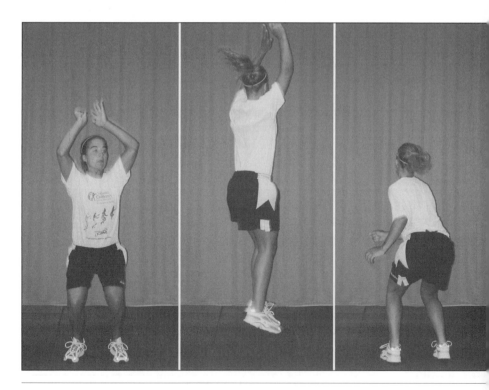

FIGURE 5.4 Plyometrics: 180° jump.

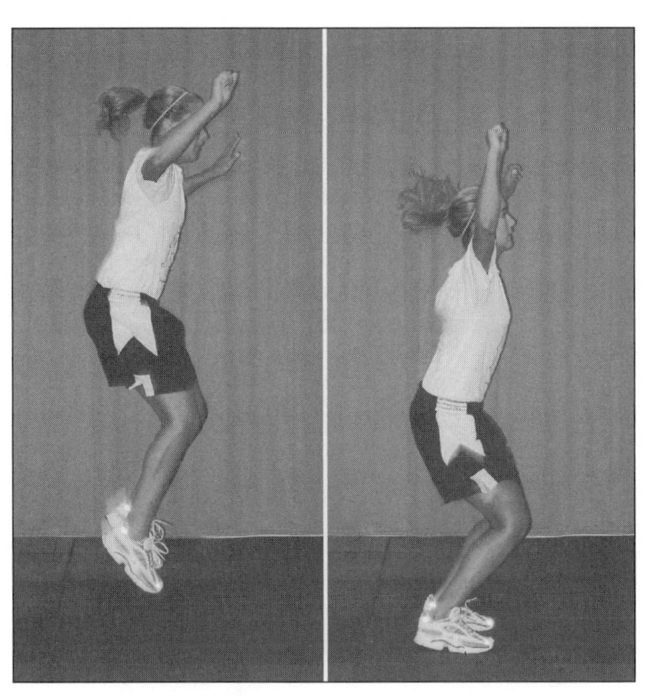

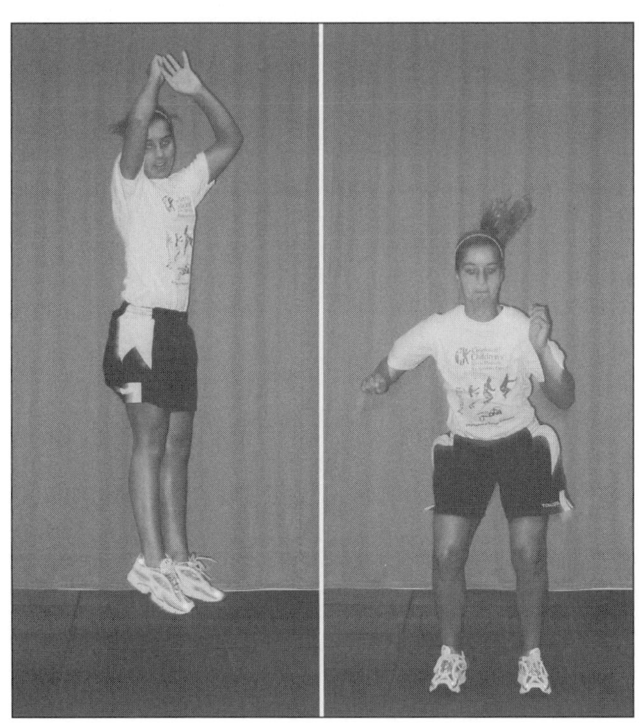

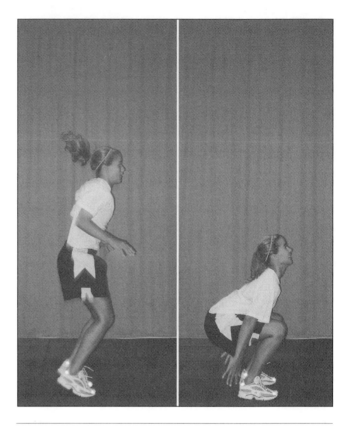

FIGURE 5.5 Plyometrics: squat jump.

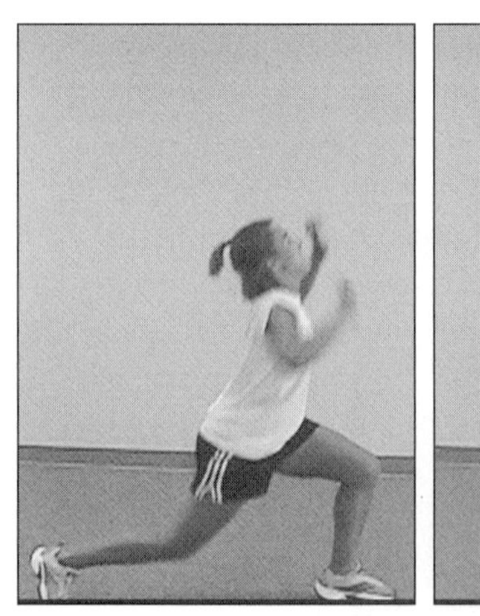
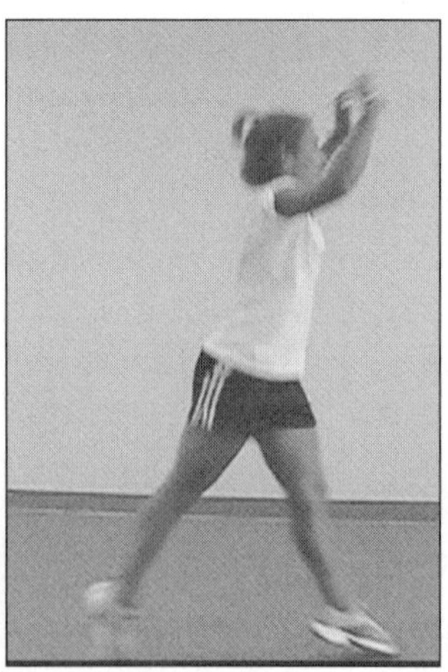
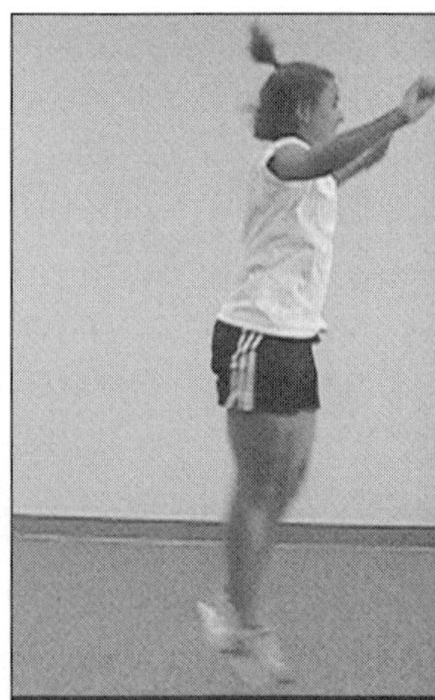

FIGURE 5.6 Plyometrics: scissors jump.

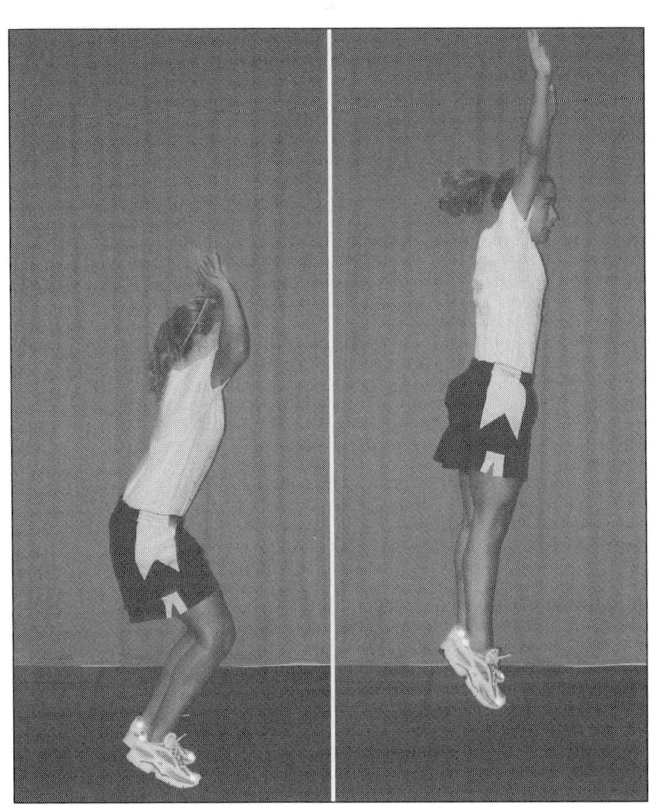

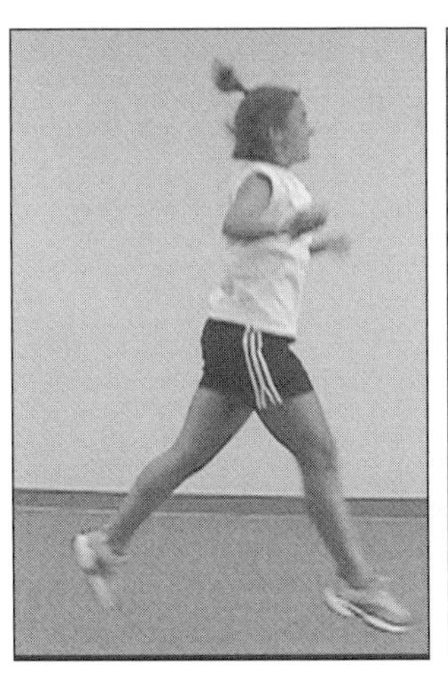

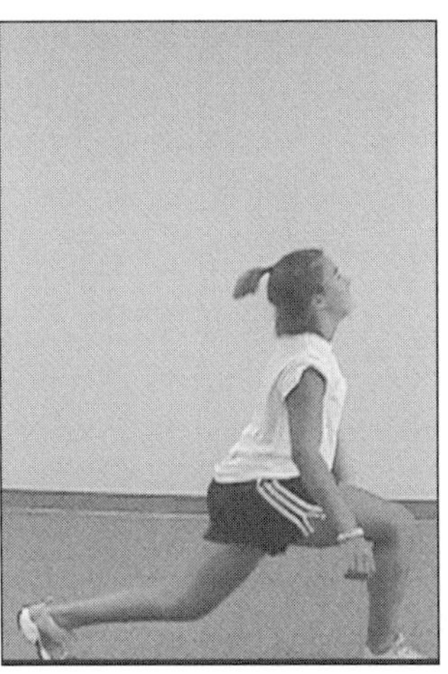

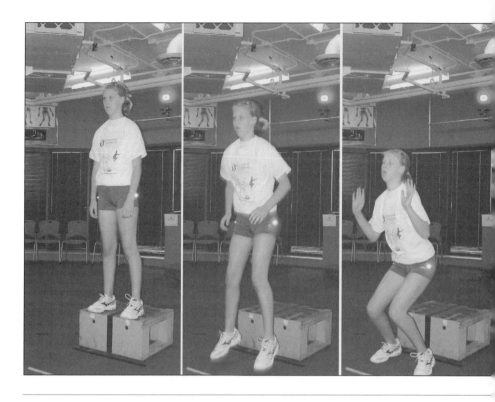

FIGURE 5.7 Plyometrics: box drop vertical jump.

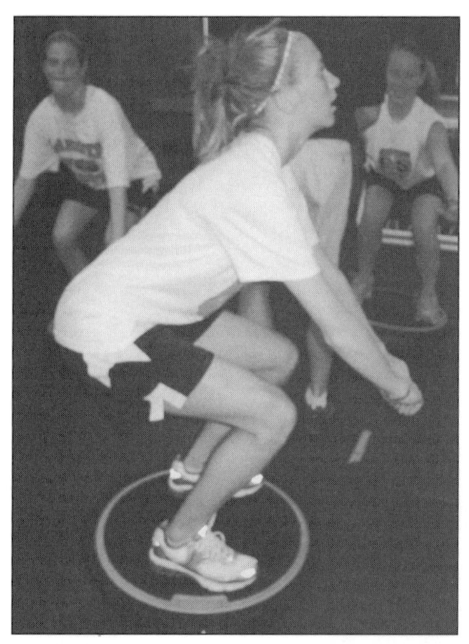

FIGURE 5.8 Balance training.

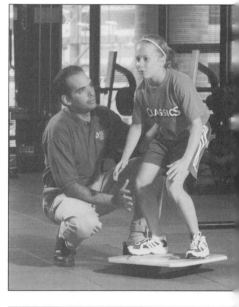

FIGURE 5.9 Balance board with biofeedback training.

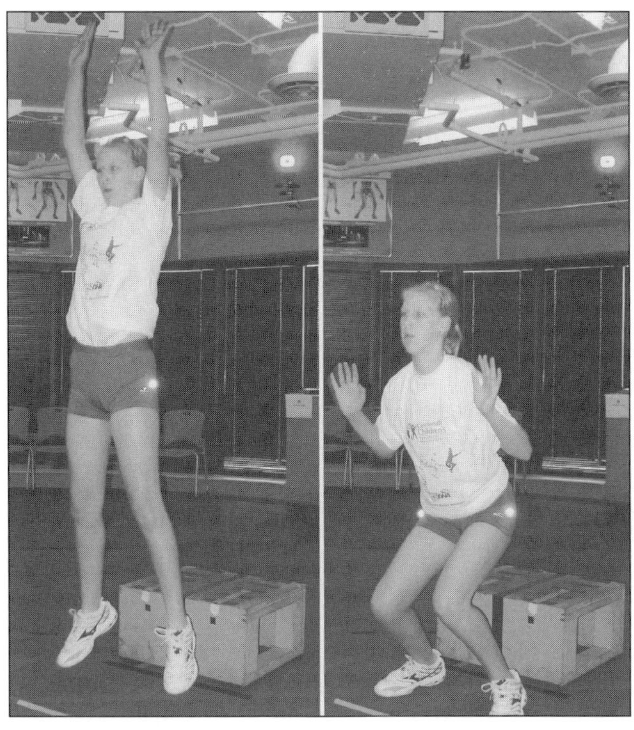

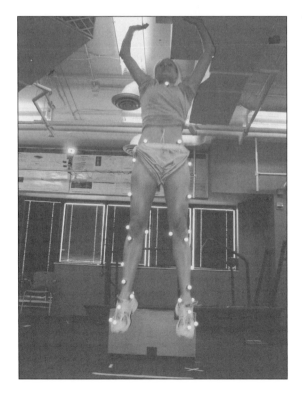

FIGURE 5.10 Box drop with biofeedback training.

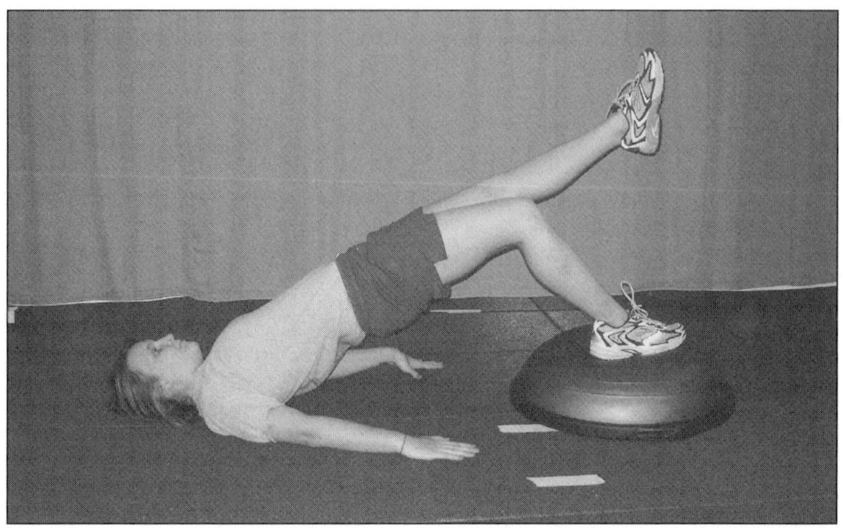

FIGURE 5.11 Core-Strength training.

young female athletes attempting to prepare for an injury-free season. Thus, if a single training component or a reduced number of components were found to alter the biomechanical risk factors related to the female athlete's increased risk of ACL injury, more effective and efficient preseason training programs could possibly be implemented.

Single-Component Training

This section deals with the potential injury prevention and biomechanical effects of utilizing a single component of training. The single training components included are plyometrics, balance, biofeedback, and strength training. There currently are no published studies incorporating a single component of training that show reduced knee or ACL injuries in female athletes.

Effects of a Plyometric Component

High-intensity plyometric movements that progress beyond footwork and agility, incorporated into an intervention, have been shown to reduce ACL injuries (Hewett et al. 1999; Mandelbaum 2002; Myklebust et al. 2003). These studies, however, combine differing levels of strength training, biofeedback, balance, and so on. Although an isolated plyometric program has not been shown to reduce knee and ACL injuries, the neuromuscular and biomechanical effects have been demonstrated by several authors (Hewett et al. 1996; Chimera et al. 2004; Irmischer et al. 2004).

Effects of Isolated Balance Training

Balance training alone may not be sufficient to produce significant ACL injury prevention effects. Wedderkopp's and Soderman's groups focused on balance training, primarily utilizing unstable wobble boards (Wedderkopp et al. 1999; Soderman et al. 2000). The interventions in these two studies were not effective, as Wedderkopp was able to reduce overall injuries, though not knee or ACL injuries, and Soderman's intervention was not effective in reducing either (Wedderkopp et al. 1999; Soderman et al. 2000). Caraffa and associates (1996) prospectively evaluated the effect of balance board exercises on noncontact ACL injury rates in male soccer players and reported significant, approximately sevenfold, decreases in ACL injury risk. However, there were several experimental design and methodological problems with this study. Soderman and colleagues attempted to replicate the Caraffa study, which had been performed in males, with female athletes; the impressive effect on ACL injury was not replicated in the female soccer players. The training consisted of approximately 20 min of balance board exercises divided into five phases. Soderman et al. compared athletes who participated in proprioceptive training prior to their competitive seasons with controls and did not observe a significantly decreased rate of ACL injuries in the trained group (Caraffa et al. 1996; Soderman et al. 2000). A possible performance benefit of balance training is improved maximum lower extremity strength and decreased side-to-side imbalances in stabilometric measures (Heitkamp et al. 2001).

Effects of Isolated Biofeedback Technique Training

Education and enforced awareness of dangerous positions and mechanisms of ACL injury can decrease ACL injury risk (Johnson 2001). Ettlinger and colleagues utilized "guided discovery" techniques whereby ski instructors viewed videotapes of ACL injuries and were encouraged to formulate their own preventive strategies using these guided discovery techniques (Johnson 2001). Anterior cruciate ligament injuries were decreased by greater than 50% with this technique (Johnson 2001). Olsen and colleagues reported that a video-based injury awareness program did not decrease injury rates in soccer (Olsen et al. 2004). Awareness programs alone, without training, may not be effective in landing and cutting sports. However, elements from Ettlinger and colleagues' ski study may be applicable to ACL injury prevention in other sports. It may be important to teach athletes to avoid positions associated with high joint loading in any sport. Henning identified three potentially dangerous maneuvers in basketball that he proposed should be modified through training to prevent ACL injury: planting and cutting, straight-knee landing, and a one-step stop with the knee extended (Griffin 2001). Henning suggested that athletes alter the plant and cut to a rounded turn, land in a more bent-knee position, utilize a three-step instead of a one-step stop, and decelerate prior to a cutting maneuver. Preliminary work that implemented these different techniques on a small sample of athletes showed a trend toward a decrease in injury rates in the trained versus the untrained study groups (Griffin 2001). However, a significant decrease was not reported.

Hewett and colleagues (1999) expanded the concept of athlete education regarding dangerous biomechanics related to injury mechanisms and utilized a trainer to provide verbal and visual feedback and awareness to an athlete during training. Verbalization and visualizations (e.g., land "straight as an arrow" and "light as a feather," be a "shock absorber," and "recoil like a spring") were utilized by trainers as verbal and visualization cues for each phase of the jump. Athletes were encouraged to perform jumps using only proper technique. As the athletes became fatigued, they were required to stop if they could not execute each jump with correct biomechanics. Myklebust and colleagues (2003) utilized partner training to provide the critical feedback. Partners encouraged each other to focus on the quality of their movements, specifically on the knee-over-the-toe position. Mandelbaum and colleagues (2005) used a training video to emphasize proper body position and movement mechanics during running and landing. The studies by Hewett et al. (1999) and Myklebust et al. (2003) specifically cited the critical analysis and feedback as contributors to the reduction of ACL injuries in their respective studies.

Effects of Isolated Strength Training

The effects of a sound resistance training component on increases in strength in female athletes have widely been documented in the literature (Ben-Sira, Ayalon, and Tavi 1995; Boyer 1990; Chilibeck et al. 1998; Fry et al. 1991). Resistance training alone has not been reported to reduce ACL injuries. However, there is inferential evidence that resistance training may reduce injury based on the beneficial adaptations that occur in bones, ligaments, and tendons following training (Fleck and Falkel 1986; Kraemer, Duncan, and Volek 1998). Lehnhard and colleagues (1996) were able to significantly reduce injury rates with the addition of a strength training regimen to a men's soccer team. They monitored injuries for two years in the absence of training and for two years with a structured strength training treatment added. While they did not observe a reduction specifically in ACL injuries, they did report a decrease in percentage of injuries that were ligament sprains. The significant reduction of ligament sprains may have been related to the reduced knee injury (43%) reported in the second year of posttrained competition (Lehnhard et al. 1996). In addition, a reduction of reported knee injuries was found in high school football when weight training was incorporated into a preseason conditioning program (Cahill and Griffith 1978). Resistance training may aid in the reduction of ACL injuries when combined with other training components; however, the efficacy of a single-faceted resistance training protocol on ACL injury prevention has yet to be determined.

Multicomponent Training

Multicomponent training may better prepare the athlete than single component training alone. The potential effects of multiple components are discussed in the next section. One important question is: are these effects combinatory? In other words, are the positive effects additive to one another? This is currently unknown. Another important question is: can we get the majority of the injury prevention effect though a single component or with an abbreviated program?

Effects of Combined Plyometric, Balance, Biofeedback, and Strengthening Components

Two studies, those of Hewett and colleagues and Mandelbaum and colleagues, have shown a reduced ACL injury rate in female athletes after a combined intervention consisting of plyometrics, balance training, biofeedback, and strength training (Hewett et al. 1999; Mandelbaum et al. 2005). In both training programs the plyometric component, which trains the muscles, connective tissue, and nervous system to effectively carry out the stretch–shortening cycle, focused on proper technique, body mechanics, and deceleration and acceleration of the center of mass of the body. Training interventions that incorporate plyometrics with safe levels of varus or valgus stress may induce more muscle-dominant neuromuscular adaptations to correct for neuromuscular imbalances in female athletes (Hewett, Paterno, and Myer 2002; Lloyd and Buchanan 2001). Such adaptations may better prepare an athlete for more multidirectional sport activities and may reduce positioning that puts high loads on the ACL (Chimera et al. 2004; Irmischer et al. 2004; Lloyd 2001). Hewett and colleagues utilized a progression of three plyometric phases with seven to nine exercises during each phase. The injury prevention program used by Mandelbaum and colleagues, an in-season warm-up modification of Hewett and colleagues' program, developed specifically for soccer, incorporated five similar plyometric exercises.

These two studies (Hewett et al. 1999; Mandelbaum et al. 2005) also incorporated functional balance training (single-leg stability), primarily utilizing hold positions from a decelerated landing, into their intervention design. These interventions elaborated on the balance board protocols by focusing on improved awareness and knee control during standing, cutting, jumping, and landing (Caraffa et al. 1996). However, there are likely advantages to incorporating both balance board and other unstable surface training devices with more sport-specific land and hold balancing techniques

As mentioned earlier, Hewett and colleagues utilized an athletic trainer to provide verbal and visual feedback and biomechanical technique awareness to athletes during training. Verbalization and visualizations such as "on your toes," "straight as an arrow," "light as a feather," "shock absorber," and "recoil like a spring" were utilized by the athletic trainer as verbal and visualization cues for each phase of the jump. Athletes were encouraged to perform jumps using only proper technique. As the athletes became fatigued, they were required to stop if they could not execute each jump with correct biomechanics. In addition, an instructional videotape depicting proper and improper technique was viewed by each subject in Mandelbaum and colleagues' study.

The strengthening components of the two programs differed in that Mandelbaum used three exercises that could be performed on the soccer field while Hewett and colleagues used eight exercises performed in a training room, gym, or clinic. Strength training may be optional for injury prevention; however, the biomechanical and strength changes observed may have been due in part to the strength training component (Hewett et al. 1996).

Effects of Combined Plyometric, Balance, and Biofeedback Components

Myklebust and colleagues (2003) reported a reduction in ACL injuries after participation in a multicomponent program consisting of plyometrics, balance exercises, and feedback. In contrast to the studies just reviewed, these studies did not use specific strengthening exercises. Mykelbust and colleagues (2003) utilized partner feedback throughout the exercises, and athletes were instructed to be aware of the quality of their movements. This protocol was more focused on balance activities, as wobble boards and balance mats were used during the exercises to provide unstable surfaces. Others have shown that this type of proprioceptive and balance training can improve postural control and that lack of postural control and stability is related to increased risk of ankle injury (Holm et al. 2004; Paterno et al. 2004; Tropp, Ekstrand, and Gillquist 1984; Tropp and Odenrick 1988). In addition, improvement in single-leg stability can be gained with a neuromuscular training intervention that incorporates perturbations into balance training on unstable surfaces (Paterno et al. 2004).

Of the six interventions, the three that reduced ACL injury rates (Hewett et al. 1999; Mandelbaum et al. 2005; Myklebust et al. 2003) all incorporated feedback techniques combined with plyometrics and balance training. Neuromuscular training that employs feedback with plyometrics and balance (and core stability) exercises adds a "neuromuscular reeducation" component to aid in decreasing ACL injury rates.

Effects of Combined Plyometric and Balance Components

The effects of the three interventions that reduced ACL injury rates appear to be relatively similar, arising from a common rationale derived from performance enhancement training and physical rehabilitation for athletes. Neuromuscular training that employs both plyometrics and balance (and core stability) drills alters active knee joint stabilization and appears to aid in decreasing ACL injury rates in female athletes.

Balance training alone may not be sufficient to produce significant knee stabilization or ACL injury prevention effects. However, when used in combination with other neuromuscular training techniques, single-leg dynamic balance training is associated with improved biomechanics and decreased injury rates. The studies by Hewett and Mandelbaum incorporated single-leg stability (functional balance) training, primarily utilizing hold positions from a decelerated landing, into their intervention design and examined the effects of a relatively comprehensive functional balance training intervention (Hewett et al. 1999; Mandelbaum et al. 2005). These findings support the integration of proprioceptive stability and balance training in ACL injury interventions. However, it appears that alone, balance drills utilizing unstable platforms may not be sufficient to reduce ACL injury risk.

Effects of a Comprehensive Program Combined With Either Plyometric or Balance Components

Recent work in our laboratory (Myer et al. 2006) compared a comprehensive program that incorporated plyometric training and excluded balance training (PLYO) with one that incorporated balance training and excluded plyometrics (BAL). These studies demonstrated that both PLYO and BAL training can reduce lower extremity valgus measures at the hip and ankle during a two-footed plyometric activity. In addition, both PLYO and BAL training can reduce lower extremity valgus measures at the knee during a single-limb dynamic stabilization task. However, in the sagittal plane, training increases in knee flexion may be dependent on the interaction between training mode and movement task. Thus, to improve knee flexion during a broad range of sport-related activities, it may be necessary to utilize both PLYO and BAL modes of training. The results of the current study do not support the exclusion of either plyometric or dynamic stabilization exercises from an injury prevention protocol.

Conclusions and Future Directions

An examination of the data extracted from the intervention studies leads to a few potentially valuable generalizations. Plyometric training combined with biomechanical analysis and technique training is common to all three studies that effectively reduced ACL injury rates. Balance training alone is likely not as effective for injury prevention as balance training combined with other types of training. One needs to consider whether the teams' or athletes' primary goal is injury prevention, performance enhancement, or both. Recent studies employing the in-season training program of Mandelbaum and colleagues demonstrated that the ACL injury reduction is not observed until later in the season in collegiate soccer, and this in-season program did not appear to change biomechanical risk factors (Gilchrist et al. 2004b; Powers et al. 2004). Finally, the most effective and efficient programs appear to require a combination of components, and the effects of these components are potentially additive.

There is evidence that neuromuscular training not only decreases the landing forces and increases balance but also decreases ACL injury incidence in female athletes. Landing biomechanics and technique, balance training, and strength training can induce neuromuscular changes and potential injury prevention effects in female athletes. However, we do not yet know which of these components may be most effective or whether their effects are combinatorial. Future directions will include assessing the relative efficacy of these interventions alone and in combination in order to achieve the optimal effect in the most efficient manner possible. Selective combination of neuromuscular training components may provide additive effects, further reducing the risk of ACL injuries in female athletes. Additional research directions include the assessment of relative injury risk using mass neuromuscular screening.

Chapter 6

Preventive Training Programs

Changing Strength Ratios Versus Positions of Muscular Efficiency

Sandra J. Shultz, PhD, ATC, CSCS

Examination of strain characteristics of the ACL reveals greater strain in weight bearing than in nonweight bearing with anterior tibial translation and across a range of valgus, varus, and external tibial rotation torques, as well as with low internal rotation torques (Fleming et al. 2001). Strain on the ACL during these motions is of particular concern in the performance of functional tasks that require an aggressive, quadriceps-dominant contraction to control the body's motion, which alone has been demonstrated to strain (in vivo) (Beynnon et al. 1997a) and injure (in vitro) (DeMorat et al. 2004) the ACL. Compared to males, females demonstrate preferential quadriceps activity (Huston and Wojtys 1996; Malinzak et al. 2001; Shultz et al. 2001), greater valgus angles (Ford, Myer, and Hewett 2003; Zeller et al. 2003; Hewett, Myer, and Ford 2004), and greater valgus-varus moments (Hewett et al. 1996; McLean et al. 1999; Malinzak et al. 2001; Chappell et al. 2002) during functional activity and testing conditions, all of which can increase strain on the ACL (Markolf et al. 1995; Fleming et al. 2001). When these forces are experienced near full knee extension (a commonly observed ACL injury mechanism) (Boden et al. 2000; Griffin et al. 2000), less anterior tibial movement is required to strain and rupture the ACL (Zavatsky and Wright 2001), and the hamstring muscles are at a mechanical disadvantage with respect to stabilizing the tibia (Renstrom et al. 1986; Hirokawa et al. 1991).

Given these strain patterns and the observed neuromuscular and biomechanical differences noted in males and females, injury prevention programs have been aimed at improving both movement strategies and neuromuscular coordination and strength patterns to reduce these injurious forces. The following discussion focuses on the potential for these programs to affect agonist–antagonist muscle strength ratios and the thigh, hip, and body core that have the potential to improve knee stability and reduce ACL injury risk.

Thigh Strength

The most fully studied strength ratio relative to knee stability is that of the quadriceps and hamstrings. Before we look at the effects of training and prevention programs on strength ratios, it is important to consider basic science and clinical studies that have examined the role of the quadriceps and hamstrings in providing joint stability and reducing mechanical loads on ligament structures.

Theoretical Background

The hamstrings play a major role, both singly and in coactivation with the quadriceps, in protecting the ACL by preventing or decreasing anterior, varus-valgus, and rotary displacement of the tibia on the femur (Markolf, Graff-Radford, and Amstutz 1978; Olmstead et al. 1986; Renstrom et al. 1986; Louie and Mote 1987; Hagood et al. 1990; Hirokawa et al. 1991; McNair and Marshall 1994; Lloyd and Buchanan 2001). With knee extension forces, a shear component acts parallel to the joint surface and creates anterior tibial translation of the tibia on the femur (Baratta et al. 1988). When the knee is flexed, the hamstrings' line of pull is primarily parallel to the joint surface and is in a favorable position for the hamstrings to counteract anterior, as well as rotary, displacement of the tibia (Baratta et al. 1988; Hirokawa et al. 1991; Gauffin and Tropp 1992; Arendt and Dick 1995). However, the effectiveness of the hamstrings in counteracting this anterior tibial displacement appears to be limited to knee flexion angles greater than 15° to 30° (Renstrom et al. 1986; Hirokawa et al. 1991). Trunk position can also influence the hamstrings' effectiveness at flexed knee angles. When the trunk is positioned directly over the knee with the center of mass leaning forward, greater hamstring coactivation occurs than when the trunk is positioned more posteriorly, with peak activity occurring between 40° and 70° of knee flexion during ascension (Wilk et al. 1996). Hence, functional positions in which the weight is forward on the balls of the feet (vs. on the heels), and in which the hip and knees are flexed, are often recommended to engage the hamstrings and improve functional stability at the knee (figure 6.1).

Although the quadriceps and hamstrings function primarily to flex and extend the knee, they also act to support varus-valgus moments. Near full extension (i.e., 0-20°), coactivation of the quadriceps and hamstrings serves primarily to increase joint stiffness and effectively reduce anterior-posterior, varus-valgus, and rotational laxity through increased tibiofemoral joint compression (Markolf, Mensch, and Amstutz 1976; Markolf, Graff-Radford, and Amstutz 1978; Olm-

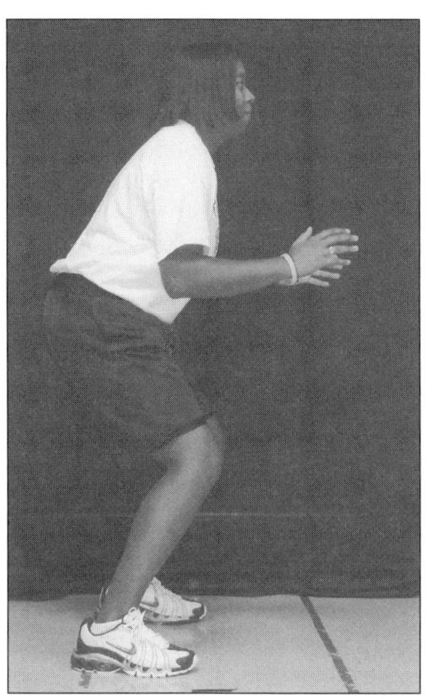

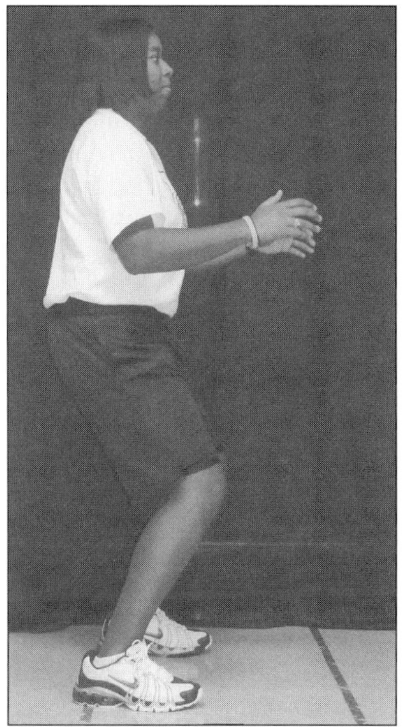

a b

FIGURE 6.1 *(a)* When the trunk is positioned directly over the knee with the center of mass leaning forward, greater hamstring coactivation occurs than *(b)* when the trunk is positioned more posteriorly.

stead et al. 1986; Louie and Mote 1987). Between 40° and 90° of knee flexion, it has been observed that cocontraction of the hamstrings and quadriceps is the primary activation strategy to support varus-valgus moments at the knee (Lloyd and Buchanan 2001). When operating independently, quadriceps activation has a greater effect on varus stability, while hamstring activation has a greater effect on valgus stability. Olmstead and colleagues (1986) reported that when the quadriceps were activated to produce a 10 Nm and 20 Nm extensor torque (equal to 8% and 15% of a maximum voluntary contraction, respectively), varus displacement was reduced by 20% and 32%, valgus displacement was reduced by 12% and 16%, and varus and valgus initial stiffness was increased by 200% and 240% and 180% and 220%, respectively. Conversely, mild to moderate hamstring torques equal to 10% and 20% of maximum contractions increase valgus stability substantially more than varus stability, with valgus displacement decreasing by 35% and 50%, respectively, and stiffness of both varus and valgus increasing by 200% and 280%.

These findings suggest that quadriceps and hamstrings play an important role in knee stability, with their effectiveness dependent on their relative coactivity and on joint and body positions. Although it is widely accepted that the quadriceps and hamstrings act as prime movers of the knee in the sagittal plane, research reports suggest that they also play a significant role in frontal and transverse plane stability. Hence, injury prevention programs that emphasize increased hamstring strength and coactivity relative to the quadriceps, as well as improved functional joint positions to increase the mechanical efficiency of the hamstrings relative to the quadriceps, should theoretically be protective of the ACL.

Effects of Preventive Training Programs on H:Q Strength Ratios

While limited studies have directly examined how hamstring-to-quadriceps strength ratios are affected through training and prevention programs, they tend to support the ability of these programs to improve hamstring function. Following a six-week preseason conditioning program that consisted of plyometrics, stretching, and isotonic strengthening (Hewett et al. 1996), two studies showed an increase in hamstring peak torque and hamstring-to-quadriceps ratio (Hewett et al. 1996; Wilkerson et al. 2004). Hewett and colleagues (1996) examined the effectiveness of a progressive jump training program on landing mechanics and lower extremity strength in female high school volleyball players. The program consisted of three 2 hr sessions per week that were designed to decrease landing forces by improving landing techniques and to increase joint stability by improving knee muscle strength. Before and after the program, the females were compared to age-, height-, and weight-matched males on vertical jump height, thigh strength, and landing forces during a volleyball block jump. Results indicated that following the six-week training program, females increased their vertical jump height by 9%; they also decreased their peak landing forces by 22% and their adduction and abduction moments by 38% and 53%, respectively. Isokinetic strength tests revealed improved isokinetic peak torque and average power at 300°/sec such that hamstring-to-quadriceps peak torque ratio improved 13% on the dominant side and 26% on the nondominant side. Posttraining strength H:Q ratios (65% compared to 51% prior to training) were similar to those in untrained males. Given the role of the quadriceps and hamstrings in supporting varus-valgus stability (Markolf, Graff-Radford, and Amstutz 1978; Olmstead et al. 1986), it is possible that the reduced varus and valgus knee moments upon landing were in part a by-product of the improved hamstring-to-quadriceps activation ratios.

Smaller but significant improvements in hamstring-to-quadriceps strength ratios were also noted by Wilkerson and colleagues in a small cohort of female collegiate basketball players following the same six-week jump training program (Hewett et al. 1996; Wilkerson et al. 2004). Eleven Division II players who participated in the jump training program along with their regular practice and training activities were compared to nine Division I players who participated in regular training and practice activities. Reciprocal, concentric peak torque for the quadriceps and hamstrings was obtained at isokinetic speeds of 60°/sec and 300°/sec. Following the training, significant improvements were found for hamstring peak torque and hamstring-to-quadriceps strength ratios at 60°/sec in the experimental group compared to the control group. Although similar improvements were found at 300°/sec, these results were not significant due to low statistical power.

A key feature of ACL injury prevention programs is eccentric loading of the hamstrings, which appears to be more effective in increasing hamstring-to-quadriceps strength ratios than traditional concentric exercises (Lee et al. 2004; Mjolsnes et al. 2004). In a study comparing traditional concentric isotonic hamstring curls to a Nordic eccentric hamstring exercise in highly trained soccer players (similar to the Russian hamstring exercise [figure 6.2] used in the Prevent Injury and Enhance Performance [PEP] program; Mandelbaum et al. 2005), only those who trained eccentrically had significant improvements in eccentric and isometric hamstring strength and in ratios of eccentric hamstrings to concentric quadriceps (Mjolsnes et al. 2004).

What is less clear is the impact of prevention programs on movement technique and body position, which may play an equally important role in improving

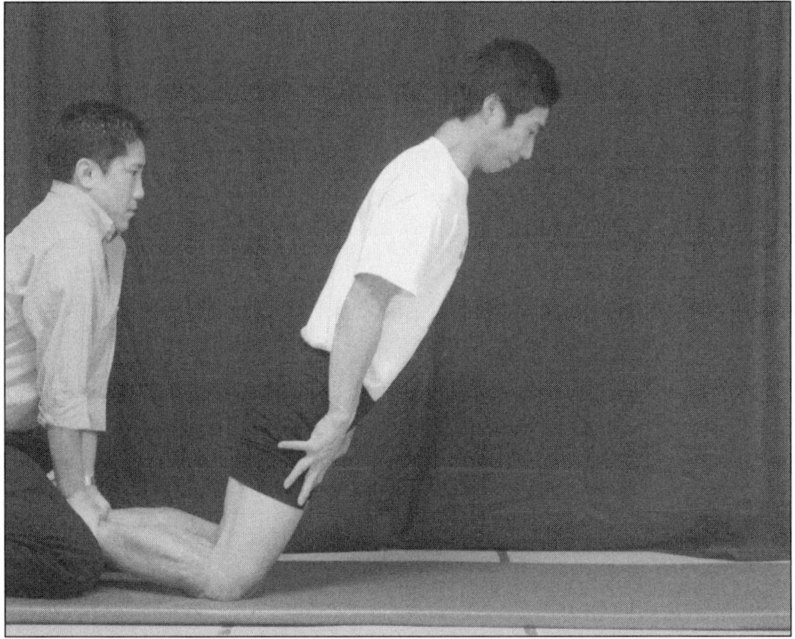

FIGURE 6.2 The Russian hamstring curl is performed during kneeling, with hands at the side. As a partner holds the ankles, the participant slowly lowers the trunk and upper body toward the ground while keeping the back straight.

hamstring-to-quadriceps functional strength ratios during sport activity. While a primary goal of ACL prevention programs is to improve movement patterns (e.g., bending the knees, getting low), research outcomes have yet to show changes in trunk position and knee and hip flexion angles during at-risk activities. Ongoing work reported by Lephart and colleagues (2002) shows promise in this regard, depicting changes in trunk position (suggestive of improved hamstring efficiency) relative to the plant leg during a cutting maneuver following an eight-week neuromuscular training program. As research on ACL prevention programs continues, functional hamstring-to-quadriceps strength ratios should be examined in relation to the body position in which the muscles are activated.

Hip Strength

The hip and pelvis serve as the attachment for muscles of the trunk as well as the lower extremity, allowing the dynamic transfer of forces between the upper torso and lower extremity. As such, the muscles about the hip and pelvis, in particular the gluteal muscles, are thought to play an important role in locomotion and postural stability. In the sagittal plane, the rise time of gluteus maximus activation has been shown to play a critical role in generating extensor moments at the hip, knee, and ankle (Bobbert and Vanzanwijk 1999), suggesting a proximal to distal activation order in the generation of lower extremity vertical movement. In the frontal plane, reflexive activation of the gluteus medius occurs, first in the contralateral and then the ipsilateral hip, in response to an inversion ankle perturbation (Beckman and Buchanan 1995). In the transverse plane, increased gluteus medius activity has been observed with an external force applied to the hip in the closed kinetic chain (Schmitz et al. 2002). Given these proximal stabilization strategies, more attention is being directed toward the strength and stability of the hip musculature as in relation to stability of the knee joint.

Theoretical Background

The role of the gluteal muscles in stabilizing the pelvis and maintaining proper hip and knee alignment in single-leg stance has been implicated in the ACL injury mechanism (Griffin et al. 2000; McClay-Davis and Ireland 2001; Zeller et al. 2003). Ireland (1999) describes a "position of no return" that is characterized by a forward flexed, adducted, and internally rotated hip; a valgus and extended knee; and an externally rotated tibia (figure 6.3). This position has been attributed to a reduction in hip abductor and extensor control, leading to uncontrolled pelvis and hip motion. The gluteal muscles function as primary stabilizers of the hip and play a critical role in maintaining a level and stable pelvis in single-leg stance (Moore 1992; Kumagai et al. 1997). While the gluteus maximus functions primarily as a hip extensor, the gluteus medius and minimus serve as the primary hip abductors and lateral stabilizers of the pelvis. Together they work to control hip rotation, with their functional importance depending on the degree of hip flexion (Lindsay et al. 1992; Delp et al. 1999). At 0° hip flexion, the gluteus minimus and anterior fibers of the gluteus medius function to internally rotate the femur; the middle and posterior fibers of the gluteus medius function to externally rotate the femur; and the gluteus maximus functions as a powerful external rotator (Joseph 1998; Delp et al. 1999). However, as the hip moves into flexion, the rotation moment arms of the gluteal muscles appear to change substantially. Specifically, the middle and posterior fibers progressively switch from external rotators to internal rotators between ~10° and 40° of hip flexion, and the anterior compartment of the gluteus maximus becomes an internal rotator while the posterior compartment has a reduced hip external rotation moment (Delp et al. 1999). Even with these significant changes in muscle function by position, comparison of isokinetic internal and external hip rotation torques suggests that internal rotation torques consistently exceed external rotation torques at both extended and flexed hip positions (Lindsay et al. 1992).

These observations suggest that, consistent with quadriceps and hamstring activation at the knee, coactivity and stability of the hip joint are dependent not only on the absolute strength and relative balance of the hip musculature, but also on the position of the hip joint at which these muscles are activated. In

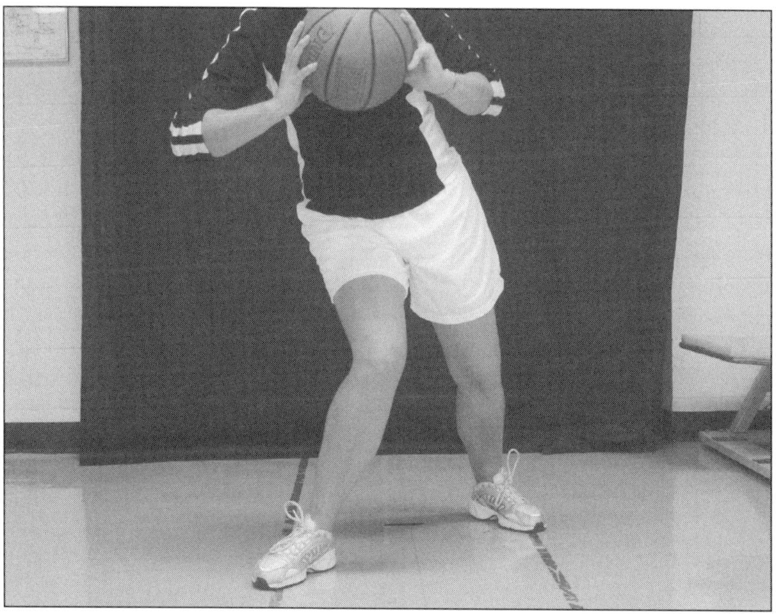

FIGURE 6.3 Body position depicting the "position of no return" described by Ireland (1999), characterized by a forward flexed, adducted, and internally rotated hip; a valgus and extended knee; and an externally rotated tibia.

particular, relative weakness of the posterior lateral hip musculature (abductors, extensors, external rotators) compared to the anterior medial hip musculature (flexor, adductors), coupled with increased hip flexion (e.g., secondary to hip flexor tightness, increased anterior pelvic tilt), may severely limit the ability of the gluteal muscles to stabilize the hip and maintain a neutral alignment of the hip and knee. Hence, ACL intervention programs that focus on increasing strength and efficiency of the posterior lateral hip musculature through multijoint strength training (e.g., squats, lunges), plyometrics, and agility training would theoretically improve lower extremity functional alignment in weight bearing, reducing rotational and valgus forces at the knee. This theory is supported by work showing decreased hip abduction and external rotation strength in females compared to males (Lindsay et al. 1992; Ferris et al. 2004; Leetun et al. 2004) and indicating that these strength deficits are related to altered knee joint biomechanics (Mascal et al. 2003; Ferris et al. 2004) and lower extremity injury risk (Ireland et al. 2003; Leetun et al. 2004).

Effects of Preventive Training Programs on Hip Strength Ratios

Unfortunately, few empirical data could be found to directly support this theoretical framework or provide evidence that these aims are being achieved. Only two studies have examined changes in hip musculature following intervention programs. In response to a six-week plyometric training program, significant increases in preparatory adductor activation, and thus an increase in preparatory adductor to abductor muscle coactivation, were noted during a vertical jump task (Chimera et al. 2004). In paralleling their findings with evidence of decreased varus and valgus moments following training (Hewett et al. 1996), the authors viewed these collective results as strong support for the role of the hip musculature in providing dynamic restraint and control of lower extremity alignment at ground contact. Although this work demonstrates the potential for improved firing patterns, data regarding changes in absolute strength or agonist–antagonist strength ratios of the hip musculature following strength, plyometric, and agility training are lacking. However, this potential also appears promising based on two case reports of subjects with patellofemoral pain, which noted improved functional and pain status, hip abductor and extensor strength, and lower extremity kinematics (reduced hip adduction, internal rotation, and knee valgus during a step-down) following progressive strength and endurance training of the posterolateral hip musculature over a 14-week period (Mascal et al. 2003). While more work is clearly needed in this area, hip strength and stability appear to be relevant factors with respect to determining the efficacy of ACL prevention programs.

Core Strength

Anterior pelvic tilt has been suggested as a predictor of ACL injury because of its effect on lower extremity postural alignment. Clinically, excessive anterior tilt of the pelvis has been associated with accentuated internal femoral rotation, genu valgus, genu recurvatum, and subtalar pronation (Loudon, Jenkins, and Loudon 1996; Hruska 1998; Chaitow and DeLany 2000). Collectively, this posture is thought to preload the ACL, increase ligamentous laxity, place the hamstrings in a lengthened and weakened position, and alter proprioception and muscular activation (Kendall and McCreary 1983; Coplan 1989; Loudon, Jenkins, and Loudon 1996; Hruska 1998). Moreover, given the changes in gluteal function with increasing hip flexion previously described (Delp et al. 1999), increased anterior pelvic tilt may contribute to weakness and inefficiency of the gluteal muscles, further accentuating a "functional valgus collapse" of the knee. While epidemiological studies are limited, various studies (most retrospective) have identified a relationship between ACL injury and excessive anterior pelvic tilt (Loudon, Jenkins, and Loudon 1996; Hertel, Dorfman, and Braham 2004), as well as a number of the concomitant lower extremity alignment faults that have been previously described (i.e., knee recurvatum, navicular drop, knee laxity) (Beckett et al. 1992; Woodford-Rogers, Cyphert, and Denegar 1994; Loudon, Jenkins, and Loudon 1996; Uhorchak et al. 2003; Hertel, Dorfman, and Braham 2004).

Theoretical Background

The lumbar spine, pelvis, and hip work together to control posture in the sagittal plane (Kendall and McCreary 1983; Gardocki et al. 2002), and can be referred to collectively as the lumbo-pelvic-hip complex. Forward or anterior pelvic tilt occurs with a combination of hip flexion and lumbosacral hyperextension, whereas posterior tilt occurs with hip extension and lumbosacral flexion (figure 6.4). Neuromuscular imbalances thought to contribute to an increase in anterior pelvic tilt and lumbopelvic instability include muscular tightness and shortening of the erector spinae and hip flexors, as well as elongation, inhibition, and weakening of the abdominal muscles and gluteals (Kendall and McCreary 1983; Hruska 1998; Chaitow and DeLany 2000). Hence, the relative balance in strength and flexibility between the back extensors and abdominal muscles, and between the hip extensors and flexors, appears to be critical in optimizing the position and stability of the pelvis.

Effects of Preventive Training Programs on Core Strength Ratios

Anterior cruciate ligament prevention programs have sought to include activities that strengthen core musculature (abdominal muscles, paraspinals, and gluteal muscles) and stretch tight hip flexors and back extensors in an effort to increase lumbopelvic stability, improve lower extremity posture, and reduce injury risk. While isokinetic data on young adults suggest that hip and trunk flexors are somewhat weaker than their respective extensors (Cahalan et al. 1989; Tis et al. 1991), no study could be found that specifically examined flexibility and strength ratios that lend optimal stability to the lumbo-pelvic-hip complex or the efficacy of preventive training programs in maximizing these ratios. Recent work by Kulas and colleagues (In press) and Ferris and colleagues (2004) supports this line of inquiry, however, showing that neuromechanical

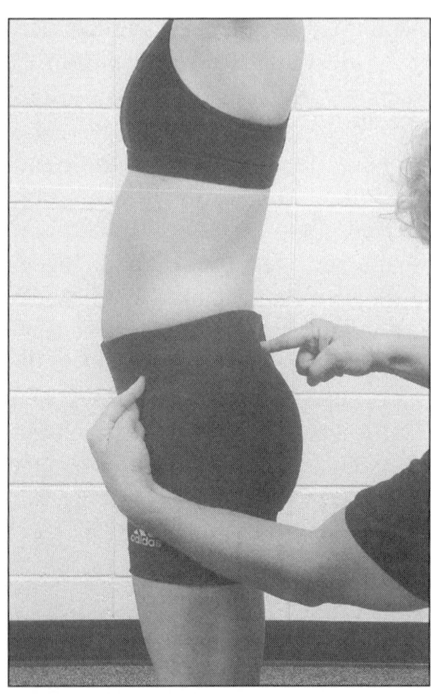

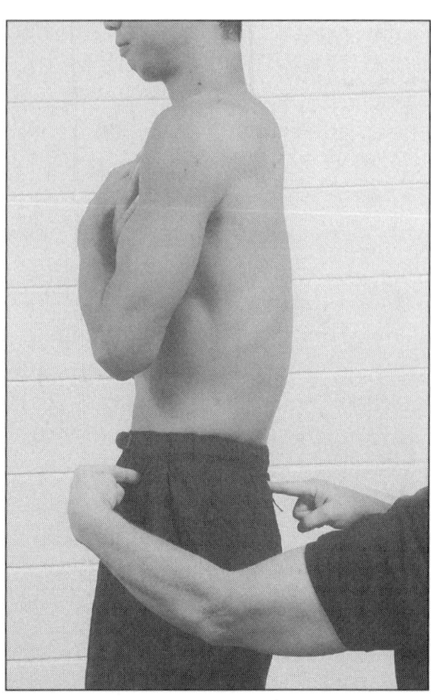

a *b*

FIGURE 6.4 *(a)* Forward or anterior pelvic tilt occurs with a combination of hip flexion and lumbosacral hyperextension, whereas *(b)* posterior tilt occurs with hip extension and lumbosacral flexion.

Reprinted, by permission, from S.J. Shultz, P. Houglum, and D.H. Perrin, 2005, *Examination of musculoskeletal injuries*, 2nd ed. (Champaign, IL: Human Kinetics), 479.

function of the abdominal muscles and posterior lateral hip musculature influences dynamic control of the pelvis and lower extremity biomechanics during landing maneuvers. As with hip strength ratios, more work is clearly needed to determine the optimal core strength ratios and their effects on positional and stabilizing effects of the lumbo-pelvic-hip complex, lower extremity biomechanics, and injury risk.

Summary

Based on studies of ACL strain patterns and the observed neuromuscular and biomechanical differences noted in males and females, injury prevention programs have sought to improve both movement strategies and neuromuscular coordination and strength patterns to reduce these injurious forces. This chapter has focused on the potential for these programs to specifically affect agonist–antagonist muscle strength ratios that have the potential to improve knee stability and reduce ACL injury risk. While there is strong theoretical support for the functional importance of adequate strength and balance of the hamstrings, posterior lateral hip, and core muscles relative to their antagonists, few empirical data are currently available to establish whether prevention programs substantially improve these strength ratios. Further, the functional importance of these strength ratios, which have been largely examined via isokinetic strength testing at isolated knee and hip angles, is unclear. Research provides strong evidence that the efficacy of the hamstrings and posterior lateral hip musculature may be largely dependent on trunk position and the knee and hip joint angles at which the muscles are activated. Hence, in addition to examining changes in absolute strength and balance of the thigh, hip, and core musculature, future studies addressing the impact of prevention programs on the body positions at which these muscle groups are activated may be equally important to our understanding of factors that lend optimal strength and stability to the knee joint during sport activity.

Chapter 7

Effect of Prevention Programs on Performance

Christopher M. Powers, PhD, PT
Christine D. Pollard, PhD, PT
Susan M. Sigward, PhD, PT, ATC

While there is evidence that various training programs can reduce the incidence of ACL injury in female athletes, dissemination and implementation of these programs remain a challenge. This may be due, in part, to the underlying motivation of athletes and their coaches to dedicate training time to programs that improve performance as opposed to injury prevention. Ireland has speculated that "injury prevention programs may be received more warmly if the program is presented with an emphasis on performance improvement as opposed to injury prevention" (Ireland 2002, p. 649).

Performance is defined in the Merriam-Webster online dictionary as the "execution of an action" or "something accomplished" (e.g., kicking or throwing a ball). The underlying components of athletic performance include strength, power, endurance, flexibility, speed, agility, balance, coordination, and reaction time (Newton, Kraemer, and Hakkinen 1999). The literature supports the use of various training programs for the improvement of specific sport skills, or the basic components of sport performance, or both (e.g., strength, power, endurance) in female athletes (Kraemer, Duncan, and Volek 1998; Kraemer et al. 2003; Myklebust 2003).

The foundation of successful ACL injury prevention programs is improvement of the basic components of sport performance. For example, injury prevention training programs have been designed to improve neuromuscular control by addressing issues of strength (Heidt et al. 2000; Hewett et al. 1999; Mandelbaum et al. 2005; Myer et al. 2005b), power (Hewett et al. 1999), flexibility (Junge et al. 2002; Mandelbaum et al. 2005), technique (Hewett et al.

1999; Junge et al. 2002; Mandelbaum et al. 2005; Myer et al. 2005b), balance (Caraffa et al. 1996; Junge et al. 2002; Myer et al. 2005b), and awareness (Junge et al. 2002; Myer et al. 2005b). The success of these programs in reducing the incidence of injury suggests that training improves these variables; however, only a handful of studies have been aimed at quantifying posttraining performance changes. A small number of studies have addressed the effects of injury prevention programs on elements of performance, including strength, balance, and agility, while others have measured changes in sport-related tasks such as vertical jump height, single-leg hop distance, and speed, with mixed results.

The purpose of this chapter is to review the literature in this area. We considered only studies that quantified changes in performance-based variables resulting from participation in a training program developed specifically for ACL injury prevention.

Performance Measure: Vertical Jump Height

Outcome: improved vertical jump height. Hewett's group (1996) was one of the first to examine how a specific injury prevention training program influences vertical jump height. At the time of their investigation, it was not known if this training program was effective at reducing the incidence of ACL injury even though it had been developed based on a review of the ACL injury literature. In a subsequent investigation, Hewett and colleagues (1999) conducted a prospective study using the same injury prevention training program and reported that females who did not participate in the program had a knee injury rate 3.6 times greater than for trained female athletes and 4.8 times greater than for untrained males. In the study that measured vertical jump height (Hewett et al. 1996), the subjects were 11 female high school volleyball players who were all right hand dominant. The authors did not report whether or not the subjects had a history of ACL injury or lower extremity injury. However, a knee exam was done before and after training. All subjects underwent 2 hr of training, three days a week for six weeks; there was no control group. The six-week training program consisted of jumping and landing exercises and included three phases. Phase I and phase II stressed technique, while phase III training focused on achieving maximal vertical jump height. Additional activities included stretching immediately before training as well as stretching and weightlifting following training.

Hewett and colleagues (1996) measured maximum vertical jump height before and after the six-week training program using a Vertec machine (Questek Corp., Northridge, CA). Each subject's standing reach was recorded at the beginning of the vertical jump height test; then subjects were instructed to perform three standing maximal-effort vertical jumps. This testing procedure was performed just before initiation of the training program and one week after completion of the program. Following the training program, subjects demonstrated a significant increase (1.5 ± 0.5 in. [3.8 ± 1.3 cm]) in average vertical jump height. The investigators considered this increase in vertical jump height a substantial performance increase that superseded the results of other training programs not specific for injury prevention but instead targeted at increasing vertical jump height.

Performance Measures: Agility, Strength, and Lunge Distance

Outcome: improved strength. A recent study by Wilkerson and colleagues (2004) used the same six-week injury prevention program reported by Hewett's group (1996, 1999) to examine how participation in such a training program influences agility, strength, and lunge distance. The experimental subjects were 11 female collegiate basketball players; eight female collegiate basketball players on a different team served as controls. The subjects had no history of ACL injury and no history of any lower extremity injury during the six months prior to the investigation. The experimental subjects participated in the injury prevention program described by Hewett and colleagues (1996) during their preseason; the program consisted of 2 hr of training three days a week for six weeks. The control subjects also participated in a preseason training program directed by their coaches for a six-week period; however, the structure of this program did not resemble that of the six-week injury prevention program described by Hewett and colleagues (1996).

Wilkerson and colleagues (2004) measured agility, strength, and lunge distance one week before the start of the six-week training program for both groups and then again at the conclusion of the training program. Agility was quantified using an infrared motion analysis system that tracked the position of the body core during performance of a T-pattern agility drill. Each subject performed three sets of the T-pattern agility drill; the first test was a practice test. Subjects wore an infrared signal transmitter, placed on a belt near their umbilicus, and were instructed to move either forward, backward, lateral right, or lateral left. These movements were guided by the appearance of targets within a virtual environment display that disappeared when the body core had been moved the proper direction and distance. To ascertain the influence of training on agility, the following variables were examined: (1) agility test duration (sec), (2) agility test average speed (m/sec), (3) agility test power (W/kg), and (4) agility test average body core vertical position (cm). In addition to agility testing, isokinetic strength testing of the hamstrings and quadriceps was conducted using a Biodex System (Biodex Medical Systems, Inc., Shirley, NY). Finally, to quantify lunge distance, subjects were instructed to lunge forward on a designated leg as far as possible and return to the starting position as fast as possible. Following training, the experimental group exhibited significantly increased hamstring strength, but neither the experimental nor the control group exhibited significant improvements in any of the other performance measures. However, the control group may not be appropriate since this group was also undergoing training. This is a potential limitation of the study.

Performance Measures: Vertical Jump Height, Single-Leg Hop, Speed, and Strength

Outcome: improved vertical jump height, single-leg hop, speed, and strength. Myer and associates (2005b) investigated whether female athletes undergoing a comprehensive neuromuscular training program designed for injury prevention could gain simultaneous performance enhancement of vertical jump height, single-leg hop distance, speed, and strength. The investigators designed an injury prevention training program based on injury prevention techniques described in the literature. The program consisted of 90 min of training, three days a week for six weeks, and included plyometrics and movement training, core strengthening, balance training, and interval speed training. While the effectiveness of this specific training program in reducing the incidence of ACL injury is unknown, the groundwork for the program was provided by an injury prevention training program that has been shown to effectively decrease ACL injury (Hewett et al. 1999). Subjects were 53 female high school athletes from various sports including basketball, soccer, and volleyball. The authors did not report whether or not the subjects had a history of ACL injury or lower extremity injury. Forty-one subjects were assigned to a training group, and 12 subjects were assigned to an untrained control group.

The first performance testing session was conducted for the control and experimental subjects one week before the initiation of training for the experimental subjects. Posttraining performance testing was conducted approximately seven weeks after their initial performance testing session. Performance testing included tests of vertical jump height, single-leg hop distance, speed, and strength. Vertical jump height was measured during a task in which the subject performed a countermovement vertical jump off both feet and grabbed a ball that was suspended overhead. Single-leg hop distance was measured as the subject stood on one leg and hopped forward as far as possible, landing on the same leg. Speed was measured as subjects sprinted a distance of 9.1 m (9.6 yd). Finally, strength was measured as the subject performed squat and bench press exercises. The strength tests were accepted if the number of repetitions completed for the exercise was eight or less. The investigators used a strength testing protocol that allowed them to predict the 1-repetition maximum (1RM) for the squat and the bench press. Following training, the experimental group demonstrated significant improvements in all of the performance tests, while the control group exhibited no significant performance changes over the six-week interval. In particular, the experimental group exhibited the following: increased vertical jump height from 39.9 to 43.2 cm (15.7 to 17 in.); increased speed from 1.80 to 1.73 sec; increased right and left single-leg hop distance by 10.4 and 8.5 cm (4.1 and 3.3 in.); increased 1RM squat by 92%; and increased bench press by 20%.

Performance Measure: Single-Limb Stability

Outcome: improved single-limb stability. Paterno and colleagues (2004) examined how a neuromuscular training program designed for injury prevention influences single-limb stability. The training program was a synthesis of exercises developed from injury prevention techniques and included balance training, hip-pelvis-trunk strengthening, plyometrics, dynamic movement training, and resistance training. Forty-one female athletes from various sports (basketball, soccer, volleyball) participated in the study, which required 90 min of training three days a week for six weeks. This study did not include a control group, and the subjects' injury histories were not reported. Prior to and immediately following the six-week training program, single-limb stability was measured using a Biodex Stability System (Biodex Medical Systems, Inc., Shirley, NY). This device allowed for the assessment of total single-limb postural stability, anterior-posterior stability, and medial-lateral stability. Following training, subjects exhibited significantly improved single-limb total stability and anterior-posterior stability; however, there were no changes in medial-lateral stability.

Performance Measures: Balance, Strength, Single-Leg Hop, Triple Jump, and Stair Hop

Outcome: improved balance. Holm and colleagues (2004) examined how an ACL injury prevention training program influences balance. They used an established training program that has been shown, over two competitive seasons, to decrease the incidence of ACL injury among elite female handball players (Myer et al. 2005b). The subjects were 35 female elite handball players from two teams. Injury histories for the subjects were reported: 19 had a history of ankle instability; four had had an ACL rupture; three had had a meniscal tear; and two had had an unknown knee injury. Six of the nine players with a history of knee injury had undergone surgery. The two teams were instructed to initially use the injury prevention training program three times a week for five to seven weeks and then once a week during the rest of their season. The focus of the training program was to improve awareness and knee control during standing, cutting, jumping, and landing. Each training session was approximately 15 min in duration and consisted of the following three types of exercise: (1) floor, (2) wobble board, and (3) balance mat exercises. Each exercise consisted of a five-step progression from easy to difficult.

Balance testing took place prior to the training (test 1) and then eight weeks (test 2) and 12 months (test 3) after the beginning of training. Balance was tested using a KAT 2000 (OEM Medical, Carlsbad, CA) balance platform device. For each testing session, subjects completed a one-leg static balance test and a two-leg dynamic balance test based on a balance protocol (Hansen et al. 2000). In addition to balance testing, functional performance tasks were examined that included a one-leg hop test and the triple jump test, in which maximal distances of the hop and jump were measured. Furthermore, performance on a stair hop test was measured as the time it took subjects to hop up 22 steps on one leg, turn around, and hop down the same 22 steps. Finally, strength of the quadriceps and hamstrings was tested using a Cybex 6000 (Cybex-Lumex, Ronkonkoma, NY). Following training, subjects showed a significant improvement in dynamic balance between test 1 and test 2 and maintained dynamic balance at one year posttraining (test 3); however, there was no change in static balance. Moreover, there were no significant improvements in the rest of the performance measures.

Summary

The results of the limited number of studies on this topic support the concept that ACL injury prevention programs may improve performance, or the basic elements of sport performance, or both; however, findings are inconsistent and not universal. All of the reviewed studies showed performance improvements. However, inconsistencies between studies are likely related to moderate sample sizes and the utilization of various training protocols that differed in focus, duration, and intensity.

With respect to sport-specific performance measures, only vertical jumping and single-limb hopping have been evaluated. More emphasis has been placed on evaluating the basic components of sport performance (e.g., balance, strength, agility). As various forms of training (not related to ACL injury prevention) have been shown to improve the basic components of sport performance, it stands to reason that ACL injury prevention programs should be able to accomplish the same results given an adequate stimulus for a particular outcome of interest. Future research should be challenged not only to evaluate the injury prevention aspects of training, but also to incorporate measures of sport performance. Such information would likely be helpful in promoting such programs to athletes, coaches, and the athletic community at large.

Chapter 8

Congruence Between Existing Prevention Programs and Research on Risk Factors and Mechanisms of Noncontact ACL Injury

William E. Garrett Jr., MD, PhD
Bing Yu, PhD

ACL-Loading Mechanisms and Risk Factors for Noncontact ACL Injury

Mechanically, ACL injury occurs when excessive loading is applied on the ACL. A noncontact ACL injury occurs when the person him- or herself generates great forces or moments at the knee that apply excessive loading on the ACL. To understand the mechanisms of noncontact ACL injuries and risk factors for sustaining noncontact ACL injuries, we have to understand the mechanisms of ACL loading during active human movements. Berns and colleagues (1992) investigated the effects of a variety of types of knee loadings on ACL strain in 13 cadaver knees. The strain of the anterior medial bundle of the ACL was recorded using liquid mercury strain gauges at 0° and 30° knee flexion. The results showed that anterior shear force on the proximal end of the tibia was the primary determinant of the strain in the anterior medial bundle of the ACL, while neither pure knee internal-external rotation moment nor pure knee valgus-varus moment had significant effects on the strain in the anterior medial bundle of the ACL. The results further showed that anterior shear force at the proximal end of the tibia combined with a knee valgus moment resulted in a significantly greater strain in the anterior medial bundle of the ACL than did anterior shear force at the proximal end of the tibia alone.

Markolf and colleagues (1995) also investigated effects of various forces on ACL loading of cadaver knees, namely, anterior shear force on the tibia and knee valgus, varus, internal rotation, and external rotation moments due to external forces on the tibia. A 100 N anterior shear force and 10 Nm knee valgus, varus, internal rotation, and external rotation moments were added to cadaver knees. The ACL loading was recorded as the knee was extended from 90° of flexion to 5° hyperextension. The results showed that an anterior shear force on the tibia generated significant ACL loading, while the knee valgus, varus, and internal rotation moments also generated significant ACL loading only when the ACL was loaded by the anterior shear force on the tibia. The results further showed that the ACL loading due to the anterior shear force combined with either knee valgus or varus moment was greater than that due to the anterior shear force alone, while ACL loading due to the anterior shear force combined with knee external rotation moment was lower than that due to anterior shear force alone. In addition, the results demonstrated that ACL loading due to combined knee varus and internal rotation moment loading was greater than that due to either knee varus moment loading or internal rotation moment loading alone; ACL loading due to combined knee valgus and external rotation moment loading was lower than that due to either knee valgus or external rotation moment loading alone. Finally, ACL loading due to the anterior shear force and knee valgus, varus, and internal rotation moments increased as the knee flexion angle decreased.

Fleming and colleagues (2001) studied the effects of weight bearing and tibia external loading on ACL strain. They implanted a differential variable reluctance transducer (DVRT) to the anterior medial bundle of the ACL of 11 subjects. Anterior cruciate ligament strains were measured in vivo when a subject's leg was attached to a knee-loading fixture that allowed independent application of anterior-posterior shear force, valgus-varus moments, and internal-external rotation moments to the tibia as well as simulation of the weight-bearing condition. The anterior shear force was applied on the proximal end of the tibia from 0 N to 130 N in 10 N increments. The valgus-varus moments were applied to the knee from –10 Nm to 10 Nm in 1 Nm increments. The internal-external rotation moments were applied to the knee from –9 Nm to 9 Nm in 1 Nm increments. The knee flexion angle was fixed at 20° during the test. The results showed that ACL strain significantly increased as the anterior shear force on the proximal end of the tibia and the knee internal rotation moment increased, while knee valgus-varus and external rotation moments had little effect on ACL strain under the weight-bearing condition.

Although quantitatively inconsistent in terms of the effects of knee valgus-varus and internal-external rotation moments on ACL loading, the three studies just discussed consistently showed that anterior shear force at the proximal end of the tibia is a major contributor to ACL loading while knee valgus, varus, and internal rotation moments may increase ACL loading when an anterior shear force at the proximal end of the tibia is applied. Accordingly, these ACL-loading mechanisms, a small knee flexion angle, and a great posterior ground reaction force may be major motor control-related risk factors for sustaining noncontact ACL injuries.

Quadriceps muscles are the major contributor to the anterior shear force at the proximal end of the tibia through the patella tendon. DeMorat and colleagues (2004) showed that a 4500 N quadriceps muscle force could create ACL injuries at 20° knee flexion. Eleven cadaver knee specimens were fixed to a knee simulator and loaded with 4500 N quadriceps muscle force. Quadriceps muscle contraction tests at 400 N (Q-400 tests) and KT-1000 tests were performed before and after the 4500 N quadriceps muscle force loading. Tibia anterior translations were recorded during the Q-400 and KT-1000 tests. All cadaver knee specimens were dissected after all tests to determine the ACL injury states. Six of the 11 specimens had confirmed ACL injuries (three complete ACL tears and three partial tears).

Decreasing knee flexion angle increases the anterior shear force at the proximal end of the tibia by increasing the patella tendon-tibia shaft angle (figure 8.1). With a given quadriceps muscle force, the anterior shear force at the proximal end of the tibia is determined by the patella tendon-tibia shaft angle defined as the angle between the patella tendon and the longitudinal axis of the tibia (Nunley et al. 2003). The greater the patella tendon-tibia shaft angle, the greater the anterior shear force on the tibia. Nunley and colleagues studied the relationship between the patella tendon-tibia shaft angle and knee flexion angle with weight bearing. Ten male and 10 female college students without known history of lower extremity injuries were recruited as the subjects. Sagittal plane X-ray films were taken for each subject at 0°, 15°, 30°, 45°, 60°, 75°, and 90° knee flexions bearing 50% of body weight. Patella tendon-tibia shaft angles were measured from the X-ray films. Regression analyses were performed to determine the relationship between patella tendon-tibia shaft angle and knee flexion angle and to compare the relationship between genders. The results showed that the patella tendon-tibia shaft angle was a function of knee flexion angle, with increased

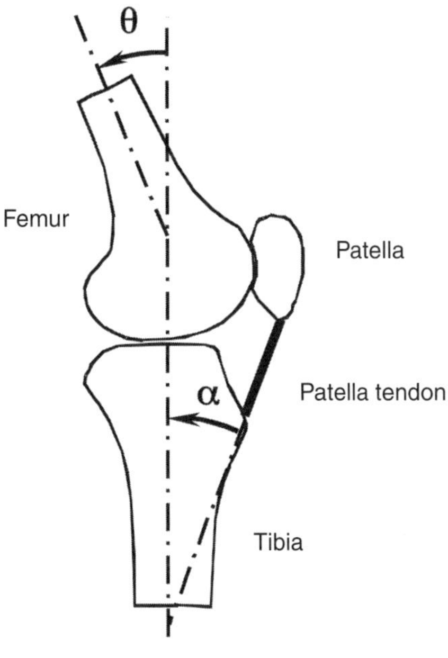

FIGURE 8.1 Definition of patella tendon-tibia shaft angle (α) and knee flexion angle (θ).

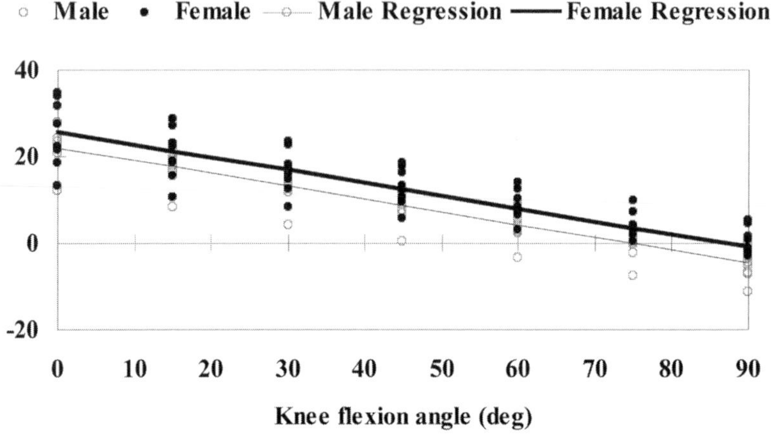

FIGURE 8.2 The effect of knee flexion angle on patella tendon-tibia shaft angle.

patella tendon-tibia shaft angle as knee flexion angle decreased, and also that, on average, the females' patella tendon-tibia shaft angle was 4° smaller than the males' (figure 8.2). The relationship between the patella tendon-tibia shaft angle and knee flexion angle obtained by Nunley and colleagues was consistent with findings from other studies on the patella tendon-tibia shaft angle under nonweight-bearing conditions (Smidt 1973; Buff, Jones, and Hungerford 1988; van Eijden et al. 1985).

Decreasing knee flexion angle also increases ACL loading by increasing ACL elevation angle and deviation angle, defined, respectively, as the angle between the longitudinal axis of the ACL and the tibia plateau and the angle between the projection of the longitudinal axis of the ACL on the tibia plateau and the posterior direction of the tibia (Li et al. 2005) (figure 8.3). The resultant force along the longitudinal axis of the ACL equals the anterior shear force on the ACL divided by the cosines of the ACL elevation and deviation angles. The greater the ACL elevation and deviation angles, the greater the ACL loading with a given anterior shear force on the ACL. Li and associates (2005) determined the in vivo ACL elevation and deviation angles as a function of knee flexion angle with weight bearing. Five young, healthy volunteers were recruited as the subjects. The ACL elevation and deviation angles at 0°, 30°, 60°, and 90° knee flexions with weight bearing were obtained using individualized dual-orthogonal fluoroscopic images and magnetic resonance image-based three-dimensional models. The results of this study showed that both ACL elevation and deviation angles increased as the knee flexion angle decreased.

The literature shows that ACL loading increases as knee flexion angle decreases. Arms and colleagues (1984) studied the biomechanics of ACL rehabilitation and reconstruction and found that quadriceps muscle contraction significantly strained the ACL from 0° to 45° knee flexion, but did not strain the ACL when knee flexion was greater than 60°. Beynnon and colleagues (1995) measured the in vivo ACL strain during rehabilitation exercises and found that isometric quadriceps muscle contraction at 15° and 30° knee flexions produced a significant increase in ACL strain, while at 60° and 90° knee flexion there was no change in ACL strain relative to that in the relaxed muscle condition. Li and colleagues (1999, 2004) investigated quadriceps and hamstring muscle loading on ACL loading and showed that the in situ ACL loading increased as knee flexion angle decreased when only quadriceps muscles were loaded and when both quadriceps and hamstring muscles were loaded. Akihiro and colleagues (2000) analyzed the forces in the ACL of cadaver knees in a simulated pivot shift test and also reported an increasing trend of in situ ACL loading with decreased knee flexion angle.

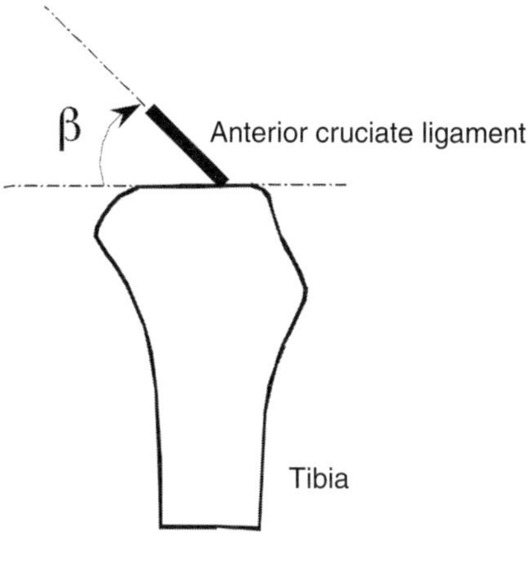

FIGURE 8.3 Definition of ACL elevation angle (β).

The literature also shows that individuals at high risk of sustaining noncontact ACL injuries have a smaller knee flexion angle during athletic tasks than individuals at low risk do. Epidemiological studies indicate that female athletes are at higher risk of sustaining noncontact ACL injuries than their male counterparts (Ferretti et al. 1992; Paulos 1992; Malone et al. 1993; Pearl 1993; Ireland 1999; Lindenfeld et al. 1994; Woodford-Rogers et al. 1994; Arendt and Dick 1995). Recent biomechanical studies demonstrated that female recreational athletes exhibited small knee flexion angles in running, jumping, and cutting tasks (Malinzak et al. 2001; Chappell et al. 2002). The literature also shows that female adolescent athletes have a sharply increased ACL injury rate after 13 years of age (Yu et al. 2002; Shea et al. 2004). In a recent biomechanical study, female adolescent soccer players began decreasing their knee flexion angle during a stop-jump task after 13 years of age (Yu et al. 2005). These results, taken together, suggest that a small knee flexion angle during landing tasks may be a risk factor for sustaining noncontact ACL injuries.

During athletic tasks, great posterior ground reaction forces due to hard landing may also be a risk factor for sustaining noncontact ACL injuries. A posterior ground reaction force creates a flexion moment relative to the knee, which needs to be balanced by a knee extension moment generated by the quadriceps muscles (Yu et al. 2006b). As previously described, quadriceps muscle contraction force adds an anterior shear force on the proximal end of the tibia through the patella tendon. The greater the posterior ground reaction force, the greater the quadriceps muscle force and the greater the ACL loading (Yu et al. 2006b). Lamontagne and colleagues (2005) recently recorded in vivo ACL strain in a hop-landing task. A DVRT was implemented to the middle portion of the anterior medial bundle of the ACLs of three subjects through surgical procedures. Subjects then performed the hop-landing task in a biomechanics laboratory. Force plate and electromyography data and in vivo ACL strain were recorded simultaneously. The results showed that the peak ACL strain occurred at the impact peak vertical ground reaction force shortly after initial contact between foot and ground. Yu and colleagues (2006b) demonstrated that peak impact vertical and posterior ground reaction forces occurred essentially at the same time. These results, taken together, suggest that a hard landing with a great posterior ground reaction force may be a risk factor for sustaining noncontact ACL injuries.

The literature also demonstrates that individuals at high risk of sustaining noncontact ACL injuries have greater posterior ground reaction forces. Chappell and colleagues (2002) studied the lower extremity kinetics as well as the kinematics of college-age recreational athletes during landings of stop-jump tasks. The results showed that female recreational athletes had greater peak resultant proximal tibia anterior shear force and knee joint resultant extension moment during landings of stop-jump tasks than did male recreational athletes. Yu and colleagues (2006b) showed that the resultant proximal tibia anterior shear force was positively correlated to posterior ground reaction force. In another investigation, Yu and colleagues (2005) studied the immediate effects of a newly designed knee brace with a constraint to knee extension during a stop-jump task. Their results showed that college-age female recreational athletes had greater posterior ground reaction force during the landing of the stop-jump task than did their male counterparts.

Although biomechanical studies have demonstrated that knee valgus moment is not a major mechanism of ACL loading, a recent epidemiological study by Hewett and colleagues (2005a) indicated that external knee valgus moment in a vertical drop-landing jump task was a predictor of ACL injuries. A total of 205 high school soccer, basketball, and volleyball players were followed for three competition seasons. Knee flexion and valgus angles at initial foot contact with the ground, as well as the maximum knee flexion and valgus angles and maximum moments during the stance phase of the vertical drop-landing jump task, were recorded prospectively for every subject. A total of nine subjects sustained ACL injuries after three competition seasons. The results of this study showed that knee abduction angle at landing was 8° greater in ACL-injured than in uninjured athletes, and that ACL-injured athletes had a 2.5 times greater peak external knee valgus moment and 20% higher peak vertical ground reaction force than did uninjured athletes. The findings further demonstrated that peak external knee valgus moment predicted ACL injury status with 73% specificity and 78% sensitivity. These results appear to indicate that knee valgus angle and moment are risk factors for sustaining ACL injuries.

Current Training Programs

Clinical studies on the noncontact ACL injury mechanism generally agree that the injury occurs during a landing from a jump or during deceleration to stop quickly or to change direction or pivot. Often there appears to be an awkward movement or an unanticipated need to alter movement (Boden et al. 2000; Olsen et al. 2004). In addition, there is often an element of apparent valgus in the coronal plane. The apparent valgus is a combination of hip adduction and internal rotation, knee flexion, and tibial external rotation. This valgus as seen in motion analysis studies may not be a true valgus force at the knee. In motion analysis studies, an apparent valgus can be created by knee flexion and hip internal rotation. Most noncontact ACL injuries do not include a medial collateral ligament injury by physical exam or magnetic resonance imaging evaluation. The dynamic valgus may include a valgus moment, which may increase strain on the ACL, and external rotation, which decreases strain on the ACL as pointed out earlier. Although we do not know how the dynamic valgus adds to the ACL injury, there certainly appears to be an association between this position and noncontact ACL injury. A recent study using a human cadaveric model suggested that the majority of the ACL load came from the quadriceps but that a valgus force did add to the ACL strain.

Clearly the kinetic factors are variables largely controlled by the central nervous system (CNS). According to current concepts of motor control, the CNS has an imprinted pattern of controlling muscle forces and their interaction with inertial, gravitational, and other forces acting on the body. The CNS contains stored patterns that control motion. These patterns are learned and with time and repetition can become relatively automatic, needing little extra input from the CNS. For example, walking and running require little extra thought. Motor learning applies to other more complex patterns such as throwing, kicking, and gymnastics.

The concept of any injury prevention program involves muscle and cardiovascular conditioning and technique training to provide motor control strategies that optimize performance and motor patterns that decrease the risk of injury. Proper coaching techniques seem to emphasize performance and often do not emphasize injury prevention. This is especially true in the younger age groups. The adolescent age group is often learning sport skills at a time when body size and muscle development are rapidly changing. This is the age group in which ACL injury is most likely. Training programs might well attend to both motor (i.e., muscle and cardiovascular systems) and motor control (the learned patterns of controlling motion).

Hewett and colleagues (2006) recently published a meta-analysis of existing neuromuscular injury prevention programs. The successful programs had several elements in common. First, the successful programs incorporated high-intensity plyometric training. Plyometric training involves landing from jumps and using the muscles controlling hip, knee, and ankle motion to absorb energy by means of eccentric contractions. Anterior cruciate ligament injury involves deceleration of the body from downward and forward motions.

Second, plyometric training should be accompanied by instruction and feedback that stress proper technique. The landings should be "soft." Soft landings are those in which the knee is flexing at the time of impact and emphasize a flexed knee position at contact and increasing total flexion. Biomechanical studies stress that the anterior tibial shear force that strains the ACL is diminished with increasing initial and total knee flexion.

Motor learning theories emphasize feedback and knowledge of results to improve technique. Onate and colleagues (2005) have stressed that feedback derived from an expert reviewer and from video-based self-examination are additive in their ability to alter favorably the biomechanics of landing. In addition, a second test at a later time confirmed that the subjects retained the technical improvement.

The third common element in the successful programs described in the meta-analysis by Hewett and colleagues (2006) is attention to balance training and core stability training. The studies by Hewett and colleagues (1996), Myklebust and colleagues (2003), and Mandelbaum and colleagues (2005) emphasized combinations of single-leg balance and single-leg landings. Myklebust and colleagues' (2003) program also used some perturbation from the training partner in team handball players. Studies, however, have shown that training programs with balance exercises alone are not effective (Soderman et al. 2000), especially for female athletes (Caraffa et al. 1996).

Strength training was used in the studies by Hewett and colleagues (1996) and Mandelbaum and colleagues (2005). The study by Myklebust's group (2003) did not have a separate element of strengthening, although the plyometric exercises themselves can lead to a strength increase.

Myer and colleagues (2004b) described a variety of exercises for modifying some commonly seen lower extremity motion patterns that are associated with risk, such as ligament dominance in landing and leg dominance and quadriceps dominance in strength. Ligament dominance in landing is defined as landing with small knee flexion angle, significant medial knee motion related to femoral adduction and internal rotation, tibial external rotation, and great impact ground reaction forces. To correct ligament dominance in landing, athletes should be shown proper athletic position with knees comfortably flexed, shoulder back, feet approximately shoulder-width apart, chest over the knees, and knees and body mass balanced over the balls of the feet. The wall jump, tuck jump, broad jump, 180° jump, and single-leg hop and hold can be used as dynamic exercises to correct ligament dominance in landing. The rationale for including these exercises in training programs for reducing risk of sustaining noncontact ACL injuries is well supported by the previously described biomechanical studies on the mechanisms of ACL injuries.

Quadriceps dominance in strength is defined as a hamstring-to-quadriceps strength ratio less than 55% (Myer et al. 2004b). Quadriceps dominance in strength can be corrected with squat jump and broad jump and hold exercises. These exercises require athletes to get into deep knee flexion angles to decrease the ability of the quadriceps to load the ACL, increase the ability of the hamstrings to unload the ACL, and improve hamstring cocontraction. Myer and colleagues (2004b), however, pointed out that the ability of the hamstring muscles to protect the ACL is limited when the knee flexion angle is small, and that the need for the hamstring muscles to protect the ACL is minimal when the knee is in deep flexion. They also noted that the squat jump and broad jump and hold exercises may cause frontal knee pain and should be used cautiously.

Leg dominance in strength is defined as a 20% difference in strength between legs (Myer et al. 2004b). Leg dominance in strength can be corrected with the tuck jump; bounding jump; and jump, jump, jump, vertical jump exercises. A single-leg balance exercise on an unstable surface may also be useful for correcting leg dominance in strength. The weaker or less coordinated leg should be emphasized during these exercises.

To be effective, prevention training must be performed often enough to achieve desired training effects on strength, neuromuscular control, and technique. The exact protocol has varied from preseason programs to in-season programs to a combination of both. A minimum frequency and duration has been identified as more than once a week for at least six weeks (Myklebust et al. 2003).

One would also think that compliance would be necessary in order for the program to be effective. Methods of assessing compliance in prevention studies have often not been rigorous. Myklebust and colleagues (2003) had the most well-developed compliance testing and demonstrated less than 30% compliance. These intervention studies have many methodological problems. Although they have shown that the programs have the potential to prevent injury, the number of participants and the number of injuries are too low for a really good epidemiological study. Better methods of monitoring compliance and exposure data are needed, and not all studies underwent proper randomization.

Future Training Program Development

Current training programs are empirical derivations from ACL injury prevention research. Additional research is needed to provide scientific support for the effectiveness of current training programs. Careful observations of conditions of ACL injury supplemented by actual motion analysis of the injuries (Olsen et al. 2004) will provide important information for understanding the injury mechanisms and the effectiveness of current training programs. In addition, prospective control cohort studies with large sample sizes are needed to gather preinjury physiological and biomechanical parameters and injury characteristics of at-risk populations to determine physiological and biomechanical predictors of ACL injuries. The results of this kind of study will form the basis for the development of specific prevention programs.

A logical way to construct a validated program would then be to test the prevention program in order to determine if the biomechanics are actually altered after an appropriate period of training. Biomechanical studies can then document retention of the alterations. Then the program should be applied to a large population. It is highly likely that prevention programs should be sport specific and even age specific. Certainly the existing programs have been designed to be specific for soccer, team handball, basketball, and volleyball. Programs have also been designed for female athletes. Although the risk of injury is clearly higher for females, the absolute number of injuries is much higher in males because of larger exposure numbers of males in sports, especially American football. There seems to be little reason to expect that any single current program is likely to prove optimal in the future.

As athletic trainers and coaches begin to think about a specific program, they should consider several very practical suggestions. Specific maneuvers that place athletes at risk for injuries should be targeted. For the most part, this means a motion that is decelerating the body in vertical and horizontal directions simultaneously. These are generally stopping, cutting, or pivoting motions, or landing from a jump with a horizontal element in addition to the straight vertical. The training program should be high intensity. It seems that the intensity should be carefully vamped up to the desired level. The landings or cutting maneuvers may be quite different for soccer, team handball, and basketball, for example.

Next it would seem important to identify techniques that can prevent injury while enhancing or at least not diminishing performance. From data presented earlier, it is clear that a flexed knee position at initial impact and active flexion should be emphasized. Hip adduction and internal rotation should be avoided. The training program should employ instruction and active feedback from a knowledgeable instructor.

Specific strength training of certain muscle groups and the core muscles will likely be beneficial and can be part of the preventive program and of normal sport-specific training. Balance training would seem to be a good component. Strength, endurance, and balance in themselves may be important because of their effects on knee flexion. For instance, muscular fatigue leads to landing with straighter knees and a resulting increase in anterior tibial shear force (Chappell et al. 2005). Muscle strength relative to body size may be an important factor that affects lower extremity motion patterns in the sagittal plane. Decreased relative strength results in decreased knee flexion angle in a stop-jump task.

If we consider a prevention program to be largely a motor control or technique issue, repetition and practice of proper technique are essential. Ideally the program should be short enough and intense enough to be easily incorporated into team practice and training sessions.

Most training programs involve exercises in which the athletes are in controlled and balanced conditions. The program developed by Myklebust's group (2003) does incorporate some perturbations that alter balance. An off-balance or awkward position is frequently seen and talked about by players who sustain an ACL injury. There may be a need for a "bail-out" strategy for an athlete in a recognized at-risk position. For instance, current training program techniques resemble safe driving techniques. The "bail-out" strategy that has not been studied might resemble strategy in driver training for handling an automobile that is out of control or spinning. Of course, devising and teaching such techniques may require new strategies that might involve a certain risk of injuries.

Finally, there are so many biomechanical and neuromuscular considerations that initially defining a prevention program surely required a leap of faith. The teams that organized the prevention programs have certainly obtained promising results and have given athletes, scientists, and the sports medicine personnel evidence that preventing noncontact ACL injuries is possible. Better intervention programs, involvement of more athletes, and better coaching techniques can possibly make an even bigger difference.

Chapter 9

Discussion, Summary, and Future Research Goals

Lars Engebretsen, MD, PhD

At a time when there is an abundance of medical meetings, journals, and papers, some might argue that the last thing we need is a new book focusing on yet another field of research. What would justify such an emphasis on a new and developing research field in medicine (Kahn 1994)? First, it must ask important questions not answered by others. Second, the new research field should have the potential to create truly new knowledge, lead to new ways of thinking, and lay the foundation for improved health for our patients. This is usually not possible without a multidisciplinary approach involving a mixture of basic scientists and clinicians. Third, research results from the new field should be publishable in respected journals, recognized and cited by peers, presentable at high-quality meetings, and fundable on competitive grant review (Kahn 1994).

Let us examine each of these issues to see if there is sufficient merit in ACL injury prevention research. First, is the field of injury prevention important? Epidemiological studies show that of injuries seen by a physician in Scandinavia, every sixth is sustained during sporting activity (Bahr, van Mechelen, and Kannus 2002). Among children, every third hospital-treated injury is the result of sport participation (Bahr, van Mechelen, and Kannus 2002). A research group within the English Football Association found that the overall risk to professional athletes is unacceptably high—approximately 1000 times higher among professional football players than for high-risk industrial occupations (Drawer and Fuller 2002). Some injury types, such as serious knee injuries, are a particular cause of concern. The highest incidence of ACL injuries is seen in 15- to 25-year-old athletes in pivoting sports such as football, basketball and handball; and the incidence is three to five times higher among women than among men (Myklebust et al. 1998). Anterior cruciate ligament injury causes longtime absence from work and sport and dramatically increases the risk of long-term sequelae—like abnormal joint dynamics and early onset of degenerative joint disease (Roos 2005). Although a massive research effort is ongoing to develop better treatment methods, we still lack evidence to suggest that reconstructive surgery of either menisci or cruciate ligaments decreases the rate of posttraumatic osteoarthritis (Myklebust and Bahr 2005). After 10 years, approximately half of the patients display signs of osteoarthritis, and it appears that the majority of patients will have osteoarthrosis after 15 to 20 years (Myklebust and Bahr 2005). Thus, whereas developing improved treatment methods for injuries in general and ACL injuries in particular remains an important goal, it may be even more important to prevent injuries.

In May 2000, a PubMed search revealed that out of 10,691 papers on athletic injury, only six involved randomized controlled trials on sport injury prevention (table 9.1). However, a similar search of the literature now reveals that sport injury prevention research is emerging as a new field in medicine. While the number of papers on athletic injuries has increased by 26% over the last five years, clinical studies and randomized controlled trials related to sport injury prevention have doubled (table 9.1). Gradually, congresses in sports medicine, orthopedics, and traumatology include an increasing number of symposia, lectures, and instructional courses on injury prevention issues. Research quality is also improving. For example, recent issues of the *British Medical Journal* have included two papers related to injury prevention: a case control study (Hagel et al. 2005) among skiers and snowboarders, indicating a 29% reduction in the risk of head injury, and a randomized controlled trial (Olsen et al. 2005) demonstrating a 47% reduction in knee and ankle injuries from a structured program of warm-up exercises in adolescent team handball players. The publication of these studies in a highly respected journal illustrates that sport injury prevention is an important public health issue.

TABLE 9.1 Results of PubMed Searches Performed[a]

Search terms	May 2000	February 2005	Increase (%)
Athletic injury	10,691	13,358	25
Athletic injury and treatment	6,606	8,525	29
• Limit: clinical trials	182	258	41
• Limit: randomized controlled trial	87	130	50
Athletic injury and prevention	2,064	2,745	33
• Limit: clinical trials	29	68	135
• Limit: randomized controlled trial	21	41	95

[a]These searches were performed in May 2000 and February 2005 on sport injury research related to prevention and treatment, respectively. The results are shown as the number of items resulting from the search terms shown.

Sport participation is also important from a public health perspective. There is no longer any doubt that regular physical activity reduces the risk of premature mortality in general and of coronary heart disease, hypertension, colon cancer, obesity, and diabetes mellitus in particular (U.S. Department of Health and Human Services 1996). The question is whether the health benefits of sport participation outweigh the risk of injury and long-term disability, especially in high-level athletes. Sarna and colleagues have studied the incidence of chronic disease and life expectancy of former male world-class athletes from Finland in endurance sports, power sports, and team sports (Sarna et al. 1993). The overall life expectancy was longer in the high-level athletes compared to a reference group (75.6 vs. 69.9 years). The same research group also showed that the rate of hospitalization was lower for endurance sports and power sports compared to the reference group (Kujala et al. 1996). This resulted from a lower rate of hospital care for heart disease, respiratory disease, and cancer. However, the athletes were more likely to have been hospitalized for musculoskeletal disorders. A follow-up study revealed that former team sport athletes had a higher risk of gonarthrosis (Kujala et al. 1995). Swedish studies also document an increased risk of hip and knee arthrosis among former football players (Roos 1998). Thus, the evidence suggests that although sport participation is beneficial, injuries are a significant side effect. To promote physical activity effectively, we have to deal professionally with the health problems of the active patient. This involves not only providing effective care for the injured patient, but also developing and promoting injury prevention measures actively.

As a first step toward injury prevention, the causes must be established. This includes information on why a particular athlete may be at risk in a given situation (i.e., risk factors) or how injuries happen (i.e., injury mechanisms). Murphy, Connolly, and Beynnon (2003) have recently reviewed the literature on the risk factors for lower extremity injuries, demonstrating that our understanding of injury causation is limited. Many risk factors have been implicated; however, there is little agreement with respect to the findings. Partly, this can be attributed to limitations in study design and the statistical methods used to assess the results. Murphy and colleagues conclude that more prospective studies are needed, emphasizing the need for proper design and sufficient sample sizes.

Risk factors are traditionally divided into two main categories: internal (or intrinsic) athlete-related risk factors and external (or extrinsic) environmental risk factors (van Mechelen, Hlobil, and Kemper 1992). However, merely to establish the internal and external risk factors for sport injuries is not enough. To establish a complete understanding of the causes, we must also identify the mechanisms by which they occur. In other words, sport injuries result from a complex interaction of multiple risk factors and events, of which only a fraction have been identified.

Therefore, studies on the etiology of sport injuries require a dynamic model that accounts for the multifactorial nature of sport injuries and in addition considers the sequence of events eventually leading to an injury. One such dynamic model was presented by Meeuwisse and colleagues (2000). This model describes how multiple factors interact to produce injury (figure 9.1).

In studies on the etiology of sport injuries, this model can be used to explore the interrelationships between risk factors and their contribution to the occurrence of injury. Meeuwisse and colleagues (2000) classify the internal risk factors as predisposing factors that act from within and that may be necessary, but are seldom sufficient, to produce injury. In their theoretical model, external risk factors act on the predisposed athlete from outside and are classified as enabling factors in that they facilitate the manifestation of injury. It is the presence of both internal and external risk factors that renders the athlete susceptible to injury, but the mere presence of these risk factors is usually not sufficient to produce injury. The sum of these risk factors and the interaction between them "prepare" the athlete for an injury to occur in a given situation. Meeuwisse and colleagues describe the inciting event as the final link in the chain that causes an injury, and such events are regarded as necessary causes. They also state that such an inciting event is usually directly associated with the onset of injury.

As shown in figure 9.1, Bahr and Holme (2003) argue that it is necessary to expand the traditional approach to describing the inciting event. First, the term

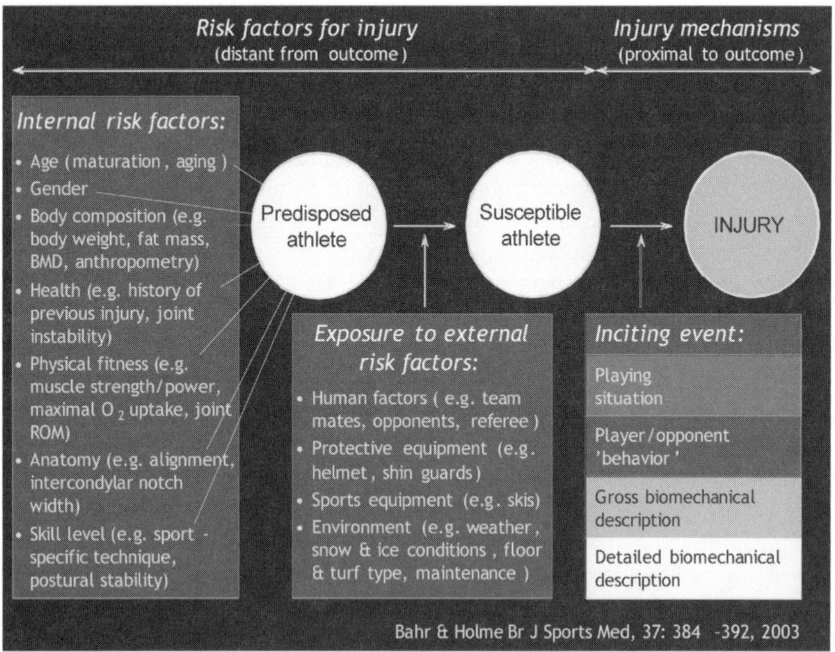

FIGURE 9.1 A dynamic, multifactorial model of sport injury etiology.

From R. Bahr and I. Holmes, 2003, "Risk factors for sports injuries—a methodological approach," *Br J Sports Med* 37: 384-392. Adapted and reproduced with permission of BMJ Publishing Group; adapted from W.H. Meeuwisse, 1994, "Assessing causation in sport injury: A multifactorial model, *Clin J Sport Med* 4: 166-170.

injury mechanism is often used to describe the inciting event in biomechanical terms only. For example, an ankle sprain could be described as resulting from an inversion injury, or an ACL injury could be described as resulting from valgus trauma to the knee. However, to be complete, the description of the injury mechanism needs to account for all of the events leading to the situation in which the injury took place (Andersen et al. 2003). Examples include the playing situation (e.g., a two-man block in volleyball), the position in the field of play (e.g., in the score box in soccer), the interaction with other players (e.g., being tackled from the side in American football), and the skill performed by the injured player (e.g., a jump shot by a team handball player). Describing an ACL injury as a noncontact or contact injury does provide meaningful information, but leaves us far from having a complete understanding of the inciting event. If patterns can be established in the events leading to an injury situation, this information can potentially be more important for preventing injuries than an exact biomechanical description of joint motion at the point of injury. Second, the inciting event can—especially for overuse injuries—sometimes be distant from the outcome. For example, for a stress fracture in a long distance runner, the inciting event is not usually the single training session when pain became evident, but the training and competition program he or she followed over the previous weeks or months.

Three main study designs are available to investigate risk factors for sport injuries: case control studies, cohort studies, and intervention studies (preferably done as a randomized controlled trial). Although the gold standard for study design is the randomized controlled trial, none of the 12 studies currently presented or published are true randomized controlled trials. This is symptomatic for this field of research, and the large majority of studies are designed as cohort studies.

In a case control study design, the approach is to compare the frequency or level of potential risk factors between a group of injured athletes and a group of injury-free athletes. Often, information on risk factors is collected retrospectively, because the approach is to identify persons with the injury of interest and then look backward in time to identify factors that may have caused it. For ACL injuries, this could mean comparing a group of patients with an ACL injury with or without surgery to a group of healthy athletes from the same sport. Three important assumptions must be met to use this approach. First, the cases that are selected must be representative for all patients with the injury in question. Second, the controls must be representative of the population of injury-free athletes. Third, the information on potential risk factors must be collected with adequate accuracy, and in the same way from cases and controls. In a study on risk factors for ACL tears, Lund-Hansen and colleagues compared injured and healthy athletes by measuring their KT-1000 (Lund-Hanssen et al. 1996). The results showed that the injured athletes had a lower strength ratio, while there was no difference in range of motion. This study illustrates another important limitation of the case control approach, that is, the inability to distinguish between risk factors and injury sequelae. Although all the subjects were tested after they had returned to full performance after their injury, it is not possible to know what the strength of the injured athletes was prior to injury. In other words, reduced strength could be a risk factor or simply a result of the injury.

In the true cohort study, all data are collected in a standardized manner prospectively in time. The approach involves measuring potential risk factors before injuries occur, after which new cases and exposure are reported during a period of follow-up. Prospective cohort studies can provide direct and accurate estimates of incidence and relative risk. The main disadvantage of the cohort study design is that study size is critical. It may be necessary to include and monitor a large number of athletes for an exceedingly long study period, particularly for less common injury types. A typical example is the Norwegian team handball study. It was not possible to plan this investigation as a randomized study since the power calculations showed that one would have needed approximately 2000 players to detect a 50% reduction in ACL injuries. Even using a pre- and postintervention comparison, one needed to include almost every team in the three upper divisions in Norway to achieve adequate statistical power. Teams in the fourth division, the only other group available for inclusion, do not practice sufficiently and play too few matches to have been used as study subjects (Mykelbust et al. 2003).

A cohort study to assess risk factors for ACL injury would involve examining a group of currently healthy athletes at baseline to test variables related to the ACL: anterior-posterior laxity, range of motion, strength deficits, landing dynamics, and so on. This cohort would then be followed prospectively to record injuries during a defined period of time, typically one or two seasons. At the end of the study, injured and noninjured athletes could be compared to examine whether there were any differences in the chosen variables.

As emphasized in the Meeuwisse model (Meeuwisse et al. 2000), the preferred approach is to use a multivariate model, to control for interactions and confounding factors. Such an approach can be used to distinguish between the effect of previous injury per se and the effect that previous injury may have through reduced strength, for example. Meeuwisse has reviewed the concepts of interaction (when two factors work together to produce a risk that is greater or less than expected) and confounding (when an association between two variables of interest could be due to the effects of a third variable) in assessment of risk factors for athletic injury, and how to distinguish between them.

The study design that can be used to examine the effect of a particular risk factor on sport injury is the intervention study. Randomized large-scale clinical trials provide the strongest evidence for both the causal nature of a modifiable risk factor and the effectiveness of modifying that factor in preventing injury outcomes (Myklebust et al. 2003). This approach involves determining if a particular intervention designed to eliminate or at least reduce a risk factor also results in a reduced risk of injury. For example, to test the association between hamstring strength and injury risk, one could select a cohort of athletes at risk and randomly assign half of them to a program of strength training for the hamstrings. The relationship between strength as a risk factor and injury risk is established if strength training improves strength and can be shown to lead to fewer injuries in the intervention group. To date, no randomized controlled study has been conducted to test the effect of potential risk factors on noncontact ACL injuries. However, as seen in chapter 5, several cohort intervention studies have been carried out with good effect. Although these are not randomized trials, they indicate that modifying strength as a potential risk factor through specific strength training may have a protective effect.

Although randomized controlled trials can provide the strongest evidence to evaluate cause-and-effect relationships, they are limited to risk factors that can be modified (e.g., through special training programs or use of protective equipment), and they are usually used to assess the effect of only one factor at a time. One can include additional factors by using more groups if the factors can be assumed to be additive on injury risk. For instance, a study could have one control group, one strength training group, one technique training group, and one group doing technique and strength training to test the effects of strength and landing techniques on ACL injuries, a 2 × 2 factorial design. The weakness of many of the current studies is that they include many possible risk factors that are not controlled. Additionally, not all risk factors are known or, if known, are difficult to eliminate or control.

Deciding when to initiate a clinical trial can also be controversial. Such trials should not be undertaken until there is a substantial body of knowledge suggesting that intervention may be effective, but not so late that conducting them would be considered unethical. Finally, it is arguably unethical to undertake a clinical trial simply to prove harm. Therefore, the first step to establish the relationship between potential risk factors and sport injuries will in most cases be to conduct a prospective cohort study.

The nature of interventions varies among the studies. Analysis of the two main forms, that is, interventions based on cognitive and psychomotor approaches, shows that both may work in some but not all settings. The best examples are probably the Vermont study on prevention of ACL injuries in ski instructors (Ettlinger, Johnson, and Shealy 1995), in which a video teaching program on fall techniques was very successful, and the study in Icelandic soccer, in which the exact same technique did not seem to work (Arnason et al. 2004). So far, the psychomotor approaches all seem to work. Only one study showed a lack of effect, probably due to lack of sufficient study size.

One unresolved issue so far is why the psychomotor interventions seem to have a major impact on injury incidence. Hewett and collegues have shown how the landing technique can be changed, but so far not whether these changes lead to a reduction of injuries (Hewett et al., 1996; Myer et al. 2005b). Improvements can be seen in many such variables—we just do not have the data to know at this stage which is the most important variable to influence.

The duration of the interventions has generally been one preseason, occasionally one full season, and in one study two full seasons. In the Norwegian study, two full seasons were necessary for statistical reasons, but this puts the research organization under much stress. Not all the studies have involved power calculations on the number of participants necessary, leading to difficulties in data interpretation. The duration of the follow-up will obviously be dictated by the power analysis.

The follow-up itself is of crucial importance, as seen from studies in which compliance is calculated. Compliance can be very low in these studies, due to many factors such as limited training facilities and time and limited interest on the part of the coach. The Norwegian team handball and youth studies have shown how important it is to know the athletes' training history, participation, and prevention exercise compliance. The authors of many studies just do not know the compliance. If compliance is low, the intervention calculations cannot be done with a sufficient amount of security. Consequently, the principal investigator in these studies must have a crew of assistants following the individuals and the teams with frequent contact points. It is crucial that compliance data be reported when the results of an intervention are presented.

Do we need prevention programs in the future? Year by year, we seem to have more information about risk factors and their relative roles. If the relative additional risk of having specific risk factors is known, some individuals will probably not participate in certain sports in which the risk factor just cannot be eliminated. On the other hand, if the effect of eliminating one risk factor after another is known, individuals may be able to participate in sports with low risk if they are compliant with their specific training program. We would like to reach a stage at which all the risk factors are known and we can assign a relative risk of an injury to individuals. During the preseason examination, individuals with risk factors will be assigned training programs that have been validated. Even if we should reach this stage, future research in this field will be necessary. The nature of sports is always changing—becoming faster and generally more stressful. Just think of the difference in alpine skiing over the last 25 years. In almost any sport, the same increase in pace is seen. Thus, risk factor research is always needed, and intervention studies are crucial.

Part III

Biomechanical and Neuromuscular Mechanisms of ACL Injuries

Timothy Edwin Hewett, PhD, FACSM

Several common differences in biomechanical motion (kinematics and kinetics), body and joint positions, and force between men and women, potentially related to the increased risk of ACL injury in women, have been noted in the literature and are detailed in the eight chapters in this section.

The following chapters deal with a number of common kinematic and kinetic differences exhibited by females either during landing from a jump (see figure III.1) or during a cutting and pivoting maneuver:

- Increased lower extremity valgus and increased knee abduction
- Increased valgus loading of the knee joint
- Reduced hip and knee flexion angles
- Adduction and internal rotation of the femur on the tibia
- Increased quadriceps activity, unbalanced by the hamstrings
- Decreased muscle stiffness around the knee joint

The clinical significance of these findings is that prevention and intervention programs should be designed to equalize and neutralize these differences. However, it should be noted that gender differences in biomechanical measures may not directly correlate to gender differences in ACL injury risk.

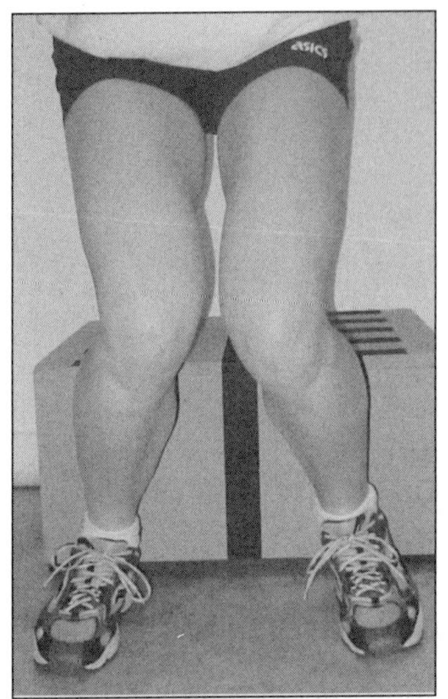

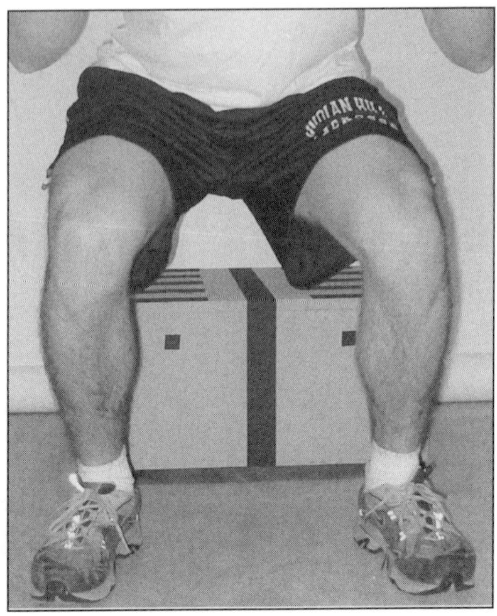

FIGURE III.1 Biomechanical differences may play a role in the gender disparity in ACL injury risk.

Chapter 10

Biomechanics Associated With Injury

Athlete Interviews and Review of Injury Tapes

Tron Krosshaug, PhD
Roald Bahr, MD, PhD

Defining "Injury Mechanisms"

A precise description of the biomechanics associated with injury—the injury mechanism—is a key component in understanding the causes of any particular injury type in sport. However, any attempt to describe the injury mechanisms raises a number of issues. A complete understanding of injury causation needs to address the multifactorial nature of sport injuries: not only the injury biomechanics, but also the risk factors associated with an increased risk of injury. Meeuwisse (1994) therefore developed a model to account for all of the factors involved. As seen from figure 10.1, while an injury may appear to have been caused by a single inciting event, it could be the result of a complex interaction between different internal and external risk factors. Internal factors like age, gender, and body composition could influence the risk of sustaining noncontact ACL injuries; thus by definition these are risk factors. External factors like shoe traction and floor friction could also modify injury risk. Olsen and colleagues (2004) recently showed an increased risk for ACL injuries on certain artificial floors, but for female players only. This indicates that there is an interaction between gender and floor friction on injury risk, which could lead us to hypothesize that there may be a difference in the characteristics of the inciting

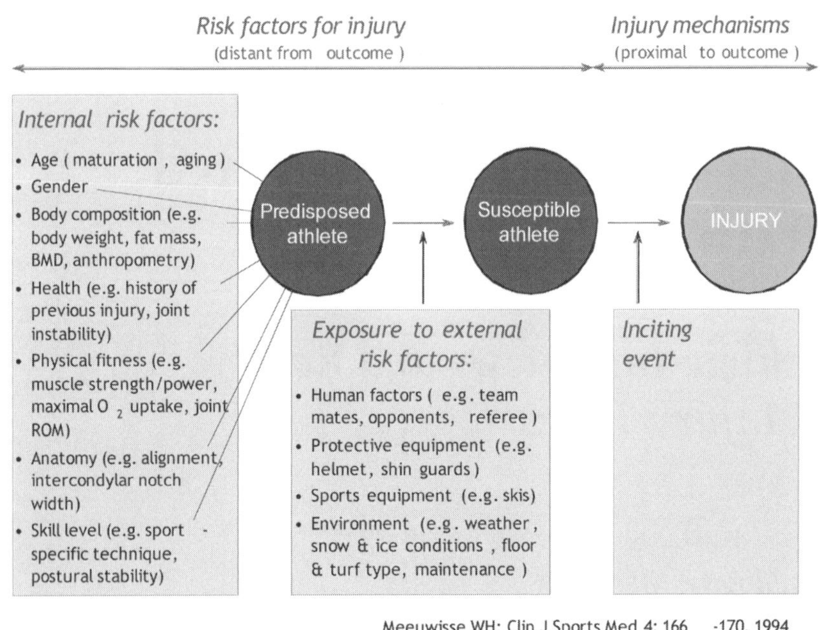

FIGURE 10.1 Meeuwisse's multifactorial model of causation in sport injuries.
From R. Bahr and I. Holmes, 2003, "Risk factors for sports injuries—a methodological approach," *Br J Sports Med* 37: 384-392. Adapted and reproduced with permission from BMJ Publishing Group; adapted from W.H. Meeuwisse, 1994, "Assessing causation in sport injury: A multifactorial model," *Clin J Sport Med* 4: 166-170.

event between genders as well. This model illustrates the need to account for all of these factors at the same time, and not examine only the biomechanics associated with injury in isolation.

Describing the Inciting Event

The term "injury mechanism" is widely used in medical literature but is not well defined. The term is being extensively used for injury descriptions on completely different levels. Some studies provide only simple characteristics such as "contact/noncontact injuries" (Arendt and Dick 1995) or "jumping/nonjumping injuries" (Paul et al. 2003). Others use terms like "sidestep cutting maneuvers," "tackle," or "long shot" (Strand et al. 1990) and "spiking" or "blocking" (Ferretti et al. 1992)—variables that are related to a specific sport (European team handball and volleyball, respectively). Still others use certain biomechanical variables to describe the mechanism of injury. The level of detail here also varies, for example "deceleration injury" (Boden et al. 2000) versus "pivot shift injury of the posterolateral tibial rim and meniscus" (Speer et al. 1992).

How widely the description of the inciting event varies can be seen from the following examples:

- "Tackle from behind" (describes a sport-specific action between two players)
- "Big jump, flat landing" (describes a sport-specific action in an individual sport)
- "Unawareness" (describes psychological aspects of the situation)
- "One-legged landing" (describes an aspect of the whole-body kinematics)
- "Phantom foot mechanism" (describes a pattern of several kinematic characteristics that leads to injury)
- "Valgus trauma" (describes the knee kinematics, kinetics, or both)
- "Anterior drawer" (describes the relative translation between femur and tibia)
- "Quadriceps drawer" (describes the relative translation between femur and tibia due to quadriceps activation)
- "Intercondylar liftoff" (describes the internal knee kinematics)

If we were to characterize the causes of injury in a situation in which a basketball player sustained an ACL injury, one explanation might be that the injury was caused by "an attacking sidestep cutting maneuver to set up for a shot." One could term this a sport-specific description of the injury. Additionally one could add that "the incident occurred to a powerful attacker, who was pushed just as he was giving all his effort to pass the opponent." Another description, with more emphasis on the biomechanical causes of the injury, might be that "the injury occurred as a result of a rapid sideways translation on a high-friction surface." A more detailed biomechanical description could be that "the injury occurred as a result of a large external valgus moment and external rotation moment in combination with a translatory shift of the tibia relative to the femur."

We suggest that the different descriptions of the inciting event could be grouped in four different description categories. Here are some examples of elements that could be relevant in each category:

1. Playing situation: attack/defense, block, tackle, guard/center/forward, jump shot
2. Player and opponent behavior: skill performed, handling the ball, pushed by opponent, attention
3. Gross biomechanical description: whole-body description, often static, of kinematics and kinetics (e.g., COM [center of mass], body rotations, external force)
4. Detailed biomechanical description: joint kinematics and kinetics (e.g., time course of angles, translations, velocities, moments, forces)

We would argue that to provide a complete understanding of the causes of injuries, a description of the inciting event needs to address the characteristics of the injury situation in each of these categories. Although it is important to have an exact and detailed biomechanical description of the injury, this is not sufficient. An account of the playing situation leading to the injury and of player and opponent movement patterns may be equally important from a prevention perspective. For instance, if all ACL injuries were caused by tackles from behind, such tackles could be banned in the rules of the game. If severe sanctions for the player and team were introduced, this should result in fewer injuries. It would then perhaps be less critical to know whether the tackles resulted in valgus or varus forces in the knee.

Research Approaches to Describe the Injury Mechanisms

As shown in figure 10.2, a number of different methodological approaches have been used to describe the inciting event. Here we limit the discussion to two possible methods: athlete interviews and video analysis. Other approaches include clinical studies (in which the clinical joint damage findings associated with an ACL tear are studied to clarify the injury mechanism, mainly through

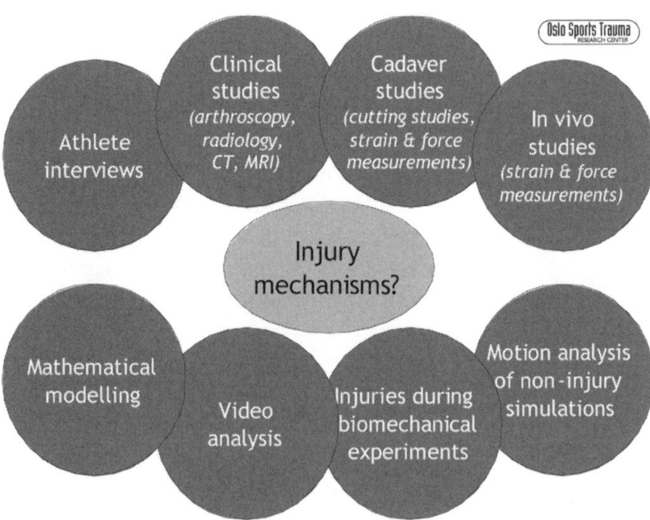

FIGURE 10.2 Research approaches to describe the mechanisms of knee injuries.
Reprinted, by permission, from T. Kroshaug et al., 2005, "Research approaches to describe the mechanisms of injuries in sport: limitations and possibilities," *Br J Sports Med* 39: 330-339.

radiography, magnetic resonance imaging [MRI], arthroscopy, or computed tomography scans), in vivo studies (measuring ACL strain or forces to understand ACL loading patterns), cadaver studies, mathematical modeling, and estimation or simulation of ACL injury situations or those "close to injury situations." In rare cases, injuries have even occurred during biomechanical experiments.

One of the most commonly used approaches in studying injury mechanisms is to use the description of the injury as reported by either the athlete, the coach, medical personnel, or others who witnessed the accident (Arnold et al. 1979). One major problem with this involves the extent to which the injured athlete or the witnesses are able to assess the sport-specific and biomechanical aspects of an injury that happened in a very brief moment in time. Another possible source of error is recall bias (Speer et al. 1995). In many cases these descriptions are "filtered" by a person writing down the description, and probably interpreting the description, for instance in the case of a physician taking notes for the medical record.

Another, perhaps more objective, source of information is video recordings of actual injury situations. However, even with extensive coverage of sports, these recordings may be difficult to collect in a systematic way, and the quality is not guaranteed. Additionally, the methods available for extracting biomechanical information from video sequences may not be adequate (Krosshaug and Bahr 2005).

Literature Search

In order to review the available literature, we searched PubMed using the following key words to identify papers using athlete interviews or video analysis to describe the injury mechanisms for ACL injuries:

- "ACL" OR "anterior cruciate ligament" OR "knee ligament"
- AND key words covering relevant motions and biomechanics (e.g., "cutting," "landing," "sidestepping," "stress," "strain," "force," "injur*," "rupture," "tear")
- NOT MeSH heading terms associated with nonrelevant sports, rehabilitation, surgery, diseases, and so on (e.g., "skiing," "bicycling," "rehabilitation," "osteoarthritis," "ligament reconstruction," "knee prosthesis")

In addition, we searched the reference lists of the identified papers, used the "Related articles" function in PubMed, and also searched the Cochrane Library database. In this way, we identified 12 papers in the athlete interview category and four papers in the video analysis category; in addition, two of the latter included questionnaire data on a larger group of cases than portrayed on the videotapes.

Athlete Interviews

Of the studies identified in the athlete interview category, six looked at noncontact sports separately, and the other six looked at mixed samples of sports (table 10.1). Studies dealing with more than one sport can be misleading unless the injury mechanisms are specified for each sport separately, as in Arendt and Dick 1995, and must be interpreted with caution. Also, in some of the studies, verification of an actual ACL rupture was not optimal, or the manner of verification was not described. Additionally, whether other ligamentous injuries had also occurred in the same injury (i.e., was the rupture "isolated"?) was not always reported.

In basketball (Arendt and Dick 1995) and team handball (Myklebust et al. 1997, 1998; Strand et al. 1990), noncontact injuries are clearly more frequent than contact injuries. Arendt and Dick's NCAA data also show that a higher proportion of the injury mechanisms in females are noncontact than in males (noncontact/contact ratios of 137/34 and 30/16, respectively). The most commonly reported injury mechanisms are landing ("jump stopping") and pivoting (twisting). Three studies presented some cases with hyperextension (Harner et al. 1994; McNair, Marshall, and Matheson 1990; Nakajima et al. 1979). Some athletes reported a "shifting sensation" between the tibia and femur (Arnold et al. 1979). Only one study (McNair, Marshall, and Matheson 1990) indicated that the knee collapsed and the athlete fell to the ground, although in that study this occurred with 22 of the 23 injuries.

In general, the injury mechanism descriptions in the athlete interview category have used widely different terminology. Categories and definitions were rarely provided, and which variables were reported seems somewhat arbitrary. Whereas some studies provided information only on contact/noncontact (Arendt and Dick 1995), others identified the sporting situation (Chong and Tan 2004; Gray et al. 1985; Strand et al. 1990), and still others (McNair, Marshall, and Matheson 1990; Feagin and Curl 1976; Harner et al. 1994) reported detailed joint kinematics. Two studies also characterized the speed of the athletes (Myklebust et al. 1997, 1998).

These studies provided very different descriptions of the injury mechanisms, probably because they were categorized according to the researcher's or surgeon's predefined criteria. Interestingly, one study (Nakajima et al. 1979), in which the injury mechanism description was written down as stated by the patient, presented 17 different descriptions. This indicates that the injury mechanism descriptions in many cases are probably filtered by the researcher who interprets the patients' statements. This may introduce bias to make the patient descriptions fit the researcher's own theory on the injury mechanism.

Nakajima and colleagues (1979) found that a large group (about 2/3) of the noncontact injuries occurred in landings, whereas Arnold and colleagues (1979) reported "internal tibial rotation" as the cause of injury in more than 80% of the injured athletes. It is noticeable that in most cases, since the reported

TABLE 10.1 Studies Presenting Injury Mechanism Data From Athlete Interviews

Reference	Methods	N	Material
Feagin and Curl 1976	Retrospective study	64 M	U.S. Military Academy between 1965 and 1971. Nearly all sports were represented.
Arnold et al. 1979	Prospective, questionnaire and interview, arthroscopy	361 M/F	78% athletic-related injuries, mean group age 21 to 26 years.
Nakajima et al. 1979	Retrospective, interview, arthroscopy	118 M/F	Most patients athletes, mean age 19 years. Most injuries occurred during athletic activities.
Wirtz 1982	Survey during and after the 1980-81 season	16 M/F	Varsity basketball athletes in Iowa high schools.
Gray et al. 1985	Prospective interview	24 M/F	Basketball-related injuries. High school senior varsity, university, and junior high teams, average age 17 years.
McNair et al. 1990	Retrospective questionnaire and interview	23	Mixed sporting activity (rugby, hockey, skiing, gymnastics, netball); level, age, and gender unknown.
Strand et al. 1990	Retrospective questionnaire	144 M/F	Norwegian team handball players, mean age 28.1 (M) and 21.4 (F) years. Recreational to elite level.
Harner et al. 1994	Follow-up with controls, interview	31 M/F	Mixed sporting activity (skiing, basketball, football, soccer, softball) and (<10%) work-related injuries. Mean age to first injury, 20.5 years (M) and 24.8 years (F). No information on skill level.
Arendt and Dick 1995	Prospective, interview	416 M/F	NCAA collegiate soccer and basketball athletes.
Myklebust et al. 1997	Prospective registration, questionnaire	87 M/F	Norwegian team handball players, top three divisions, mean age between 19.4 and 25.1 years in the different divisions.
Myklebust et al. 1998	Prospective registration, personal interview	28 M/F	Elite Norwegian handball, mean age 21.4 (F) and 23.4 (M) years.

(continued)

TABLE 10.1 (continued)

Reference	Methods	N	Material
Boden et al. 2000	Retrospective questionnaire, interview	90 M/F	Basketball, football, and soccer were the most common activities, mean age 26 years. Recreational, varsity, and intramural levels.
Olsen et al. 2004	Prospective cohort study, personal interview	32 F	The three upper divisions in Norwegian female handball, mean age 21 years.
Chong and Tan 2004	Retrospective telephone interview	13 F	8 experienced athletes—netball, rugby, tae kwon do, roller hockey; 5 inexperienced—squash, kick boxing aerobics, volleyball, wakeboarding, and touch rugby. Age 13 to 38 years.

injury characteristics are not very precise, they rarely exclude other characteristics. A landing injury can also very well have included internal rotation, and an internal rotation injury can very well have occurred in a landing. Another common description is "deceleration mechanisms" that could include stopping, sidestepping, and landing, since all these can be characterized similarly based on biomechanical features. As already mentioned, the categories are seldom well defined, which makes interpretation difficult.

In most of the studies, the injuries were reported to have occurred with a relatively straight knee (Arnold et al. 1979). McNair and colleagues (1990) also reported that 10 of the 23 injured athletes recalled a knee flexion angle between 0° and 20°. In basketball (77%) (Arendt and Dick 1995), in European team handball (90-95%), and in soccer (57%) (Arendt and Dick 1995), of ACL injuries are classified as noncontact. In basketball, landings seem to be the most frequently reported injury mechanism (Gray et al. 1985), whereas in team handball, sidestep cutting injuries are more common (Myklebust et al. 1997).

Video Analysis

Although video analysis may seem to be a more reliable way of examining injury mechanism compared to interviews, current methods for estimating kinematics from uncalibrated video sequences are inadequate (Krosshaug and Bahr 2005). None of the studies listed in table 10.2 used methods other than simple visual inspection to extract kinematic information from the videos. It is inherently difficult to interpret segment attitudes and to calculate joint angles in three planes simply through visual inspection. In two of the studies, a consensus approach was used, but this method was not validated. Finally, these methods

TABLE 10.2 Studies Presenting Injury Mechanism Data From Athlete Videos

Reference	N	Methods
Boden et al. 2000	27	Videos obtained from professional and collegiate teams—football (53%), basketball (30%), soccer (9%), and volleyball (4%)
Ebstrup and Bojsen-Moller 2000	3 (15)	Prospective collection of videos from Danish indoor ball games
Teitz 2001	54	Retrospective multicenter video analysis—20 basketball, 18 football, and 9 soccer injuries
Olsen et al. 2004	20	Retrospective and prospective video collection—women's Norwegian or international handball competition

cannot produce continuous estimates of joint angles and positions, which are necessary for detailed biomechanical analyses of the injury mechanisms—for example, joint angle time histories, velocities, and accelerations.

The degree to which a two-camera recording improves these estimates in such a visual inspection approach is not currently known. A recent study by Krosshaug and Bahr (2005) indicates that the use of several camera views increases the accuracy in a model-based image-matching technique to extract human motion from uncalibrated video images. Also, video quality and the viewing angle relative to the athlete will determine what variables are more reliable (Krosshaug and Bahr 2005). Another source of error is the determination of the point of injury. Although Teitz and colleagues (2001) stated that they could determine the "precise point of injury," no methodological details were given. In contrast, Boden and colleagues (2000) stated that finding the exact moment of ACL disruption was impossible.

Two of these studies were prospective, and in one, the authors (Olsen et al. 2004) stated that MRIs had been taken. Unfortunately, the associated findings (meniscal injuries and bone bruises) were not reported. The studies seem to agree that the knee was relatively straight; at least no flexion of more than 30° was reported. The same was reported from the interview studies. On the other hand, while Boden and colleagues (2000) reported an inconsistency between the questionnaires and videos in terms of the description of the kinematics, Olsen and colleagues (2004) reported good agreement. Also, there does not seem to be a complete consensus among the studies regarding the injury mechanisms. Boden's group reported that the amount of internal and external rotation in the videos at the time of injury was minimal, whereas Olsen and colleagues (2004) and Ebstrup and Bojsen-Moller (2000) emphasized the role of internal-external, as well as valgus, rotation. Teitz (2001) did not report varus-valgus or internal-external angles. Authors of two of the studies stated that most of the injuries occurred in high-speed situations. This implies that the forces involved were relatively high. This is also further emphasized by the estimated weight distribution in the study by Olsen and colleagues (2004), in which all except one injured athlete had at least 80% of the weight distribution on the injured leg.

Although several of the interview studies note hyperextension as an injury mechanism in ball and team sports, no such incident was reported among the 60 ACL injury videos analyzed in these four studies.

One of the studies (Teitz 2001) indicated that a center of gravity posterior to the knee was an important factor; none of the other studies presented similar findings. It is difficult to understand the rationale behind this theory, as one would normally expect that in the braking phase, the leg is indeed placed in front of the body in order to generate a ground reaction force vector that will prevent the body from gaining too much forward angular momentum, thereby falling. Since it is not possible to determine the ground reaction force vector and its angle from viewing a video, it is also questionable whether the hip joint moment is flexor dominated as suggested.

Conclusions

- Studies based on athlete interviews are fraught with significant methodological limitations. It is difficult to interpret the injury situation in the first place; recall and reporting bias may be important additional factors; and nonstandardized variables and criteria are used.
- Only a few studies use video analysis; the cases are few, and these have been analyzed using visual inspection alone.
- The proportion of noncontact injuries seems to be greater among females than males.
- Only "crude" descriptions are given in the existing studies, but the following biomechanics are suggested to be associated with noncontact ACL injuries in ball and team sports:

    1. Injuries seem to occur most often in landing, cutting, and other similar deceleration movements on a relatively straight leg.
    2. Although some hyperextension injuries are reported in interviews, none were seen in any of the noncontact injuries from video analysis.
    3. Internal rotation seems like a mechanism of injury, but the studies suggesting this mechanism are limited in their methodological approach; thus more evidence is necessary to fully support the hypothesis.
    4. Valgus-external rotation also seems to be a likely mechanism of injury, but here as well, the obvious lack of good studies prevents us from forming decisive conclusions.

Chapter 11

Clinical Biomechanical Studies on ACL Injury Risk Factors

Laura J. Huston, MS

Noncontact ACL injuries occur when the joint moment developed at the knee overcomes the static and dynamic restraint system. Several differences between men and women related to biomechanical motion (kinematics and kinetics), body and joint positions, and force have been noted in the literature that may render women susceptible to this injury. Based on recent research from a number of institutions, it appears that the most prevalent kinematic and kinetic differences females exhibited either when landing from a jump or during a cutting and pivoting maneuver are the following:

- Reduced hip and knee flexion angles
- Increased knee valgus
- Internal rotation of the femur on the tibia
- High quadriceps activity, unbalanced by the hamstrings
- Inadequate trans-knee muscle stiffness

Background

The last five years have seen an unprecedented advancement in both the number and quality of scientific studies examining the (dynamic) movements postulated to invoke a noncontact ACL injury. At the time of Hunt Valley I in 1999, the most notable advances in the field came from identifying the types of movements that were most likely to be involved in a noncontact ACL injury—movements sustained either during a cutting or sidestep maneuver or in landing from a jump (Arendt, Agel, and Dick 1999; Boden et al. 2000; Colby et al. 2000; Delfico and Garrett 1998; Miyasaka et al. 1991; Moul 1998; Murphy, Connolly, and Beynnon 2003; Olsen et al. 2004; Uhorchak et al. 2003). Both scenarios include a sudden deceleration that may or may not be combined with a rapid directional change. A number of studies have since been published on the potential relationship between lower extremity biomechanics and electromyographic (EMG) patterns demonstrated during these “high-risk” movements and the well-documented gender disparity in ACL injury rates.

From a clinical biomechanical standpoint, we have progressed from using simple static models to using sophisticated 3-D dynamic musculoskeletal models that are capable of feeding kinematic and kinetic data gathered from in vivo testing into musculoskeletal modeling and computer simulations (termed “patient-specific modeling”). These dynamic patient-specific musculoskeletal models have great potential for predictive clinical applications in orthopedics (Reinbolt et al. 2005).

The goal of this chapter is to synthesize the body of knowledge that has been published in the area of clinical biomechanical studies relating to ACL injury risk factors. These clinical studies can be subdivided into the following categories: (1) kinematics and kinetics, (2) body position, and (3) muscular differences.

Kinematic and Kinetic Differences

Numerous published studies have identified kinematic and kinetic patterns that potentially place females at increased risk for ACL injury (Hewett et al. 1996; Biscevic et al. 2005; Colby et al. 2000; Decker et al. 2003; Fagenbaum and Darling 2003; Ford, Myer, and Hewett 2003; Ford et al. 2005; Haas et al. 2005; Hewett et al. 2005b; Kernozek et al. 2005; Lephart et al. 2002b; McLean et al. 1999; McLean, Huang, and van den Bogert 2005; Padua et al. 2004; Pollard, Davis McClay, and Hamill 2004; Salci et al. 2004; Sigward and Powers 2006; Urabe et al. 2005; Zeller et al. 2003). In addition, it has been stressed that the landing performance differences between males and females also require scrutiny beyond the kinematic level in order to advance understanding of the etiology of selection by the genders of a distinct energy absorption strategy during landing (Decker et al. 2003).

Jump Landings

Landing from a jump is one of the primary noncontact mechanisms for ACL injury in female basketball and volleyball players (Ferretti et al. 1992; Gerberich et al. 1987; Kirkendall and Garrett 2000). During landing, the lower extremity functions to decelerate and control the downward momentum through joint flexion. However, if the joint angle upon impact is small, higher forces are transferred through the joints. Similarly, if the lower extremity fails to continue its downward momentum, the muscles surrounding the knee joint do not have the opportunity to dissipate the induced loads (Nigg 1985). Thus, knee flexion angle produced in response to ground impact may be a significant factor in ACL injury.

Hip, Knee, and Ankle Flexion Angles

Consensus from controlled laboratory experiments indicates that females land in a more erect position upon ground contact, thus predisposing the ACL to potentially greater loads (Decker et al. 2003; Huston, Vibert, and Wojtys 2001; Lephart et al. 2001, 2002; Onate et al. 2003; Padua et al. 2004; Salci et al. 2004). The exception is the work by Fagenbaum and Darling (2003), indicating that women landed with greater knee flexion angles than their collegiate male counterparts.

In a study by Lephart and colleagues (2001), females had significantly less maximum knee flexion and greater femoral internal rotation and tibial external rotation upon landing (figure 11.1). Nigg (1985) and Stacoff and colleagues (1988) reported that landing with a straighter knee position upon ground contact leads to progressively greater peak vertical ground reaction forces (Nigg 1985; Stacoff, Kaelin, and Stuessi 1988). As compensation for this lack of initial knee flexion, Decker and colleagues (2003) and Kernozek and colleagues (2005) found that females subsequently exhibit greater ankle range of motions throughout the landing phase. They suggested that this compensatory landing pattern is an attempt to dissipate the large external forces over a wider range of joint motion (Decker et al. 2003). Self and Paine (2001), studying landings with four different ankle strategies, found that the strategy with the largest ankle plantarflexion position at ground contact demonstrated the most shock absorption and reduction of the peak vertical ground reaction force. Therefore,

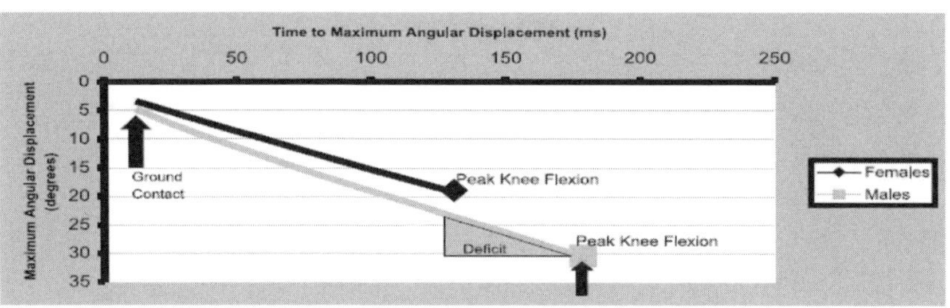

FIGURE 11.1 Gender differences seen in a landing task, from ground contact to peak knee flexion.

females may compensate for a more erect posture upon landing from a jump by employing a balancing muscular strategy by the ankle plantarflexor muscles, resulting in similar peak vertical ground reaction forces to males.

Joint Absorption Strategy

The preferred energy absorption strategy during landing seems to differ between genders (Devita and Skelly 1992; McNitt-Gray 1993; Schot, Dufek, and Bates 1991; Zhang, Bates, and Dufek 2000) (table 11.1). Studies have shown that the ankle plantarflexor, knee, and hip extensor muscle groups in males generally contribute 22%, 41%, and 38% to the total energy absorption (table 11.1; McNitt-Gray 1993; Zhang, Bates, and Dufek 2000), compared with 40%, 41%, and 19% in the strategy generally preferred by females (Devita and Skelly 1992; Schot, Dufek, and Bates 1991).

TABLE 11.1 Literature Review of Gender-Specific Lower Extremity Shock Absorption Contributions During Soft or Normal Landings From a Height of 60 cm

Authors	Subjects	Landing height (cm)	Landing style	Ankle %	Knee %	Hip %
		FEMALE LANDERS				
Schot et al. 1991[a]	5 female, 4 male intercollegiate athletes	60	Natural	43	45	12
Devita and Skelly 1992	8 female intercollegiate athletes	59	Soft	37	37	25
Decker 2003	9 female recreational athletes	60	Natural	35	47	18
		MALE LANDERS				
McNitt-Gray 1993	6 male recreational athletes	72	Natural	30	33	37
Zhang et al. 2000	9 male recreational athletes	62	Soft	14	44	42
Zhang et al. 2000	9 male recreational athletes	62	Natural	21	46	34
Current study	12 male recreational athletes	60	Natural	29	41	30

[a]Predominantly female subject population.

Collectively, the results of these studies indicated that while the knee was the preferred primary shock absorber for both genders, the females preferred to use the ankle musculature for impact attenuation while the males preferred to employ the hip extensor muscles.

Knee Valgus

Females have also been shown to exhibit greater knee valgus angles following a jump landing (Ford, Myer, and Hewett 2003; Ford et al. 2005; Padua et al. 2004). Ford and colleagues (2003) first reported gender differences in valgus knee motion during jump-landing maneuvers using a high school population of basketball players. They found that although females demonstrated slightly more valgus knee motion at the point of initial ground contact compared to males (5.9° vs. 3.3°), valgus angles for females were significantly greater at the point of maximum knee flexion (females, 27.6° vs. males, 16.1°). Their conclusion was that athletes with increased valgus knee motion likely exhibit decreased joint control in the coronal plane and that these decreases in dynamic knee joint control may place them at an increased risk of knee injury. In a follow-up study, Ford and colleagues (2005) confirmed this finding in a group of height- and weight-matched male and female collegiate basketball and soccer athletes. The female athletes demonstrated increased lower extremity coronal plane excursion while performing single-leg drop landings in both the medial and lateral directions.

Knee abduction angles upon landing have subsequently been shown to be strong predictors of ACL injury risk (Hewett 2005). Hewett and colleagues (2005) reported that knee abduction angles at landing were 8° greater in ACL-injured than in uninjured athletes (figure 11.2). These injured athletes had a 2.5 times greater knee abduction moment and 20% higher ground reaction force ($P < 0.05$). The knee abduction moment predicted ACL injury status with 73% specificity and 78% sensitivity; dynamic valgus measures showed a predictive r^2 of 0.88.

These views are supported by the work of Kernozek and colleagues (2005), who similarly reported frontal plane kinematic differences between males and females. This group found that females exhibited greater peak knee valgus positions during landing than males, and that after individual body mass was accounted for, females generated smaller internal knee varus moment at the time of peak valgus knee angulation.

Development Changes During Maturation

Interestingly, there has been increasing evidence in the literature demonstrating developmental differences in knee kinematics and kinetics during landing and potential effects of maturation on injury risk (Hewett, Myer, and Ford 2004; Yu et al. 2005; Haas et al. 2005). Most landing studies have historically focused on kinetics, neuromuscular activity, and kinematics in the sagittal plane without regard to maturation. However, there is a paucity of information on the landing control

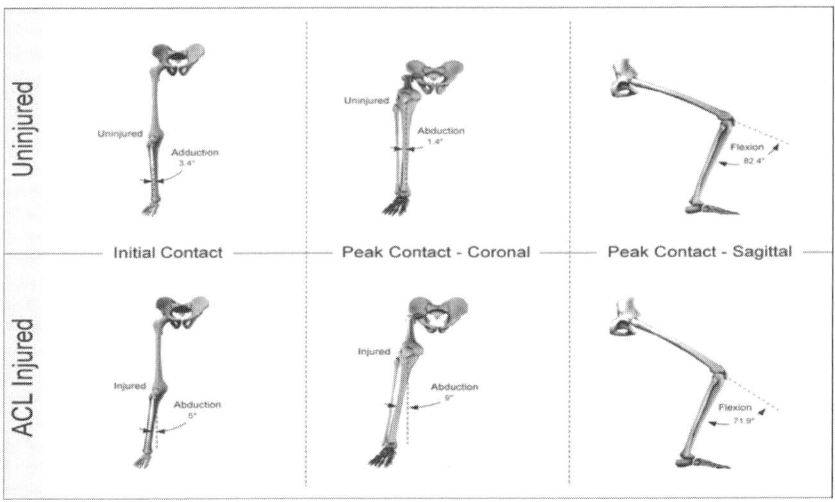

FIGURE 11.2 Biomechanical model depicting mean knee joint kinematics during a drop vertical jump at initial contact and maximal displacement in ACL-injured and uninjured groups (n = 9 knees and n = 390 knees, respectively). Left: coronal plane view of knee abduction angle at initial contact. Center: coronal plane view of maximum knee abduction angle. Right: sagittal plane view of maximum knee flexion angle.

Reprinted, by permission, from T.E. Hewett et al., 2005, "Biomechanical measures of neuromuscular control and valgus loading of the knee predict ACL injury risk in female athletes: A prospective study," *Am J Sports Med* 33(4): 492-501.

strategies in preadolescent female sport participants. Studies by Hewett and colleagues (2004), Barber-Westin and colleagues (2005), Haas and colleagues (2005), and Yu and colleagues (2005) have addressed lower extremity biomechanical differences between prepubescent and postpubescent female recreational athletes to determine whether maturation may influence injury risk. Hewett and colleagues (2004) theorized that, unlike males, females do not have a "neuromuscular spurt" to match their growth spurt. Moreover, their rapid increase in size and weight at or near the time of puberty, in the absence of increased neuromuscular power and neuromuscular control, may increase the risk of ACL injury.

Hewett and colleagues (2004) reported that following the onset of maturation, female athletes landed with greater total medial motion of the knees and a greater maximum lower extremity valgus angle than did the male athletes. The girls demonstrated decreased flexor torques compared with the boys, as well as a significant difference between the maximum valgus angles of their dominant and nondominant lower extremities after maturation. Yu and colleagues (2005) found that males and females have similar knee flexion angles at ground contact before the age of 12 and that females have decreased knee flexion angles after age 13 (Yu et al. 2005). Barber-Westin and colleagues (2005) reported that a high percentage of the prepubescent athletes studied had a distinctly valgus lower limb alignment during the drop-jump test and a lack of lower limb symmetry during hop tests—indices that have been hypothesized to increase the risk for knee ligament injuries in older athletes. Haas and colleagues (2005) reported that the postpubescent participants in his study exhibited reduced knee flexion at initial foot–ground contact, increased mediolateral knee joint forces, and reduced knee extensor moments. He concluded that the older female participants may have been utilizing landing strategies that become injurious when changes in the skeletal architecture occurring after the onset of menarche interact with these strategies.

Sidestep and Cutting Maneuvers

Beginning in 1999, researchers began to quantify kinematic characteristics in more realistic athletic scenarios, in hopes of mimicking true ACL injury-producing situations. The sidestep and cut maneuver, commonly seen in pivoting sports such as basketball and soccer, were mimicked in controlled laboratory settings in hopes of identifying characteristic precursor movements that could be later linked with potential ACL injury-producing movements.

Hip, Knee, and Ankle Flexion Angles

Select gender differences have been identified during sidestepping in several recent studies (Ford et al. 2005; Hewett, Myer, and Ford 2004; Malinzak et al. 2001; McLean, Huang, and van den Bogert 2005; Pollard, Davis McClay, and Hamill 2004; Sigward and Powers 2006). In general, women were found to have less knee flexion (Hewett, Myer, and Ford 2004; Malinzak et al. 2001), greater knee valgus (Ford et al. 2005; Hewett, Myer, and Ford 2004; Malinzak et al. 2001; McLean, Huang, and van den Bogert 2005), greater quadriceps activation (Malinzak et al. 2001), and lower hamstring activation (Malinzak et al. 2001) in comparison to the men. In addition, Pollard and colleagues (2004) reported significantly less peak hip abduction in the females compared with the males. Otherwise, there were no gender differences in selected peak hip and knee joint kinematics and moments: Male and female collegiate soccer players demonstrated similar hip and knee joint mechanics while performing a randomly cued cutting maneuver.

Knee Valgus

Utilizing 3-D high-speed video and ground reaction force data, McLean and colleagues (2005) found that females displayed significantly larger maximum knee abduction (10.2 ± 2.9°) during sidestepping compared with males (7.2 ± 0.9°). In addition, females demonstrated significantly larger mean variability in internal-external tibial rotation (3.6 ± 0.7°) compared with males (1.9 ± 0.7°). The authors hypothesized that this increased knee abduction seen in females (figure 11.3), in combination with the increased variability in tibial rotation, may contribute to females' increased risk of ACL injury.

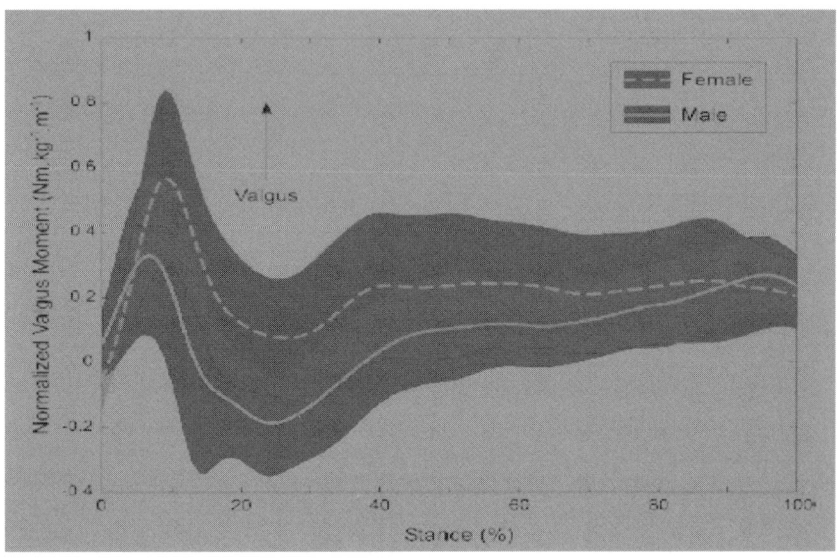

FIGURE 11.3 Effect of gender on mean (+SD) normalized (height × mass) external knee valgus moment demonstrated during sidestep stance.

Reprinted from *Clinical biomechanics*, Vol. 20, S.G. McLean, X. Huang, and A.J. van den Bogert, "Association between lower extremity posture at contact and peak knee valgus moment during sidestepping: Implications for ACL injury," pages 863-870, Copyright 2005, with permission from Elsevier.

Ford and colleagues (2005) compared knee and ankle joint angles between males and females during an unanticipated cutting maneuver. Females exhibited greater knee abduction (valgus) angles than males. Gender differences were also found in maximum ankle eversion and maximum inversion during stance phase. The investigators hypothesized that the gender differences in knee and ankle kinematics in the frontal plane during cutting may help explain the gender differences in ACL injury rates. These views were supported by the work of Sigward and Powers (2006), who similarly reported that females experienced increased frontal plane moments and decreased sagittal plane moments during early deceleration. Furthermore, increased quadriceps activity and smaller net flexor moments reported by the group at Cincinnati Children's suggest less sagittal plane protection (i.e., increased tendency toward anterior tibial translation).

Anterior Tibial Translation

Chappell and colleagues (2002) focused on anterior tibial translation in 3-D kinematic and kinetic takeoff and landing patterns, and found that the landing phase generates larger anterior knee shear forces compared with the takeoff phase. Their results suggested that females exhibit greater proximal tibia anterior shear forces as well as larger knee extension and valgus knee moments during the landing phase compared with males.

Femoral and Tibial Rotation

In 2001, Lephart and colleagues reported that females exhibited significantly greater femoral internal rotation and tibial external rotation upon landing than males. Similarly, Padua and colleagues (2004) had subjects perform a standardized jump-landing task and found greater peak tibial internal rotation among the female subjects compared with the males. McLean and colleagues (2005) also found that females demonstrated significantly larger mean variability in internal-external tibial rotation (3.6 ± 0.7°) compared with males (1.9 ± 0.7°). They hypothesized that this increased knee abduction seen in females, in combination with the increased variability in tibial rotation, may contribute to the increased risk of ACL injury.

Conversely, Pollard and colleagues (2005) reported that the pattern variability was decreased in females compared to males, showing 32% less thigh rotation, 40% less abduction-adduction, and 44% less knee flexion-extension and hip rotation variability. They suggested that these less flexible coordination patterns decreased the ability of females to adapt to external perturbations incurred during play.

Interestingly, inferences have been drawn regarding excessive foot pronation and the increased incidence of ACL injury (Loudon, Jenkins, and Loudon 1996; Shultz et al. 2001). In 1996, Loudon and colleagues examined the correlation between static postural faults in female athletes and the prevalence of noncontact ACL injury. Seven variables were measured in a group of 20 ACL-injured females and 20 age-matched controls: standing pelvic position, hip position, standing sagittal knee position, standing frontal knee position, hamstring length, prone subtalar joint position, and navicular drop test. A conditional stepwise logistic regression analysis revealed that the factors of knee recurvatum, an excessive navicular drop, and excessive subtalar joint pronation were significant discriminators between the ACL-injured and noninjured groups. In 2001, Shultz and colleagues (2001) took static measurements of Q angle and navicular drop to determine their influence on muscular response times and activation patterns. They found that the pronators (or subjects who had excessive navicular drop) responded significantly faster than the neutral group. Since excessive pronation has been found to increase internal tibial rotation in stance, the authors concluded that lower limb alignment would influence neuromuscular timing and activation patterns (Shultz et al. 2001). Collectively, these findings may have implications regarding potential ACL risk factors in addition to rehabilitation techniques in physical therapy.

Muscular Differences

Muscles serve as the primary active stabilizers of the knee during functional loading conditions, protecting against injury. Certain combinations of knee muscle forces can rupture the ACL, while others offer protection. The need to suddenly arrest, change, or increase body momentum during high-risk activities requires large quadriceps muscle forces, typically generated through lengthening contractions. Large quadriceps muscle forces can cause anterior tibial translation via patellofemoral loading and can increase ACL strain, while the hamstrings function synergistically with the ACL to resist anterior translations of the tibia. It has already been demonstrated in vitro that powerful isolated lengthening quadriceps contractions with the knee fixed in flexion can rupture the ACL (DeMorat et al. 2004; Dikeman 1998), while balanced quadriceps, hamstring, and gastrocnemius cocontractions may prevent such injuries (MacWilliams et al. 1999; Shultz and Perrin 1999a). Additionally, in vitro, in vivo, and computer modeling work by a number of investigators has shown that ACL strain is significantly affected by the balance of muscle activity in the quadriceps and hamstring muscles (Bach and Hull 1998; Berns, Hull, and Patterson 1992; Beynnon and Fleming 1998; Draganich and Vahey 1990; Dürselen, Claes, and Kiefer 1995; Pandy and Shelburne 1997; Renstrom et al. 1986; Shultz and Perrin 1999a; Torzilli, Deng, and Warren 1994).

Differences in control of the knee musculature have been observed between male and female athletes, through both altered muscle activation patterns and reduced muscle stiffness generation.

Altered Muscle Activation Patterns

A number of groups have postulated that muscle activation patterns differ between male and female athletes (Colby et al. 2000; DeMont and Lephart 2004; DeMorat et al. 2004; Hewett 2005; Kibler et al. 2001; MacWilliams et al. 1999; Malinzak et al. 2001; More et al. 1993; Myer, Ford, and Hewett 2005; Shultz and Perrin 1999a; Urabe et al. 2005). These laboratory studies show that female athletes have muscle activation patterns in which suboptimal hamstring muscle activation is coupled with predominant quadriceps activation. Huston and Wojtys (1996) found quadriceps-dominant muscle-stabilizing responses to anterior tibial translation when compared to male and female nonathlete controls. Malinzak and colleagues (2001) and Urabe and colleagues (2005) reported that female recreational athletes had greater quadriceps muscle activation and lower hamstring activation than their male counterparts (Malinzak et al. 2001; Urabe et al. 2005). White and colleagues (2003) found quadriceps coactivation ratios significantly higher in collegiate female athletes compared to their male counterparts.

Kibler and colleagues (2001) recruited skilled male and female collegiate athletes and put them through a plant and side-cut maneuver at a self-selected maximum velocity. Their female subjects were found to have significantly longer activation durations in the rectus femoris muscle group, a pattern that the authors suggested is suboptimal for knee stabilization. Conversely, Fagenbaum and Darling (2003) studied male and female collegiate athletes and observed similar muscle activation patterns between the two groups.

Collectively, these studies have shown that compared to males, females generally employ a neuromuscular strategy defined by significantly greater quadriceps activation and significantly less hamstring activation during high-risk athletic maneuvers. This decreased neuromuscular control of the lower extremity in women may decrease dynamic knee stability, increase the potential for greater ACL strain, and account for a greater likelihood of ACL injury.

Inadequate Muscle Stiffness

Active muscle stiffness is essential for the maintenance of joint stability and can be voluntarily controlled through muscle recruitment. Under an active state, the primary determinant of musculotendinous stiffness is the number of cross-bridges formed in parallel. Unfortunately, reduced effective stiffness may contribute to the gender bias in risk of musculoskeletal instability.

Five controlled laboratory studies comparing knee stiffness in noninjured healthy males and females showed significantly decreased stiffness in the female cohort (Granata, Padua, and Wilson 2002; Heise, Bohne, and Bressel 2001; Kibler et al. 2001; Wojtys, Ashton-Miller, and Huston 2002; Wojtys et al. 2003). Heise and colleagues (2001) quantified hopping on a force platform at a preferred frequency while EMG data and vertical ground reaction force data were recorded. Leg stiffness was found to be significantly higher in males (24.6 kN/m) compared with females (18.9 kN/m). Men activated their lower extremity muscles significantly earlier than women, which may partly explain why men exhibited higher leg stiffness. In summary, differences in leg stiffness between men and women were accompanied by differences in muscle preactivation times. Kibler and colleagues (2001) found longer activation duration in muscles that initiated and maintained knee (gastrocnemius) and lower extremity stiffness (gluteus) in male college athletes compared to female college athletes. The consequences of this may lead to increased anterior tibial translation and decreased knee stiffness in females. Granata and colleagues (2002) measured the transient motion in response to an angular perturbation in males and females. Females have been found to demonstrate significantly reduced muscle stiffness in both the quadriceps and hamstring muscles, exhibiting 56% to 73% of the effective stiffness of males (Granata, Padua, and Wilson 2002) (figures 11.4 and 11.5). These gender differences were not attributable to voluntary muscle activation, reflex response, coactivation, or passive muscle stiffness properties.

Wojtys and colleagues conducted two different studies in males and females (Wojtys, Ashton-Miller, and Huston 2002; Wojtys et al. 2003). The percentage increase in shear knee stiffness in response to an anteriorly directed perturbation of the knee in males was significantly greater (379%) than in females (212%) (Wojtys, Ashton-Miller, and Huston 2002). In the second study, male and female cohorts were matched for height, weight, body mass index, shoe size, and activity level (Wojtys et al. 2003). The ability of the knee to resist angular perturbation at the foot, causing internal rotation, was measured. Males had more stiffness (218%) than females (178%), and females from pivot sports had the least increase in knee stiffness (Wojtys et al. 2003). The influence of

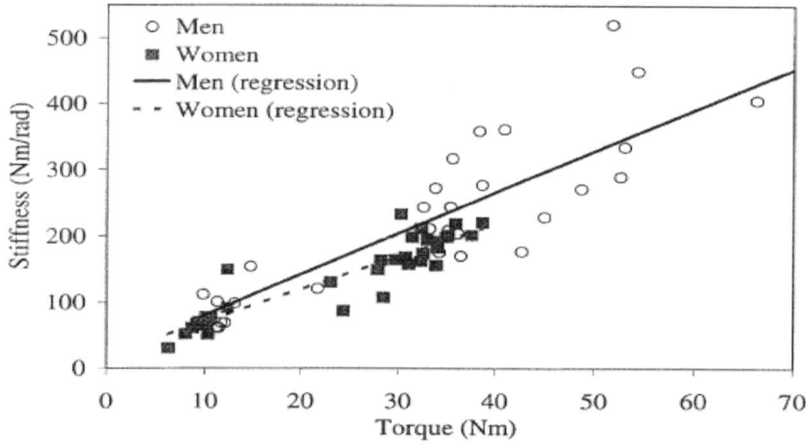

FIGURE 11.4 Stiffness for the quadriceps. Linear regressions between stiffness and torque for the male and female populations are significantly different in slope. Men: K = 6.21T + 18.1; r^2 = 0.77. Women: K = 0.99T + 19.6; r^2 = 0.83.

Reprinted from *Journal of electromyography and kinesiology,* Vol. 12, K.P. Granata, D.A. Padua, and S.E. Wilson, "Gender differences in active musculoskeletal stiffness. Part I-Quantification in controlled measurements of knee joint dynamics," pages 119-126, Copyright 2002, with permission from Elsevier.

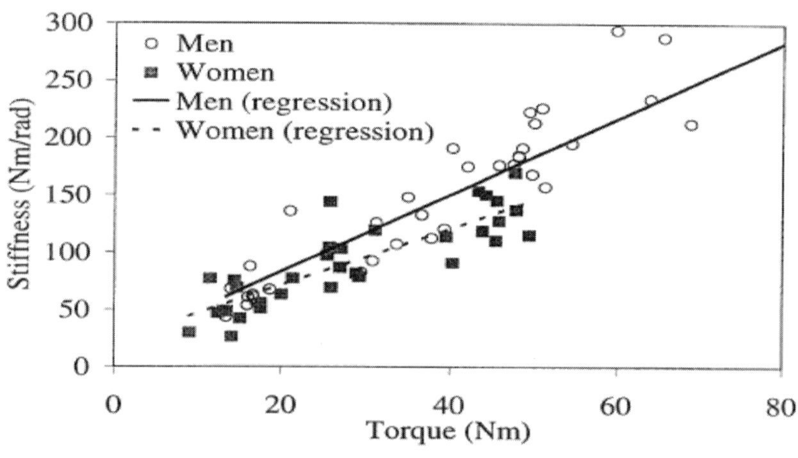

FIGURE 11.5 Stiffness for the hamstrings. Linear regressions between stiffness and torque for the male and female populations are significantly different in slope. Men: K = 3.34T + 16.9; r^2 = 0.78. Women: K = 2.47T + 22.1; r^2 = 0.73.

Reprinted from *Journal of electromyography and kinesiology,* Vol. 12, K.P. Granata, D.A. Padua, and S.E. Wilson, "Gender differences in active musculoskeletal stiffness. Part I-Quantification in controlled measurements of knee joint dynamics," pages 119-126, Copyright 2002, with permission from Elsevier.

muscle activation on this force-versus-displacement ratio suggests potential gender differences in the stiffness of the recruited muscles.

In summary, female leg muscles conservatively exhibit 20% less resistance to dynamic stretch than in age- and size-matched males (Heise, Bohne, and Bressel 2001; Wojtys, Ashton-Miller, and Huston 2002; Wojtys et al. 2003; Granata, Wilson, and Padua 2002). The relative deficiencies of this population of female athletes in generating protective muscle resistance to minimize anterior tibial translation and external tibial rotation are quite apparent; these shortcomings may subject the ACL to higher levels of hazardous forces during athletic activities.

Conclusions

The mechanics of ACL injury, with an emphasis on the kinematics and kinetics that may predispose females to noncontact ACL tears, has been a focus of research in the sport biomechanics community. In general, ACL injuries are thought to be associated with abnormal loading of the knee. Females, on average, have knee motion and muscle use patterns in athletic maneuvers that frequently bring them close to body positions in which noncontact ACL injuries occur. Controlled laboratory studies have repeatedly shown that females, compared with males, appear to land a jump, cut, and pivot with less knee and hip flexion, increased knee valgus, increased internal rotation of the hip, increased external rotation of the tibia, less knee joint stiffness, and high quadriceps activity relative to hamstring activity. Females also exhibit "leg dominance"—that is, an imbalance between muscular strength, flexibility, and coordination between their lower extremities; and such imbalances are associated with an increased risk of injury. Documenting these neuromuscular differences provides a basis for future research and aids in current rehabilitation and intervention programs.

Chapter 12

Effects of Neuromuscular Training on Lower Extremity Motion Patterns

Bing Yu, PhD
Marlene DeMaio, MD

Combined Training Programs Including Plyometrics

A literature review of the effects of plyometric, strength, and balance training on lower extremity motion patterns during athletic tasks was performed. Hewett and colleagues (1996) investigated the effects of a plyometric training program on peak vertical ground reaction force in landing after a volleyball block jump. They provided 11 high school volleyball players with a six-week jump-landing training program. The program emphasized appropriate posture and body alignment, minimum excessive side-to-side and forward-backward movements, soft landing with increased knee flexion motion, and preparation for the next jump. The training program was divided into three phases: the technique phase with emphasis on basic techniques, the fundamental phase with emphasis on strength and power, and the performance phase with emphasis on maximum vertical jump height. Nine height-, body weight-, age-, and playing experience-matched male high school volleyball players were used as a control group. The authors reported a 22% decrease in peak vertical ground reaction force and a 50% decrease in knee valgus-varus moments after training. Peak external knee extension moment did not significantly change after training.

Irmischer and colleagues (2004) investigated the effects of a nine-week, low-intensity and low-volume plyometric training program on peak vertical ground reaction force and rate of development of peak vertical ground reaction force during a vertical jump-landing-jump task. They studied 14 female athletes in a training group and 14 female athletes in a control group. The training program included only plyometric and dynamic stabilization exercises. The subjects in the training group attended the training program twice a week for nine weeks. The authors found that the training group significantly decreased their peak vertical ground reaction force during landing and the rate of development of the peak ground reaction force.

In another study, Lephart and associates (2005) compared the effects of a plyometric training program and a basic resistance training program on lower extremity neuromuscular and biomechanical characteristics. Twenty-seven female high school athletes were randomly assigned to either a plyometric or basic resistance training group. The training program for each group was divided into two phases. In the first four weeks (phase I), both groups trained with flexibility, balance, and resistance exercises. In the second four weeks (phase II), the plyometric training group trained with flexibility, plyometric, balance, resistance, and agility exercises while the basic resistance training group trained with flexibility, balance, and resistance exercises. Subjects in both programs increased quadriceps muscle strength and also increased hip and knee flexion angles and decreased hip and knee flexion motion during landing in a jump-landing task. No significant differences in posttraining lower extremity motion patterns between training programs were observed.

Myer and colleagues (2005b) evaluated the effects of a comprehensive neuromuscular training program on the lower extremity motion patterns in a drop-landing vertical jump task. The program consisted of several sets of plyometric exercises, a set of resistance exercises, a set of balance exercises, and speed exercises. Fifty-three female high school basketball, volleyball, and soccer players participated in this study. Subjects significantly decreased the maximum valgus (28%) and varus (38%) moments for their right knee during the stance phase of the drop-landing vertical jump task. Subjects also showed a trend toward decreases in maximum knee valgus and varus moments for the left knee. This study showed that the combination of multiple injury prevention exercise components in a comprehensive program improved performance and modified lower extremity motion patterns.

Balance and Proprioception Training Programs

Holm and colleagues (2004) conducted a study on proprioception, balance, and muscle strength training and lower extremity function of female team handball players. They had 27 elite team handball players from two professional teams complete a training program in five to seven weeks. The main exercises were floor exercises focused on landing technique and wobble board and balance mat exercises focused on balance control. Each exercise progressed from easy to difficult. Subjects attended the training program three times a week for five to seven weeks, and then once a week for the remainder of the season. The results showed that subjects significantly decreased their two-leg dynamic balance index, which may suggest an improvement in ability to maintain dynamic balance. The decreased two-leg dynamic balance index was retained one year after the start of the training program. The results also showed that left knee isokinetic flexion strength at 240°/sec was significantly increased after training. This increase was retained one year after the start of the training program.

Paterno and colleagues (2004) also studied the effects of balance training in young female athletes. They recruited 41 healthy female high school athletes as subjects and provided a six-week neuromuscular training program that included (1) balance training and hip-pelvis-trunk strengthening, (2) plyometrics and dynamic movement training, and (3) resistance training exercises. The single-leg postural stability of each subject was evaluated using a Biodex Stability System before and after the training program. This study showed that the subjects significantly improved anterior-posterior stability control but not medial-lateral stability control for both the right and left legs after the training program. The results also demonstrated that subjects had better postural stability control with their right leg than with their left leg.

Plyometric Versus Balance and Proprioception Training Programs Myer et al. (2006a) further studied the effects of plyometric exercise and of dynamic stabilization and balance exercises on the lower extremity motion pattern. They separated the plyometric components and the balance exercises in their comprehensive training program (Myer et al. 2005b) into two individual training programs and compared the effects of these two programs on lower extremity motion patterns in two drop-landing tasks. Eighteen female high school volleyball players were randomly assigned to either a plyometric or a balance training group. Both plyometric and balance training programs included a set of resistance exercises. All subjects significantly decreased hip adduction angle and ankle eversion angle during a drop vertical jump task and knee abduction angle during a medial drop-landing task. Additionally, subjects in the plyometric training group significantly increased knee flexion angle during the drop vertical jump task but did not significantly change knee flexion angle during the medial drop-landing task (figures 12.1 & 12.2). In contrast, subjects in the balance training group significantly increased knee flexion angle during the medial drop-landing task but did not significantly change knee flexion angle during the drop vertical jump task (figure 12.3). The knee valgus and varus moments before and after training were not compared in this study.

Landing Technique Training Programs

Landing technique training may also assist in altering lower extremity motion patterns. Prapavessis and McNair (1999) studied the effects of instruction in landing techniques on peak vertical ground reaction force during a vertical drop landing. Ninety-one subjects were randomly assigned to a training group with sensory feedback or a training group with augmented feedback. The purpose of training was to reduce the vertical ground reaction force during landing and to determine if sensory feedback reduces landing force. Subjects in the sensory

Maximum Knee Flexion Angle (deg)

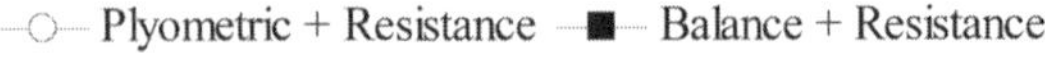

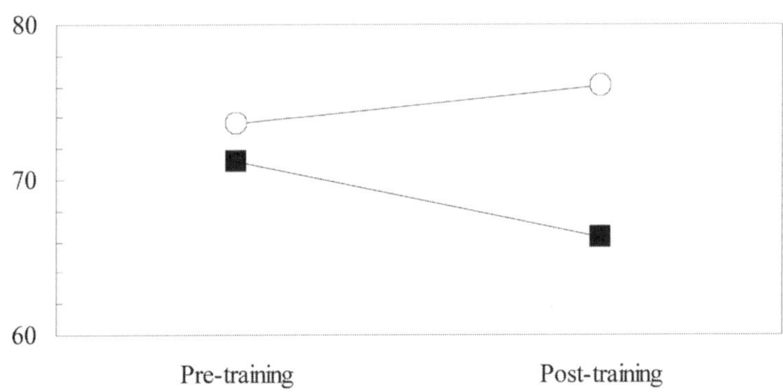

FIGURE 12.1 Effects of plyometric and balance training programs on maximum knee flexion angle during a vertical drop-landing jump task. Subjects significantly increased knee flexion angular displacement after plyometrics plus resistance training, but did not significantly change this knee kinematic measure after the balance plus resistance training program.

Adapted, by permission, from G.D. Myer et al. 2006, "The effects of plyometric versus dynamic stabilization and balance training on lower extremity biomechanics," *Am J Sports Med* 34(3): 445-455.

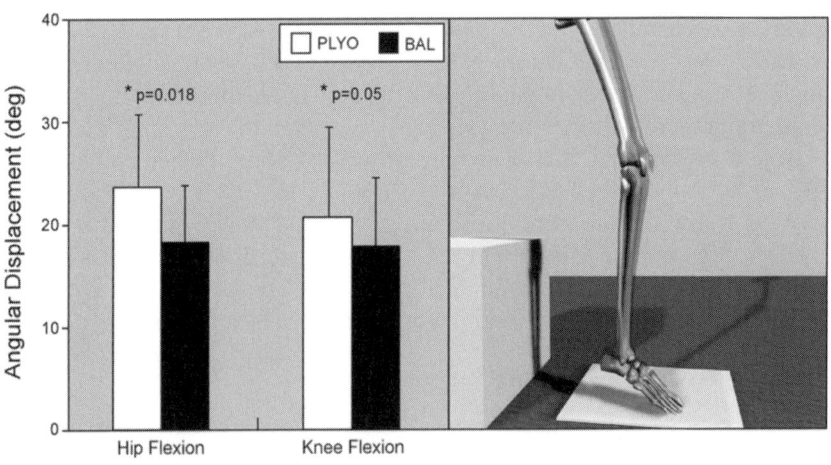

FIGURE 12.2 Increased knee flexion angle with both plyometric and balance training.

Adapted, by permission, from G.D. Myer et al. 2006, "The effects of plyometric versus dynamic stabilization and balance training on lower extremity biomechanics," *Am J Sports Med* 34(3): 445-455.

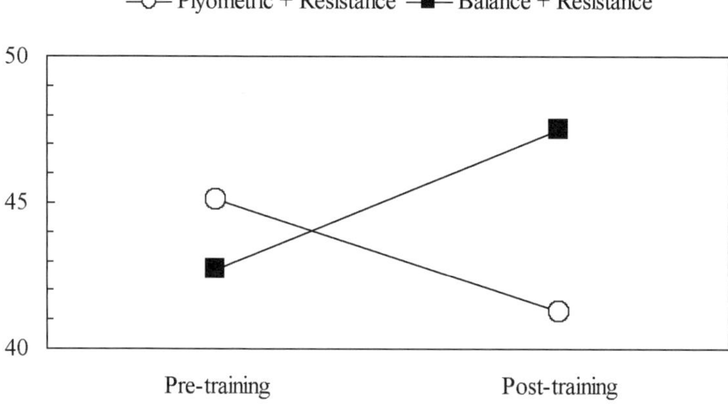

FIGURE 12.3 Effects of plyometric and balance training programs on maximum knee flexion angle during a medial drop-landing task. Subjects significantly increased their maximum knee flexion angle during the medial drop-landing task after the balance plus resistance training program, but did not significantly change this knee kinematic measure after the plyometric plus resistance training program.

Adapted, by permission, from G.D. Myer et al. 2006, "The effects of plyometric versus dynamic stabilization and balance training on lower extremity biomechanics," *Am J Sports Med* 34(3): 445-455.

feedback group were instructed to use their experience in their first landing as feedback to modify their landing techniques, while subjects in the augmented feedback group were given verbal instructions to modify their techniques to reduce vertical ground reaction force during landing. The results showed that subjects in the augmented feedback group significantly reduced their peak vertical ground reaction force during the landing after receiving feedback. In another study, McNair and colleagues (2000) further compared the effects of different feedback techniques on peak vertical ground reaction force during landing. They reported that verbal technical instructions and use of the sound of landing as feedback (auditory feedback) to modify landing techniques had the same effects in reducing peak vertical ground reaction force during landing. They also reported that the auditory feedback group reduced ground reaction forces and landing imagery techniques did not.

Onate and colleagues (2005) investigated the effects of using video images as feedback in landing technique training to reduce peak ground reaction force. Fifty-one subjects were randomly assigned to three training groups and a control group. The three training groups were designated expert technique feedback group, self-technique feedback group, and combined technique feedback group. The expert technique feedback group used a video image of an expert in landing as feedback to modify landing techniques to reduce ground reaction force. Subjects in the self-technique group used a videotape of their own landing techniques as feedback. Subjects in the combined technique feedback group used video images of an expert as well as their own landing techniques as feedback. All training groups and the control group increased their knee flexion motion and reduced peak vertical ground reaction force during a vertical drop landing after the training period and also retained the training effects. The results further demonstrated that the self-technique feedback group and combined technique feedback group increased knee flexion motion and reduced peak ground reaction force during landing more than did the expert technique feedback group and the control group.

Future Study of Training Programs Considerable research efforts have been directed toward determining the effects of training on lower extremity motion patterns. These pioneer studies provide preliminary understanding of training effects on lower extremity motion patterns and support the current concept of prevention of noncontact ACL injuries. This concept is based on two major hypotheses: (1) Altered lower extremity motion patterns are a risk factor for noncontact ACL injuries, and (2) lower extremity motion patterns in athletic tasks can be modified through training (Griffin et al. 2000). The current literature on training effects demonstrates that lower extremity motion patterns can be modified through certain types of physical and technical training programs. This forms the theoretical basis for future development of training programs to reduce the risk of sustaining noncontact ACL injuries.

The current literature regarding training effects on lower extremity motion patterns also forms the basis for future studies on this topic. Although this literature demonstrates that lower extremity motion patterns can be modified through physical and technical training, the specific training effects on lower extremity motion patterns remain unclear. The studies by Hewett and colleagues (1996) and Irmischer and colleagues (2004) indicate that plyometric training can reduce peak vertical ground reaction force during vertical drop landing. The study by Lephart and colleagues (2005), however, appears to suggest that plyometric exercises have little effect on peak vertical ground reaction force during vertical drop landing. The study by Myer and colleagues (2006a) showed differing effects of plyometric and dynamic stabilization on knee range of motion in different landing tasks (figures 12.1-12.3).

Further, most of the training programs studied consisted of multiple types of exercises, which prevents us from understanding the training effects of specific types of exercises on motion patterns. For example, the plyometric training program and the balance training program compared by Myer and colleagues (2005b) both had a resistance training component, while the plyometric training program and the resistance training program compared by Lephart and colleagues (2005) both had flexibility and balance exercise components. The inclusion and combination of different types of exercises in training programs make it difficult to differentiate the effects of different types of exercises on motion patterns.

In addition, although studies show that training modified lower extremity motion patterns in selected athletic tasks, the relevance of these altered patterns to risk of sustaining noncontact ACL injuries is not clear. The published literature shows that training programs improved dynamic balance (Holm et al. 2004); increased hip and knee flexion angles (Myer et al. 2006; Onate et al. 2005); and decreased knee valgus and varus moments (Myer et al. 2005b), peak vertical ground reaction force (Hewett et al. 1996; Prapavessis and McNair 1999; Irmischer et al. 2004; Onate et al. 2005), and knee flexion moment (Lephart et al. 2005) during landing tasks. The effects of the improved dynamic balance and the changes in lower extremity kinematics and kinetics on ACL loading have not been established experimentally. The gap between observed training effects on lower extremity motion patterns and reduction of the risk of sustaining noncontact ACL injuries still needs to be filled.

The training effect of a specific type of exercise on lower extremity motion patterns should be established with appropriate experimental designs in future studies. Appropriate control groups are important for determining the effect of specific types of exercises on lower extremity motion patterns or for comparing the effects of different types of exercises on these patterns. To determine the effects of specific types of exercises, an ideal control group should have no exercise at all, while each experimental group should have only one type of exercise. In the situation in which an ideal control group without any training is not feasible, the control group should have a basic set of exercises that each experimental group also performs. For a comparison of the effects of different types of exercises on lower extremity motion patterns, each comparison group should perform only one type of exercise if a no-exercise control group is not used. Appropriate experimental designs will assist in interpretation of the results and in determination of the actual effects of exercises on lower extremity motion patterns.

The relevance of training programs to reduction of the risk of sustaining noncontact ACL injuries can be established when the mechanisms and risk factors have been identified. Van Mechelen and colleagues (1992) described a four-step model of sport injury prevention research (figure 12.4). The first step is to identify the magnitude of the injury problem by determining the injury incidence and severity. The second step is to establish the etiology and mechanisms of the injury. The third step is to introduce prevention measures. The fourth step is to assess prevention measures by reevaluating the injury incidence and severity. Establishing the etiology and mechanisms of the injury is a critical step in this injury prevention research model (Bahr and Krosshaug 2005). This includes obtaining information on why a particular athlete or a group of athletes may be at risk in a given situation (risk factors) and on how injuries happen (injury mechanisms) (Bahr and Krosshaug 2005). This information is extremely important for developing evidence-based training programs to reduce the risk of sustaining a given sport injury and for understanding training effects. In the prevention of noncontact ACL injuries, although tremendous efforts have been made to establish the mechanisms of noncontact ACL injuries and to identify the risk factors, the injury mechanisms and risk factors are not perfectly clear. This means that future research is still needed to elucidate the effects of existing training programs or to develop new training programs to effectively reduce the risk.

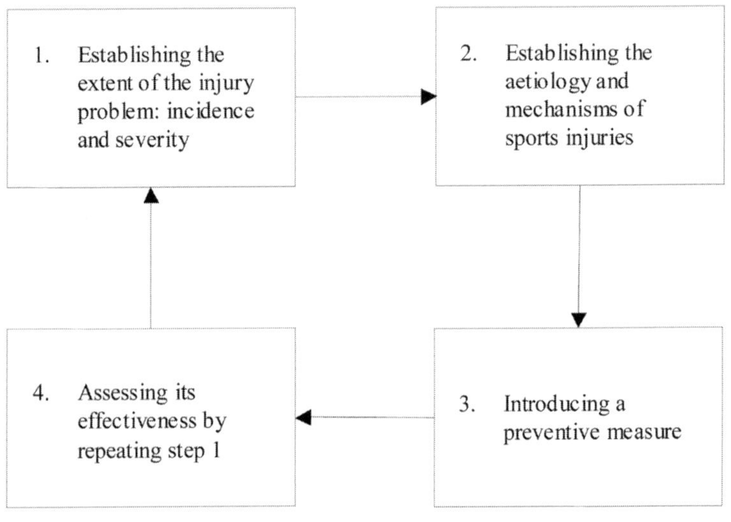

FIGURE 12.4 A four-step model of sport injury prevention research described by van Mechelen and colleagues (1992).

Adapted, by permission, from W. van Mechelen, H. Hlobil, and H.C. Kemper, 1992, "Incidence, severity, aetiology and prevention of sports injuries. A review of concepts," *Sports Medicine* 14(2): 82-99.

Chapter 13

Sport-Specific Injury Mechanisms Associated With Pivoting, Cutting, and Landing

Mary Lloyd Ireland, MD

> The athlete jumps, then lands awkwardly in an upright position perhaps a million times, but that one unfortunate time—pop goes the ACL. It only takes 70 milliseconds. (Yasuda et al. 1992)

Almost 80% of ACL injuries result from a noncontact mechanism (Noyes et al. 1983). Common positions of injury have been determined from observation of injury tapes (Boden et al. 2000). Seventy percent of ACL injuries occur during landing from a jump. Most are in the deceleration phase, which includes landing from a jump, decelerating to a stop or a change of direction (McLean et al. 1999).

In a prospective study, Hewett and colleagues (2005) evaluated neuromuscular control for 205 athletes playing the high risk sports of soccer, basketball, and volleyball. Nine of the 205 females had ACL injuries and were noted to have a different knee posture with knee abduction angle increased by 8°, 2.5 times greater knee abduction moment, and higher ground reaction forces with stance times 16% shorter. The overall result was an increase in motion force and more quickly acquired moments. This increase in dynamic valgus and hip abduction loads increases risk of ACL injuries. Development and implementation of neuromuscular control programs are necessary to reduce risk of lower extremity injury (Hewett et al. 2005).

In a study analyzing sidestep maneuvers, the ACL-injured knee position was valgus and rotation. Females had significantly larger valgus angles (McLean et al. 1999). McNair noted that ACL injuries occur when the knee is in an almost fully extended position, with the tibia rotating on the femur. Schematically, the femur internally rotates on a fixed tibia (figure 13.1) (Olsen et al. 2004; McNair et al. 1990). In a cadaver study of 37 knees, internal tibial torque was greatest in extension or full flexion. In skiing, the most dangerous position for ACL tears is full extension or full flexion when internal tibial torque is at a maxium.

The quadriceps activity and rotated femoral tibial position with knee extended are typical in ACL tears. Typically the knee is in an extended position as the athlete lands from a jump or sidesteps or changes direction abruptly. It is difficult for reviewers of videotapes to agree totally on factors such as degrees of hip and knee flexion, knee angle, and valgus versus varus tibial rotation. However, the consensus of experts reviewing recorded ACL injuries was that the knee was in valgus relative to an extended knee and hip and that body momentum was backward. The consensus of the researchers reviewing the injury video was that the knee was most frequently less than 30° flexed in valgus, with external rotation of the foot relative to the knee. The center of gravity is behind the knee on landing a jump or stopping a run (Teitz 2001). The question remains: When does the ACL tear occur?

The mechanism of ACL injury is caught with video during live action and not in gait labs live action. On the field, movement patterns can be planned or reactive and influenced by external forces, including time left in the game, score, playing offense versus defense, fear or anticipation of someone coming in to block or steal

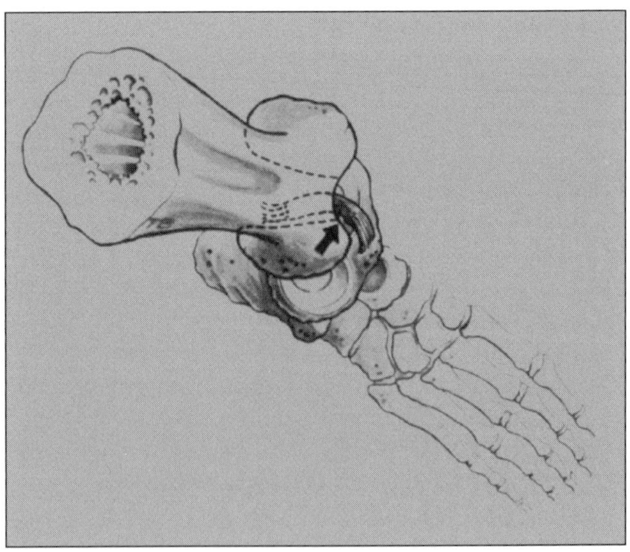

FIGURE 13.1 Possible mechanism of ACL rupture. Tibial rotation added to forceful quadriceps contraction in a valgus position may cause impingement of the ACL on the femoral condyle.

Illustration by Tommy Bolic. Reprinted, by permission, from R. Bahr, S. Maehlum, (eds.), *Idrettsskader* (Oslo, Norway: Gazette Bok.)

the ball. Attempts to combine athlete's recollection of ACL injury and video analysis are helpful. Bahr advocates a multifactorial approach to understand all factors contributing to an ACL injury (Bahr and Krosshaug 2005). This includes player interview, inciting events, and description of body and joint alignment. Thirty-five healthy high school basketball athletes (18 males and 17 females) underwent analysis of knee during planned and reactive jump start tasks in three different directions (Sell et al. 2006). Lateral jumps were found to be more dangerous than stop jumps. Compared to males, female subjects in reactive jumps had less knee flexion, greater maximum knee valgus, and greater shear forces and knee moments. Reactive jumps were different than planned jumps, suggesting problems in comparison of basic gait lab situations to playing field scenarios. In the design of research projects, the appropriate tasks as done in the sport must be included, for example directional reactive versus planned tasks (Sell et al. 2006).

Gender Comparisons

Athlete interviews should be detailed and should employ the standard vocabulary of assessment of sport injuries. This includes external and internal factors and history of the specific conditions experienced by the athlete at the time of the ACL tear. Specifically, the athlete describes the playing situation, field position, player and opponent behavior, whole-body joint kinematics, and kinetics of the injury (Olsen et al. 2004). In sports demanding rapid direction change, the mechanism of injury by athlete description or observation is predictable. The athlete is not hit directly on her knee but is perturbed or agitated as she goes to do a complex task, usually in a game. Even the other athletes on the court or field know the ACL injury drill—rapidly decelerate, feel or hear a pop, fall down on back, grab knee to chest, then scream.

The 70 millisecond time frame for tearing the ACL, as well as the unlikelihood that video is running in a frontal sagittal plane to allow analysis of body and leg position and subsequent forces, makes it difficult to determine the exact time at which the ACL tears and the position of the upper body, lumbar spine, hip, knee, ankle, and foot. Coaches teach athletes to stay in a get-down or flexed knee, hip position in basketball for guarding or for jumping. Landing lighter in a more flexed hip and flexed knee position protects the ACL. In video analysis of athletes tearing their ACL, in basketball the athlete is typically upright, with all weight on the injured limb, and the foot is fixed typically in pronation, resulting in limb malrotation. In extension, the knee dislocates, and the tibia is anteriorly translated and internally rotated, then self-reduces as the athlete flexes the knee. This standing pivot shift maneuver correlates well with the magnetic resonance imaging bone bruise pattern of the midlateral femoral condyle and posterolateral tibial plateau. The concept of position of safety and position of no return is based on observation of mechanism of injury (Ireland, Gaudette, and Crook 1997) (figure 13.2).

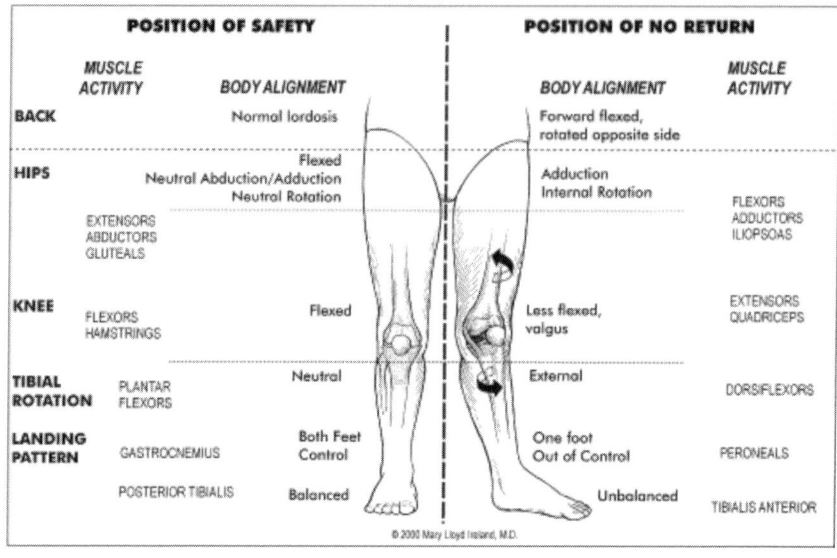

FIGURE 13.2 This diagram shows the "position of no return." This term refers to an awkward out-of-control landing with the leg pronated in valgus angulation, the body more upright and the leg in pronation and external rotation, and the knee in valgus angulation, which places the ACL at risk of tearing. In the high-risk landing position, the trunk is upright; the pelvis is more anteriorly rotated and subsequently the lower extremity is malrotated, the knee is in valgus, and ACL injury is more likely. The safety position is more flexed, with the body over the knees and knees over feet with greater balance and control.

The knee is the victim of poor proximal position of the lumbar spine and hip in sports demanding rapid stops and momentum changes. In an upright posture, the awkward landing drives more distal limb malrotation (femur internal and adducted, knee valgus). Due to the joint position and 70 milliseconds time to tear the ACL, the muscles which work to protect the ACL fail and anterior tibial translation occurs. The ACL protective muscles are the two joint hamstrings and hip abductors and external rotators. The two joint muscle quadriceps and hip adductors and flexors contribute to ACL tear. ACL injuries rarely occur in weak lower extremity muscled individuals.

Definitions of Mechanism of Injury

There are four ACL injury mechanisms: noncontact-perturbated, totally noncontact, contact, and skiing. In skiing, the mechanism is unique to that sport, typically involving falling backward after landing from a jump, with quadriceps contraction causing anterior tibial translation (Ettlinger, Johnson, and Shealy 1995; Johnson and Ettlinger 1982; McConkey 1986; Speer et al. 1995). The tail of the ski points in the direction of the foot (phantom foot ACL injury mechanism). The position is hips below knees, upper body downhill, and weight on inside edge of downhill ski (figure 13.3) (Ettlinger, Johnson, and Shealy 1995).

The contact mechanism and sudden ACL tear in an athlete, out-of-the-blue, running-downfield noncontact are more common mechanisms of ACL

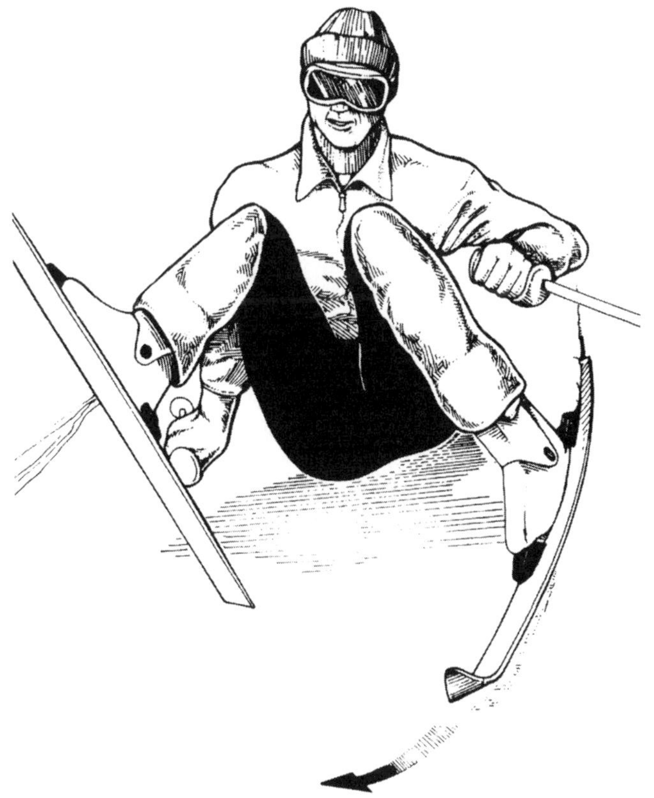

FIGURE 13.3 "Because this injury involves the tail of the ski, a lever that points in a direction opposite that of the human foot, we have termed this mechanism of injury the phantom-foot ACL injury mechanism and believe it to be the most common and insidious ACL injury scenario in alpine skiing today. In all the cases we have observed in our video analysis, the skier is off balance to the rear, with all his or her weight on the inside edge of the tail of the downhill ski and the uphill ski unweighted. The hips are below the knees with the upper body generally facing the downhill ski. The uphill arm is back and the injury is sustained in each case by the downhill leg."

Illustration courtesy of Vermont Safety Research.

tear. Anterior cruciate ligaments are most commonly torn in a noncontact way with perturbation or agitation from an external or internal force. Athlete description is key. Someone is guarding the athlete, going to block him, run down the ball—and awkward movement results in an ACL tear. The perturbation is an agitation or distraction from some external or internal influence. If mechanisms are documented, specific instruction on movement in the sport and strengthening and proprioception preparation programs can be designed for each sport.

Soccer

The typical soccer mechanism of injury involves a rapid change in direction, the cleat rapidly engaging the field, and valgus knee rotation at the hip. Obviously no jumping is involved (Heidt et al. 2000). More often than in basketball or team handball, the athlete may be just running downfield and tear the ACL without any external perturbation forces. Certainly in soccer there is a foot dominance, and specific athlete description of the mechanism of injury should include the planted foot, the kick foot, and the perturbating factors in that particular play.

Three hundred female soccer athletes underwent a seven-week preseason conditioning program and then were followed for injuries during the season. Although there were not enough ACL injuries to reach statistical significance, lower extremity injuries were significantly reduced in the trained versus the untrained group ($P = 0.0085$) (Heidt et al. 2000). Anterior cruciate ligament injuries in soccer are reported to occur due to several factors: equipment (type of shoe and shin guards), playing surface (grass vs. artificial turf), rules (sportspersonship and adherence to rules), and player factors (joint instability, muscle tightness, conditioning, and rehabilitation) (Ekstrand and Gillquist 1983). Assessment of these factors should be documented in preparticipation physicals, as well as injury mechanism, to allow better analysis of causes of lower extremity injuries.

Team Handball

In studies by Myklebust on mechanisms of ACL injury in 115 male and female handball athletes, 95% and 89% of players reported that no player-to-player contact was associated with their injuries (Myklebust et al. 1997, 1998). Injuries occurred in a movement that they had done numerous times before. We need a standardized, more detailed questionnaire for the athletes regarding the perceived mechanism and playing conditions in order to stratify the factors contributing to ACL injury, at least from the athlete perspective.

Detailed video analysis of injury mechanisms for 20 athletes sustaining ACL injuries in team handball was reported by Olsen and colleagues (2004). The evaluators were three physicians and three national team coaches. The injury mechanism was forceful valgus collapse with the knee close to full extension, combined with external or internal rotation of the tibia. The variables assessed in the video were foot and knee position at foot strike, time of ACL rupture, movement direction at the time of injury, and weight distribution of percentage body weight on injured leg. The two main injury situations were plant and cut (12 cases); four of these were two-footed and eight were one-footed push-offs and one-legged landing from a jump (four cases). The proposed mechanism of ACL rupture was foot planted with tibia in external rotation and femoral internal rotation with quadriceps contraction (see figure 13.1). In fewer degrees of flexion, the quadriceps and knee moments can result in anterior tibial translation and hence the mechanism of standing pivot shift. The question posed by Olsen is whether the valgus collapse observed in the videos is actually the cause of the injury or whether it occurs after the ACL is torn. Most likely when the knee is in extreme valgus, in an action much like that of a whip, the femur internally rotates on a planted foot, and the tibia externally rotates. Whether the quadriceps musculature causes the tear or the biomechanical forces (including tibial slope and anterior shear) cause the pivot shift remains controversial.

Basketball

The incidence of ACL injuries in female compared to male basketball athletes at the collegiate level from 1989 to 2002 was 3.38 (female-to-male ratio) and for soccer was 2.75 (NCAA 2002). At Kentucky Sports Medicine, over a 14-year period of ACL reconstructions performed on basketball players, 67% of the females were high school age and 39% of the males were high school age. In the postcollege age group (>23 years), 41% were males and only 6% were females (Crook and Ireland 2005). In basketball athletes, there is a 3% failure rate and a 6% rate of ACL injury on the opposite side (personal communication, unpublished Kentucky Sports Medicine data).

The easiest sport in which to capture ACL tears on video is basketball. Unfortunately, the cameras on courts and fields do not show frontal and sagittal planes as in the laboratory. The athlete in figure 13.4 rebounds from a shot and comes down awkwardly, thinking about turning back to put up another shot, and is perturbated by the defender. Injury has definitely occurred by the fourth frame and possibly already by the third frame. In the "position of no return," a combination of moments in torque with the hip adducted and internally rotated, foot planted in a rapid stop in this poor body position creates the situation for ACL injury. Neuromuscular control cannot occur rapidly enough to prevent ACL tear (Ireland, Gaudette, and Crook 1997). The relationship of hip strength, specifically abduction, external rotation to lower extremity injuries and patellofemoral pain has been reported (Ireland et al. 2003).

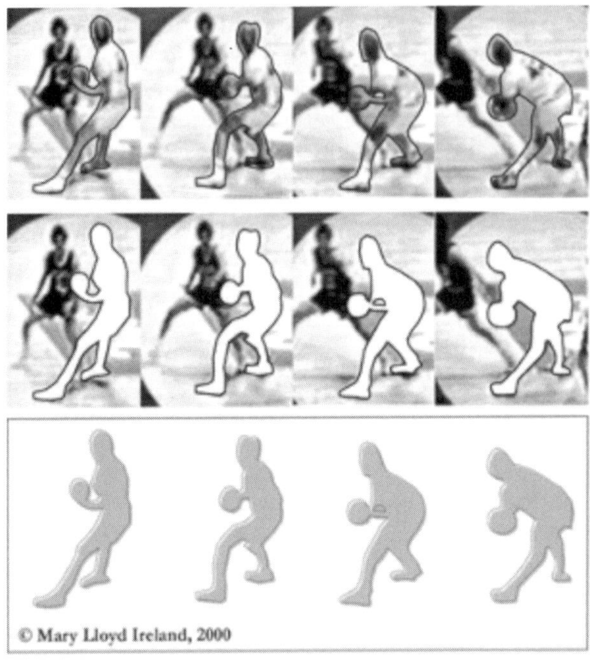

FIGURE 13.4 Analysis by videotape—basketball athlete. Injury to the left knee as observed from the back and left side of the athlete. She has just rebounded and stops to change direction to avoid the defending player. She lands in an upright position with less knee and hip flexion, and forward-flexed lumbar spine. After the ACL fails, she falls forward and knee valgus rotation and flexion increase. She is unable to upright herself and regain pelvis control to avoid ACL injury.
© 2000 Mary Lloyd Ireland, MD.

Gender Differences

Collegiate athlete numbers continue to rise (table 13.1). Unfortunately, the rate of noncontact ACL injury in females remains significantly higher in sports demanding rapid stops, cuts, and change in direction (basketball, soccer, team handball; Ireland 2005). When one looks at the NCAA participants and includes football, ratios are 1.3:1. If football is excluded, ratios are 1:1.

Conclusions

The work of Hewett's group (1999) was instrumental in our understanding of knee injury patterns. Further research needs to be done so that coaches can better understand the cues players need to hear during practice (jumping straight as an arrow, landing light as a feather). Analysis of injury must include

TABLE 13.1 2003-2004 NCAA Participants[a]

	Women	M:W ratio	Men	Men playing football	M (football): W ratio	Men w/o football	Total
Div I	69,768	1.2	86,826	25,363	0.9	61,463	156,594
Div II	31,725	1.5	46,662	14,206	1.0	32,456	78,387
Div III	61,259	1.4	83,821	20,411	1.0	63,410	145,080
Total	162,752	1.3	217,309	59,980	1.0	157,329	380,061

[a]Overall numbers and gender ratios—with and without men's football.

body position, momentum, joint position, activity on court or field, and joint angles of flexion-extension and rotation.

The question remains: What are the risk factors for ACL injury? Until the risk factors can be determined and ranked, prevention programs, although they do appear to be working, remain the black box. If the factors responsible for ACL tears are unknown, then we cannot state what has changed. Prospective studies on risk factors are necessary to answer this question.

The literature on risk factors with prospective study designs has been reviewed (Murphy, Connolly, and Beynnon 2003). The risk factors for lower extremity injury were divided into extrinsic and intrinsic. The extrinsic factors evaluated were level of competition, skill level, shoe type, ankle bracing, and playing surface; the intrinsic factors were age, days of the menstrual cycle, previous injury and inadequate rehabilitation, aerobic fitness, body size, limb dominance, flexibility (generalized joint laxity and ankle and knee joint laxity, muscle tightness, range of motion), muscle strength, imbalance, reaction time, limb girth, anatomic alignment, and hand and foot morphology. Regarding ACL injuries, the risks are being female, having had a previous ACL injury followed by inadequate rehabilitation, having a narrow femoral intercondylar notch width, competing in games compared to practice sessions, and wearing edge-type cleats compared to other cleat designs. More multiple-center prospective studies are needed to determine the risk factors.

A better understanding of ACL mechanisms will allow specific strengthening and proprioception programs to be analyzed for relative risk. A risk ratio from ranking of risk factors can then be established. Coaches can then better understand positions of safety and implement strengthening programs to avoid the risky positions and situations leading to ACL injury. Several ACL research retreats have been held. In these retreats, researchers present their work and participate in a think tank to assess the present knowledge base—what we know and what we don't know (McClay-Davis and Ireland 2001, 2003). These ACL research retreats have focused on the gender bias. Hunt Valley I and II have helped elucidate factors involved in ACL injuries from the basic science to the clinical level (Griffin and Gael 2000; Griffin et al. In press-a).

Chapter 14

Effects of Muscle Firing on Neuromuscular Control and ACL Injury

Timothy Edwin Hewett, PhD, FACSM
Bohdanna T. Zazulak, DPT, MS, OCS
Gregory D. Myer, MS, CSCS

Deficits in dynamic neuromuscular control of joint stability in all planes of motion along the entire lower extremity kinetic chain may contribute to differences in ACL injury rates between female and male athletes. The contribution of relative muscle activation levels to this important clinical dilemma is not yet delineated. Lack of dynamic neuromuscular (active restraint) control of the knee is an important contributor to ACL (passive restraint to tibiofemoral motion) injury in female athletes (Hewett et al. 2005a). Anterior cruciate ligament injury likely occurs under conditions of high dynamic loading of the knee joint when active muscular restraints do not adequately dampen joint loads, subjecting the passive restraints to increased loads (Beynnon and Fleming 1998). Decreased neuromuscular control of the joint may place increased stress on the passive ligament structures, exceeding the failure strength of the ligament (Markolf, Graff-Radford, and Amstutz 1978; Li et al. 1999). Neuromuscular recruitment patterns that compromise active joint restraints subject passive joint restraints to greater load, decrease dynamic knee stability, and increase risk of ACL injury (Li et al. 1999; Besier et al. 2001a; Besier et al. 2001b).

Female athletes demonstrate different neuromuscular strategies than do male athletes when performing activities that are related to ACL injury (Rozzi et al. 1999; Wojtys, Ashton-Miller, and Huston 2002; Zazulak et al. 2005; Myer et al. 2005; Olsen et al. 2004). These gender differences in muscle recruitment strategies may affect dynamic knee stability. Preplanned neuromuscular engrams may facilitate the desirable feedforward recruitment of the musculature that controls knee joint positioning during landing and pivoting maneuvers (Besier et al. 2001a; Besier et al. 2001b). Imbalanced or inappropriately timed neuromuscular firing may lead to lower extremity alignment during athletic maneuvers that puts the ACL under increased strain and risk of injury in female athletes (Myer et al. 2005; Malinzak et al. 2001; Chappell et al. 2002; Ford, Myer, and Hewett 2003; Hewett, Myer, and Ford 2004; McLean and Huang 2004; Hewett et al. 2005a).

Altered neuromuscular timing and recruitment may lead to the dynamic lower extremity valgus commonly observed in female athletes during tasks related to ACL injury (Malinzak et al. 2001; Chappell et al. 2002; Ford, Myer, and Hewett 2003; Hewett, Myer, and Ford 2004; McLean, Huang, et al. 2004; Hewett et al. 2005a). Measures of dynamic valgus (knee abduction torque) predict noncontact ACL injury risk in female athletes with a sensitivity of 73% and a specificity of 78% (Hewett et al. 2005a). In addition, computer simulation modeling demonstrates that lower extremity valgus loads at the knee are high enough to rupture the ACL (McLean, Huang, et al. 2004). Thus it appears salient to determine the neuromuscular control strategies that facilitate dynamic lower extremity valgus alignment in female athletes. Once this has been determined, the potential interventional protocols can be instituted to help improve neuromuscular control strategies in high-risk female athletes.

Dynamic neuromuscular restraints to lower extremity joint motion include both feedforward and feedback motor control loops (Lephart et al. 2002b). Feedforward neuromuscular activation may preactivate muscles around the joint prior to excessive loading. This mechanism may appropriate forces and decrease stress on the passive restraints at the knee (Beard et al. 1993). Feedback or reactive motor control strategies alter muscle activation in response to situations that load the lower extremity joints (Dyhre-Poulsen et al. 1991). Females may demonstrate a longer latency period (i.e., electromechanical delay) between preparatory and reactive muscle activation than males (Winter and Brookes 1991). Preparatory muscle activity can stiffen joints prior to unexpected perturbations and may counteract increased latency in muscle activation (Dietz et al. 1981; Dyhre-Poulsen et al. 1991; Beard et al. 1993; Wojtys and Huston 1994).

Neuromuscular training that reproduces loads similar to those encountered during competitive sports may assist in the development of both feedforward and reactive muscle activation strategies to protect the knee joint from excessive load (Greenwood and Hopkins 1976; Dietz et al. 1981; Dunn et al. 1986; Dyhre-Poulsen et al. 1991; Winter and Brookes 1991; Thompson and McKinley 1995). Plyometric exercises teach athletes to respond to rapid loads with preparatory muscle tone prior to the joint load from the initial momentum. However, it may not be possible to modify the stretch receptors to activate in a preparatory way. They are sensitive to stretch that occurs when the joint begins to load during a plyometric activity. On the other hand, this stretch receptor mechanism may be in play if the antagonist at the joint is activating early to induce stretch. Balance and core stability exercises may facilitate the production of neuromuscular engrams that help the athlete to rapidly react to unwanted motions or unanticipated perturbations.

If neuromuscular training can increase neuromuscular control of the joint and decrease knee and ACL injury risk, it is likely that the mechanisms underlying the increased risk are neuromuscular in nature. Several prospective studies have demonstrated that neuromuscular training in athletes has the potential to decrease knee injuries in general and ACL injuries in particular (Hewett et al. 1999; Wedderkopp et al. 1999; Heidt et al. 2000; Soderman et al. 2000; Mandelbaum et al. 2005). Intensive short-term neuromuscular training may induce a "neuromuscular spurt" that may otherwise be absent in adolescent females (Hewett et al. 1996; Hewett, Myer, and Ford 2004; Myer et al. 2004a; Myer et al. 2004b). Training and strength differences may account for only a portion of the increased incidence of knee injury in female athletes, yet lowering these high figures by even a percentage could have a significant effect on the number of noncontact ACL injuries. Such training, if effectively implemented on a widespread basis, could help to significantly decrease the number of athletes injured each year.

Differences in EMG Activation Levels Between Males and Females

The evidence for altered muscular activation and timing relative to ACL injury risk in female athletes compared to male athletes may be summarized and categorized into segments and planes of the kinetic chain, which include proximal, anterior-posterior, medial-lateral, and distal lower extremity.

Proximal

Asymmetry of proximal muscle activation may alter the position of the knee in female athletes during landing and cutting. Decreased activation of the trunk and hip musculature may lead to high-risk lower extremity alignment that may decrease the potential for appropriate muscular response to joint load.

Asymmetry of proximal muscle activation may alter the position of the knee in female athletes during landing and cutting. Decreased activation of the trunk and hip musculature may lead to high-risk lower extremity alignment that may decrease the potential for appropriate muscular response to joint load. Zazulak et al. (AOSSM Specialty Day Meeting, San Diego California, 2005) prospectively measured 277 collegiate athletes (140F, 137M) for core stability and subsequently tracked three years for knee injury. Active trunk repositioning and trunk displacements in response to quick force release were measured. Deficits in trunk proprioception and trunk displacement were observed in females with knee, ligament, and ACL injuries compared to uninjured females. These findings suggest female athletes have decreased core stability and are at increased risk of knee injury.

Lephart and colleagues (2002b) reported that females have increased hip internal rotation during landing. Increased hip internal rotation with associated knee valgus may increase strain on the ACL (Markolf et al. 1995; Beynnon and Fleming 1998). Zazulak and colleagues (2005) reported lower gluteal electromyographic (EMG) activity in females compared to males during landing (figure 14.1). The proximal stabilizing muscles, specifically the gluteals, control lower limb alignment and aid in energy absorption during landing (Delp et al. 1999; Zazulak et al. 2005).

Chimera and colleagues (2004) evaluated the effects of plyometric training on muscle activation patterns during jump exercises and reported increased firing of the hip adductor muscles during the prelanding phase. The experimental group demonstrated greater preparatory adductor to abductor muscle activation. However, increased hip adductor activation would likely increase the propensity for lower extremity valgus alignment at landing. Therefore, this training regime may have done more harm than good. Other contradictory data are reported in the literature regarding proximal (hip) control of the knee

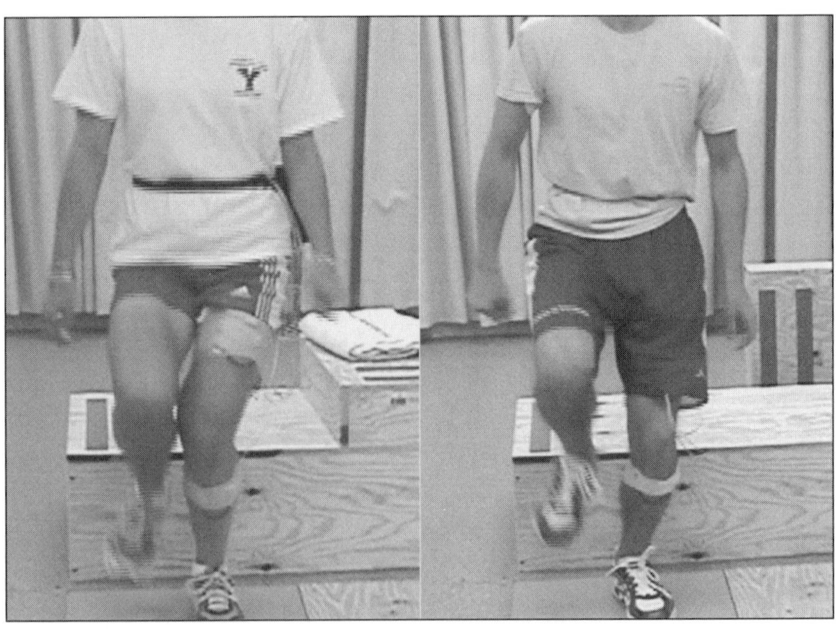

FIGURE 14.1 Visual representation of the landing maneuver tested in the study by Zazulak and colleagues (2005). Female (left) and male (right) subjects completing drop landings from 30.5 cm (12 in.) box height.

joint. Padua and colleagues (Padua 2006) found differences in trunk kinematics between male and female athletes at both the elite and recreational levels. These authors reported that the trunk was more extended in females and suggested that females should bend the trunk more during sporting activities. However, increased trunk flexion may not be a more mechanically advantageous position for female athletes to assume. These findings provide evidence for the role of hip muscular activation in dynamic restraint and control of lower extremity alignment.

Anterior-Posterior

Female athletes demonstrate increased activation of the quadriceps relative to the antagonistic hamstring musculature (Malinzak et al. 2001; Wojtys et al. 1996). This disproportional recruitment of the quadriceps musculature increases anterior shear force at the low knee flexion angles that occur during high-risk landing and pivoting movements (Markolf et al. 1995; Myer et al. 2005). The quadriceps, through the anterior pull of the patellar tendon on the tibia, contribute to ACL loading when knee flexion is less than 45° (Renstrom et al. 1986; Markolf et al. 1995). Training interventions that improve muscular cocontraction during dynamic tasks may facilitate joint compression, which may protect the ACL against anterior drawer (Imran and O'Connor 1997).

Zazulak and colleagues reported increased peak quadriceps activity in females compared to males, as shown in figure 14.2 (Zazulak et al. 2005). Decreased balance in strength and recruitment of the flexor relative to the extensor musculature is observed in female athletes and may contribute to their greater risk of ACL injury (Hewett et al. 1996). Improved strength of knee flexors may balance contraction of the quadriceps during landing, helping the athlete to

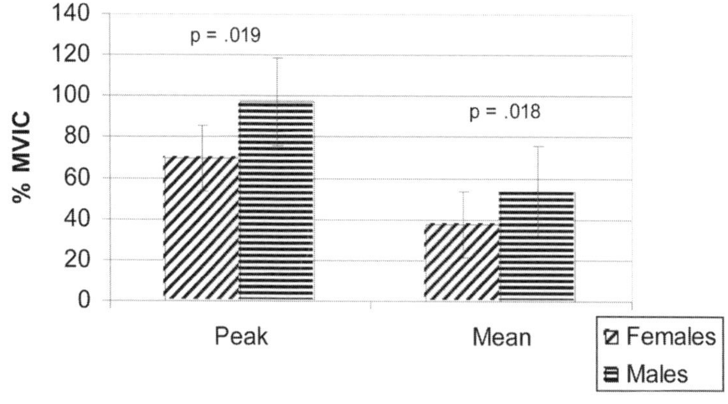

FIGURE 14.2 Rectus femoris precontact ensemble peak and ensemble mean EMG values, females versus males (means ± 1.96 SE).

better control high knee extension and abduction torques (Hewett et al. 1996). Appropriate hamstrings recruitment may prevent the loads necessary to rupture the ACL during maneuvers that place the athlete at risk for an injury.

Urabe and colleagues recently (2005) reported that hamstring:quadriceps (H:Q) ratios were greater in male compared to female athletes. In agreement with Zazulak and colleagues (2005), they found that increased quadriceps activity was not balanced by antagonistic hamstring activity in the female athlete. Padua and colleagues (2005) further support the quadriceps-dominant muscle activity pattern in female athletes. These authors reported that during hopping there was greater quadriceps activity and a decreased hamstrings-to-quadriceps coactivation ratio in females compared to males (Padua, Distefano, et al. 2005). This decreased relative hamstrings to quadriceps activity may play an important role in dynamic lower extremity alignment, especially related to control of valgus and varus loads at the knee (Lloyd 2001).

Medial-Lateral

Joint compression through muscular cocontraction allows valgus loads to be carried by articular contact forces, thus protecting the ligaments (Lloyd 2001). Decreased medial joint compression may limit passive resistance to dynamic knee valgus, predisposing the female knee to medial femoral condylar liftoff and increased loads on the ACL (Kim et al. 1995; Lloyd 2001; Ford, Myer, and Hewett 2003). Rozzi and colleagues (1999) reported that female athletes demonstrate a disproportionate (four times greater) firing of their lateral hamstrings than medial hamstrings during landing. Myer and colleagues (2005) demonstrated a decreased ratio of medial to lateral quadriceps recruitment in females (figure 14.3). Thus an unbalanced or low ratio of medial to lateral quadriceps recruitment may combine with increased lateral hamstring firing to compress the lateral joint, open the medial joint, and increase anterior shear force (Rozzi et al. 1999; Sell et al. 2004; Myer et al. 2005).

Together, these neuromuscular imbalances may increase the potential for dynamic valgus when athletes are in high-risk positions (Ford, Myer, and Hewett 2003; Ford et al. 2005). Repeated performance of the high-risk maneuvers with insufficient neuromuscular control and dynamic valgus may lead to the valgus collapse and ACL rupture (Teitz 2001; Boden et al. 2000; Hewett et al. 2005a). Markolf and colleagues (1995) showed that muscular contraction can decrease both the valgus and varus laxity of the knee threefold. Thus, interventions designed to improve balance with synergistic and antagonistic recruitment strategies may aid with active control of medial-lateral joint loads at the knee. Myer and colleagues (2006b) demonstrated that both plyometric and dynamic stabilization training were effective at improving balance in knee flexor relative to knee extensor strength. The improved balance in lower extremity strength may have been related to the concurrent improvement in medial-lateral ground reaction force control and decreased lower extremity valgus control in the coronal plane (Myer et al. 2006a, 2006b). Improved

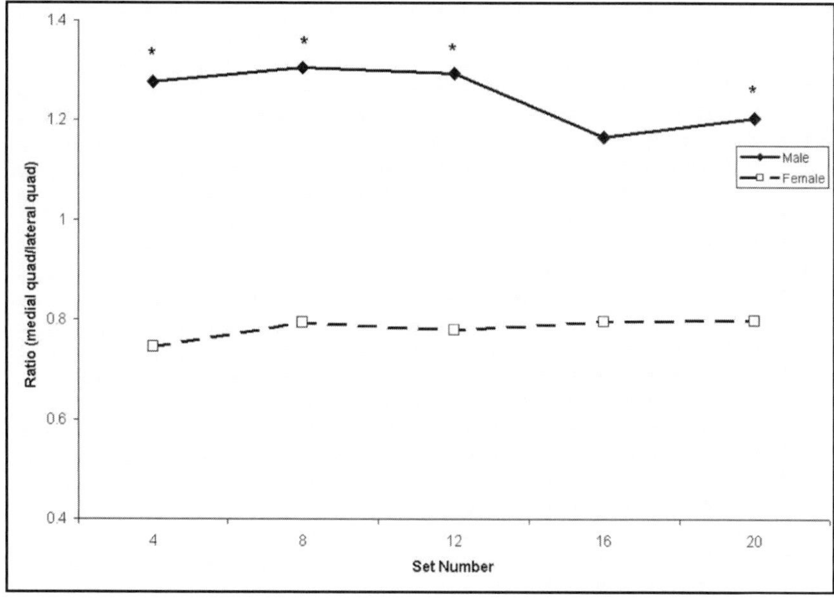

FIGURE 14.3 Root mean square ratio of medial to lateral quadriceps activation during performance of exercise sets. Females demonstrated significantly decreased medial-lateral quadriceps activation.

coronal plane control may reduce injury risk in female athletes (Hewett et al. 1999, 1996, 2005a).

Distal

Recruitment of the ankle and calf musculature may play an important role in the dynamic stabilization of the knee joint (Besier et al. 2001a; Beynnon and Fleming 1998; and Nyland 1997). At relatively low knee flexion angles the soleus appears to act as an agonist of the ACL. However, at low knee flexion angles, in the range of 5° to 10°, the gastrocnemius may function as an antagonist to the ACL. At greater knee flexion angles, both of these muscles may function as agonists to the ACL. For example, Besier and colleagues (2001a) reported selective activation of the medial knee musculature, including the medial gastrocnemius, that was associated with increased valgus and external rotation moments during sidestep maneuvers. Padua and colleagues (2005) observed greater soleus activity in female athletes during hopping. In addition, Nyland and colleagues (1997) concluded that compensatory gastrocnemius muscle activity increased dynamic knee stabilization following quadriceps fatigue. However, following injury, ACL-deficient females may demonstrate decreased activation of the lateral gastrocnemius prior to limb loading (DeMont et al.

1999). The role that distal musculature plays in loading and or protecting the ACL is still unclear and remains a fertile area for future research.

Lower extremity muscle activation generally follows a distal to proximal firing pattern (Nashner 1977; Shultz et al. 2000). Shultz and colleagues (2000) evaluated the protective neuromuscular response and activation patterns to an imposed perturbation during weight-bearing stance (i.e., a sudden forward and either internal or external rotation moment of the trunk and femur). The gastrocnemius fired faster than the hamstring, which fired faster than the quadriceps. This activation pattern is similar to the postural response reported by Nashner, specifically a distal to proximal firing pattern, with the distal muscles preceding the proximal muscles by 10 to 15 msec. This distal to proximal firing pattern may have a significant effect on dynamic lower extremity joint alignment, as it may provide the initial response's ground reaction force vectors at contact during landing or cutting. Myer and colleagues (2006a) utilized neuromuscular training to reduce ankle eversion angles, which were matched with improved proximal control of lower extremity valgus alignment during the same landing task.

Timing of Muscle Firing

Electromyographic studies demonstrate gender-related differences in the timing of muscle activation during athletic movement (Wojtys et al. 1996; Rozzi et al. 1999; Besier et al. 2001a; Besier et al. 2001b; Cowling and Steele 2001; Besier et al. 2003; Myer et al. 2005; Zazulak et al. 2005). Zazulak and colleagues (2005) reported increased peak quadriceps activity in females during the precontact phase of landing. Greater rectus femoris activity was observed in females compared to males (see figure 14.2). Increased activation of the quadriceps musculature in females may increase strain on the ACL during landing. Increased quadriceps activity, combined with decreased hamstring activity, may alter muscular energy absorption during landing and may increase ground reaction forces and torques associated with increased risk of ACL injury (Hewett et al. 2005c).

Huston and Wojtys reported that female athletes have a slower response of hamstring activation to anterior stress on the ACL (Huston and Wojtys 1996). However, Cowling and Steele reported gender differences in muscle activation strategies in the hamstring musculature that contradict the findings of Huston and Wojtys (Cowling and Steele 2001). They found that males activated their semimembranosus muscle later than females in the prelanding phase and reached peak activity before females. Besier and colleagues (2001a) examined a sidestep cut at two different angles under both preplanned and unanticipated conditions. They found increased varus-valgus and internal-external knee moments during unanticipated movements and suggested that there may be increased potential for noncontact knee injuries during unanticipated sport movements.

Lower extremity muscle activation during cutting may be different between preplanned and unanticipated conditions (Besier et al. 2003). Besier and colleagues (2003) also reported that activation patterns during cutting maneuvers are initiated prior to load in preparation for varus-valgus and internal-external rotation moments at the knee. They found that the unanticipated sidestep condition increased muscle activation 10% to 25%, with the greatest increase before initial contact. Anterior cruciate ligament injuries may occur too quickly for reflexive or voluntary muscular activation; however, preactivation may reduce the probability of injuries caused by unexpected perturbations. The lower extremity musculature may be 40% to 80% activated at the time that the foot touches the ground (Neptune et al. 1999).

Core muscle activity occurs prior to extremity muscle activity during athletic tasks. Hodges and Richardson (1997) demonstrated that trunk muscle activity occurs before the activity of the lower extremity musculature. Specifically, the transversus abdominis was the first muscle to fire in preparation for lower extremity movement, immediately followed by the multifidus. The authors concluded that the central nervous system creates a stable foundation for movement of the lower extremities through cocontraction of the transversus abdominis and multifidus muscles. Cholewicki and Van Vliet (2002) reported that all the musculature of the trunk, including abdominal as well as back muscles, contribute to core stability with the relative contributions of each muscle continually changing throughout an athletic task. Zazulak and colleagues recently identified neuromuscular deficits of the trunk as prospective predictors of knee, ligament, and ACL injury in collegiate athletes (Zazulak et al., forthcoming). Decreased core muscle activity and control may place the lower extremity in high ACL risk position of increased hip adduction and femoral internal rotation and lower extremity valgus during athletic maneuvers.

There is evidence that neuromuscular training may alter lower extremity muscle activation in female athletes (Hurd et al. 2006). Hurd and colleagues examined the effects of perturbation training on the EMG activity of vastus lateralis, medial and lateral hamstrings, and medial gastrocnemius. Knee stiffness, as measured by muscle cocontraction, was calculated and reported during gait. These authors reported increased relative hamstrings to quadriceps activity and increased active knee stiffness during walking following the perturbation training protocol. The increased knee stiffness was a result of increased hamstring and gastrocnemius activity and altered timing of the firing of these muscles. However, it will be necessary to examine more extensively the contributions of these muscles during dynamic tasks similar to those that place the ACL at increased risk of injury.

Summary and Conclusions

Sex differences are observed in male and female EMG firing patterns. Decreased neuromuscular control of the trunk and lower extremity in females may increase the potential for valgus lower extremity position and increased ACL injury risk.

Identification of these neuromuscular imbalances has the potential for both screening for high-risk athletes and targeting interventions for specific deficits. Dynamic neuromuscular training can increase active knee stabilization and decrease the incidence of ACL injury in the female athletic population (Hewett et al. 1996, 1999; Myklebust et al. 2003; Myer et al. 2005b). Training may facilitate neuromuscular adaptations that provide increased joint stabilization and muscular preactivation and reactive patterns that protect the athlete's ACL from increased loading (Lloyd and Buchanan 1996; Solomonow and Krogsgaard 2001; Myer et al. 2005).

In conclusion, there is evidence that neuromuscular training alters muscle firing patterns as it decreases landing forces and reduces ACL injury risk in female athletes. Future directions will be to utilize EMG analysis to assess the relative efficacy of these interventions in order to achieve the optimal effect in the most efficient manner possible. Selective combination of neuromuscular training components may provide additive effects, further reducing the risk of ACL injuries in female athletes. Additional research directions include the assessment of relative injury risk utilizing mass neuromuscular screening. The development of screening and intervention protocols may lead to the reduction of ACL injury incidence in female athletes via identification of the high-risk female athlete subgroup that demonstrates decreased hip and increased quadriceps muscle firing, as well as to correction of these neuromuscular control deficits.

Chapter 15

Epidemiology and Mechanisms of ACL Injury in Alpine Skiing

Bruce D. Beynnon, PhD
Carl F. Ettlinger, MSME
Robert J. Johnson, MD

The Epidemiology of Alpine Skiing Injuries

There has been a decrease in the overall incidence of injuries in alpine skiing over time, and this is attributed to advances in the ski-binding-boot system. The overall incidence of ski injuries in North America has decreased from 5 to 8 injuries per 1000 skier days before the 1970s (Johnson, Pope, and Ettlinger 1974), to 3 to 4 injuries per 1000 skier days in the early and mid-1980s (Johnson, Ettlinger, and Shealy 1989; Shealy 1985) and to between 2 and 3 injuries per 1000 skier days in the late 1980s and early 1990s (Johnson, Ettlinger and Shealy 1997, 1993; Shealy 1993; Warme et al. 1995). In contrast, the incidence of severe knee injuries has increased dramatically since the early 1970s (Johnson, Ettlinger, and Shealy 1993; Johnson and Pope 1991). Although the medial collateral ligament (MCL) is the most frequently injured ligament of the knee, the ACL is injured in approximately 20% of all skiing injuries (Johnson, Ettlinger, and Shealy 1997; Johnson 1988; Warme et al. 1995). In our ongoing cohort study of injury trends associated with recreational alpine skiing at a moderately sized ski area in central Vermont, United States, we observed a 52% decline in the overall injury rate between 1972 and 2002 (Johnson, Ettlinger, and Shealy 2004). The majority of the decline was attributed to an 82% reduction in the incidence of lower extremity injuries such as fractures and sprains. In 1994, grade I and grade II knee sprains, usually involving the MCL, decreased by 64%; however, during the same time period, serious grade

III knee sprains, usually involving the ACL, increased significantly (228%). In a more recent study between 1990 and 2002, it was found in northern Vermont that there has been a statistically significant decrease in the risk of sustaining an ACL injury (Ettlinger, Johnson, and Shealy 2005). At its worst in the early 1990s the ACL injury rate was approximately 1 in 1900 skier visits and even though the rate has decreased significantly it is still 1 in 2747 skier visits.

Among competitive alpine skiers, we observed that the proportion of females to males sustaining a knee injury was 2.3 to 1 (Stevenson et al. 1998). In addition, in a recent study (1999-2002), female recreational skiers were 3.3 times more likely to have sustained an ACL disruption than their male counterparts (Johnson, Shealy, and Ettlinger 2005). There is no doubt that rupture of the ACL is one of the most common serious medical problems associated with recreational and competitive alpine skiing (Johnson, Ettlinger, and Shealy 1997).

It has been shown by our group that sprains and fractures of the lower leg are related to measurable or observable qualities of the release system (ski bindings) whereas injuries to the ACL are not (Ettlinger, Johnson, and Shealy 2005; Diebert et al. 1998; Ettlinger, Johnson, and Shealy 1995; Johnson, Ettlinger, and Shealy 2003; Shealy, Ettlinger, and Johnson 2003; Ettlinger, Johnson, and Shealy 2003). Currently, modern ski equipment does not have the capability to reduce the risk of ACL injuries sustained by downhill skiers.

While the high rate of ACL injuries associated with alpine skiing is discouraging, there is reason to be optimistic that these serious injuries can be reduced through education programs. A recent study by our group showed that the risk of ACL injuries among experienced skiing professionals (ski patrollers and ski instructors) can be reduced by 62% through participation in the ACL Awareness Training Program (Ettlinger, Johnson, and Shealy 1995). Attempts to adapt this program to the general skiing population are being made, but the effects of these efforts to date have not been completely successful.

ACL Injury Mechanisms Associated With Alpine Skiing

Through analysis of the Vermont database and with the aid of videotapes of skiers experiencing ACL injuries, the most common ACL injury mechanisms in alpine skiing have been identified (Ettlinger, Johnson, and Shealy 1995; Johnson 1988; Elmqvist and Johnson 1994). They can be divided into two categories, the boot-induced anterior drawer mechanism and flexion-internal rotation.

Boot-Induced Anterior Drawer Mechanism of ACL Injury

In the boot-induced anterior drawer injury mechanism, the ACL is torn when the top of the ski boot drives the tibia anterior relative to the femur (Ettlinger 1986). This produces an anterior-directed force on the tibia relative to the femur

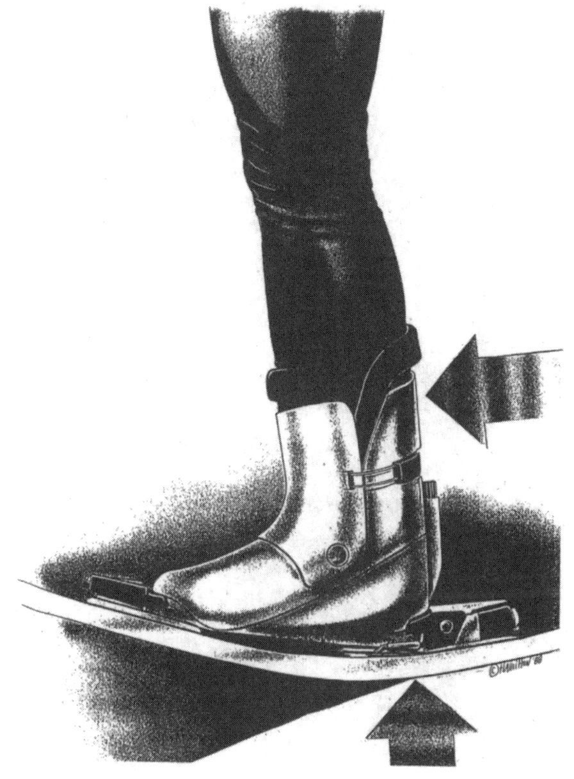

FIGURE 15.1 The boot-induced anterior drawer injury mechanism in alpine skiing.
Illustration courtesy of Vermont Safety Research.

(i.e., an "anterior drawer" that can disrupt the ACL; figure 15.1). This injury mechanism is sustained during hard landings following a jump by off-balance skiers (Ettlinger 1986; Ettlinger, Johnson, and Shealy 1995); it is common among freestyle skiers but quite unusual in recreational skiers. During the landing the knee is in extension and therefore, because of the fixed dorsiflexion of the modern ski boot, the tail of the ski first contacts the snow. As the foot is driven flat to the snow with the knee in extension, the posterior aspect of the top of the boot produces an anterior-directed force to the back of the calf, resulting in an ACL disruption. Fortunately this injury mechanism is relatively rare, accounting for very few of the 2430 alpine skiing-induced ACL injuries our group has evaluated (Johnson, Shealy, and Ettlinger 2005).

Flexion-Internal Rotation ("Phantom Foot" Mechanism of ACL Injury)

In flexion-internal rotation, the most common of ACL injury mechanisms, the skier typically loses balance and sits far backward (figure 15.2) (Ettlinger

1986). Because of deep knee flexion, the hips are placed below the level of the knees; the upper body generally faces the downhill ski; the uphill ski is unweighted; weight is placed on the inside edge of the downhill ski; and the uphill (opposite) hand is placed on the snow surface. This results in a sudden internal rotation of the tibia on the hyperflexed knee. The magnitude of this moment is sufficient to produce an ACL tear while the properly set and optimally functional binding is not exposed to forces high enough to result in a release. This has been termed the "phantom foot" injury mechanism in reference to the rear body of the ski, which protrudes behind the foot and produces the torque that results in injury.

For these two mechanisms, the design of the boot directly contributes to the injury (Ettlinger 1986). In the past, when boot tops were more flexible, they permitted plantarflexion about the ankle, and severe knee ligament sprains occurred less frequently (Elmqvist and Johnson 1994; Kannus and Johnson 1991; Ettlinger 1986). The reason may be that skiers were able to unload their knees by transmitting force through their buttocks rather than their knee while the knee was in this hyperflexed position.

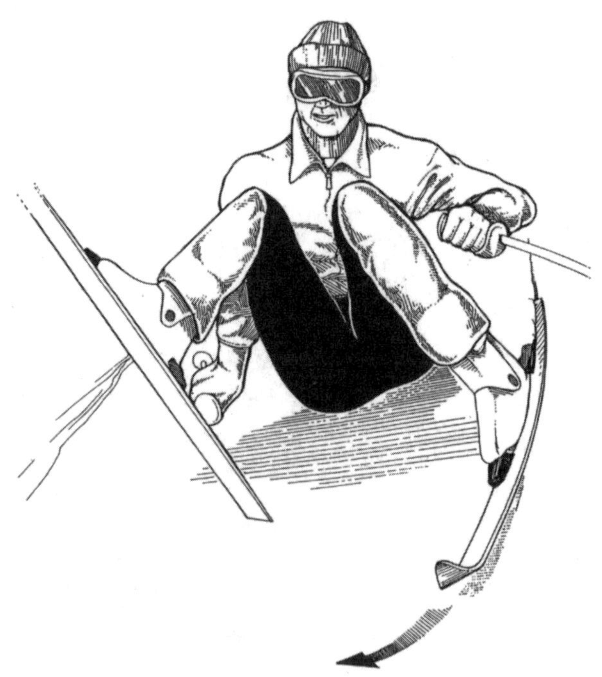

FIGURE 15.2 The flexion-internal rotation injury mechanism of ACL injury ("phantom foot" injury mechanism).

Illustration courtesy of Vermont Safety Research.

Other Suggested Knee Ligament Injury Mechanisms Produced During Alpine Skiing

Many other knee ligament injury mechanisms have been proposed, but we have been unable to assemble video footage of these mechanisms (Marshall and Johnson 1977; Freudiger and Friederich 2000; Barone, Senner, and Schaff 1999; Young 1981; Ekeland and Thoreson 1987; Feagin et al. 1987; Bally and Del Pedro 1990; Bruce, Cross, and Pinczewski 1989; Rossi, Lubowitz, and Guttmann 2003; McConkey 1986; Geyer and Wirth 1991). Thus, we can assume that these mechanisms are either rare or rarely recorded. Likewise, it is clear from various publications addressing ACL injury mechanisms that interpretations vary widely concerning what is seen on film of injuries occurring and what is reconstructed from interviews with patients about how they believe they were injured. Our attempts to reconstruct the injury mechanism from patient interviews revealed that such interpretations are very unreliable, even when the interviews are done immediately after the injury (Johnson, Shealy, and Ettlinger 2005).

It has been proposed that valgus-external rotation of the knee is an ACL injury mechanism. In this apparently relatively common mechanism, the medial edge of the anterior portion of the ski engages the snow, and the skier is propelled forward by his or her forward momentum as the tibia is abducted and externally rotated in relation to the femur. The long moment arm of the ski creates torque about the knee. It is hypothesized that the primary ligament injured in such a fall is usually the MCL; however, in approximately 20% of these cases the ACL is also torn (Ettlinger, Johnson, and Shealy 1995; Johnson 1988; Jarvinen et al. 1994). We have seen a decrease in grade I and II sprains of the knee primarily involving the MCL, which may indicate that appropriate binding function (proper release of the toe piece) has resulted in a decreased risk of these injuries (Ryder et al. 1997).

It has also been proposed that forward falls resulting in hyperextension, or a combination of internal rotation and hyperextension of the knee, may result in disruption of the ACL and perhaps the lateral structures of the knee (Marshall and Johnson 1977; Elmqvist and Johnson 1994; Rossi, Lubowitz, and Guttmann 2003). However, we have not seen any videos confirming that this mechanism occurs and have interviewed very few injured skiers who believed this had happened to them.

Some researchers believe that another mechanism occurs when skiers are down and sliding with the principal axis of the ski perpendicular to the long axis of the body and the skier's direction of travel (Chambat et al. 1997). At that point, the skier can suddenly catch the outside edge of the downhill ski; this creates a sudden jerk that lifts the tibia up suddenly and therefore puts the knee in internal rotation, resulting in an ACL disruption.

It has also been proposed that a forceful quadriceps contraction may injure the ACL as the skier is trying to regain balance from an off-balance position to the rear (McConkey 1986; Geyer and Worth 1991). When the knee is near extension, contraction of the quadriceps muscle will produce an anterior-directed intersegmental shear force that acts to translate the tibia anteriorly, relative to the femur (Beynnon et al. 1992). Although the ACL is influenced by the forces produced by contraction of the thigh muscles, there is some controversy as to whether a forceful quadriceps contraction can disrupt the ACL (Aune, Schaff, and Nordsletten 1995; Chiang and Mote 1993). In fact, the quadriceps muscle may even protect the ACL from injury with the knee in deep flexion, because the orientation of the patella tendon produces a posterior-directed intersegmental force on the tibia that acts to translate the tibia in a posterior direction relative to the femur (Aune, Cawley, and Ekeland 1997).

Summary

Anterior cruciate ligament disruption remains one of the most common serious medical problems associated with recreational and competitive alpine skiing. Currently, the most common ACL injury mechanism is the "phantom foot," which occurs when the ski produces internal rotation of the tibia relative to the femur on the hyperflexed knee. To date, the only effective means of reducing the high rate of ACL injuries has been the ACL Awareness Training Program, which has been shown to work among experienced skiing professionals.

Chapter 16

Noncontact ACL Injuries in Dance and Skating

Carol C. Teitz, MD

Anterior cruciate ligament injuries are conspicuously absent in dancers and skaters. A literature review of injuries in dancers and skaters was conducted starting with PubMed. PubMed was searched using ACL-dance, ACL-ballet, ACL-skating, and ACL-hockey. In addition, the bibliographies of the articles obtained were searched for additional references not found in the PubMed search. Fourteen articles concerning patterns of injuries in dancers were reviewed, including 3541 theatrical, ballet, modern, and aerobic dancers (Bowling 1989; Bronner and Brownstein 1997; Bronner, Ojofeitimi, and Rose 2003; Byhring and Bo 2002; Evans et al. 1996; Garrick, Gillien, and Whiteside 1986; Garrick and Requa 1993; Nilsson et al. 2001; Quirk 1983; Rothenberger, Chang, and Cable 1988; Rovere et al. 1983; Solomon and Micheli 1986; Solomon et al. 1995; Washington 1978). Two ACL injuries were reported in Broadway theatrical dancers and one in a modern dancer (sex not reported) (0.1%) (Bronner and Brownstein 1997; Washington 1978) (see table 16.1). Twelve articles concerning patterns of injuries in skaters were reviewed; the skaters included 643 figure, 150 speed, and thousands of in-line skaters (Brock and Striowski 1986; Dubravcic-Simunjak et al. 2003; Garrick 1982; Kjaer and Larsson 1992; Lam et al. 1997; Mulder 2002; Nguyen 2001; Quinn et al. 2003; Smith and Micheli 1982; Smith and Ludington 1989; Tan, Seldes, and Daluiski 2001; Williamson and Lowden 1986). Two reports of ACL injuries were found in figure skaters (one male and one female) (0.31%) (Nichols et al. 1998) (see table 16.2). An additional article dealt with rehabilitation of a female ice hockey athlete with an ACL tear (Tyler and McHugh 2001).

The articles just cited included dancers and skaters of varying levels of expertise from recreational to professional. The articles originated in the United States, Canada, England, Australia, Hong Kong, Norway, and Sweden. Contact was also made in 2004 with Dr. Angela Smith and Dr. James Garrick. Each

TABLE 16.1 Knee Injuries Reported in Dancers

Authors	No. of subjects	No. injured	No. of injuries	% Knee
Bowling 1989	141		67	10
Bronner and Brownstein 1997	30	12		8
Bronner et al. 2003	42			(1 ACL)
Byhring and Bo 2002	51			
Evans et al. 1996	313			
Garrick et al. 1986	411	327		
Garrick and Requa 1993	200	104	309	
Nilsson et al. 2001	98		390	11
Quirk 1983	664			17.3
Rothenberger et al. 1988	725			9.2
Rovere et al. 1983	218	185	352	3.2
Solomon and Micheli 1986	164	164	229	20.1
Solomon et al. 1995	70	64	137	11.7
Washington 1978	146		414	14.7 (2 ACL)

TABLE 16.2 Knee Injuries Reported in Skaters

Authors	No. of subjects	No. injured	No. of injuries	% Knee
Brock and Striowski 1986	60		14	
Dubravcic-Simunjak et al. 2003	469		124	8
Garrick 1982	70			
Kjaer and Larsson 1992	8			
Lam et al. 1997	43			
Mulder 2002		65,000		4-10
Nguyen 2001		245	331	10
Quinn et al. 2003	95	61	111	23
Smith and Micheli 1982	19			31.57
Smith and Ludington 1989	44	29	49	9.2
Tan et al. 2001				
Williamson and Lowden 1986	74,676		203	3.45

authored many of the figure skating and dance articles. Dr. Smith stated that fewer than 12 ACL injuries have been noted in skaters in the last 10 years. Dr. Garrick was aware of two ACL injuries in male dancers (dancing the same role) not reported in the literature. I have treated one male ballet dancer for an ACL injury

What "protects" the ACL in these athletes? Based on our current knowledge about noncontact ACL injuries, the following hypotheses should be considered.

Muscular Control

Single-Leg Work

One component of current ACL tear prevention programs is strengthening of hip abductors and external rotators to protect the knee from valgus and internal rotation deformity associated with ACL injury (Griffin et al. 2000). Dancers and skaters perform many movements on one leg. Skaters also land most jumps on one leg. Single-leg work demands strong hip abductors. Hamilton and colleagues (1992) compared hip abductor strength in professional ballet dancers with that in "normals" in the Cybex database. They found male dancers to have 18% stronger abductors and female dancers to have 21% stronger abductors than normals.

Many centers report that quadriceps dominance can lead to noncontact ACL injury in women (Huston and Wojtys 1996; Yu et al. 2002). Although dancers and skaters have what appear to be well-developed quadriceps muscles, they often develop overuse injuries of the quadriceps mechanism. Kirkendall and Calabrese (1983) noted that quadriceps torque at 30°/sec in female ballet dancers was 70% of weight-predicted norms for athletes. Hamilton also measured quadriceps:hamstring torque ratios and found that in female dancers, the Q:H ratio was normal (Hamilton et al. 1992). Chmelar and colleagues (1998) compared hamstring strength in dancers to that in basketball players and runners, showing that dancers have hamstring muscle strength similar to that of basketball players, despite the dancers' lower body weight, but have weaker hamstrings than runners. However, the hamstring-to-quadriceps ratio was 17% greater in dancers than in either athletic group because of the dancers' relatively weaker quadriceps and relatively stronger hamstring muscles (Chmelar et al. 1998).

Ball-of-Foot Work

Wojtys and Huston (1994) noted delayed firing of the gastrocnemius muscles in patients with ACL-deficient knees who underwent an anterior tibial translation stress test, and pointed out that the gastrocnemius muscle may also stabilize the knee joint. Dancers, no matter which type of dance they engage in, typically spend a majority of time on the ball of the foot. Working in this way leads to very strong ankle plantarflexors. Hamilton and colleagues (1992), studying a professional ballet company, found 44% stronger plantarflexors in males and 33% stronger plantarflexors in females compared with normals.

Lower Limb in External Rotation

In video analyses of athletes sustaining noncontact ACL tears, Teitz and Hutchinson and their colleagues noted that the position of the lower limb at the moment of ACL tear includes thigh adduction and internal rotation relative to the tibia and valgus knee angulation (Teitz 2001; Hutchinson, Williams, and Ireland 2002). Almost all dance forms, except for aerobic dance, emphasize external rotation of the lower limb originating at the hip joint (Teitz 2002). In skating, the limb that has just pushed off also is pushed into an abducted and externally rotated position at the hip (Tyler and McHugh 2001).

Shoe–Surface Interface

Another potential etiologic factor in noncontact ACL injuries is the shoe–surface interface. In field sports, cleats increase the friction and fixation of the shoe to the turf or grass. In gym sports, the shoes are designed to provide some traction on the floor to allow sudden starts and stops. In contrast, skating, by definition, is gliding on a surface. Therefore skates of various types are all designed to have a low coefficient of friction between the skate and the surface that it contacts, whether that surface is ice, wood, or cement. Dr. Smith (personal communication, 2004) noted that some of the few ACL injuries reported in skating occurred when the skate blade caught a rut in the ice. Ballet slippers and pointe shoes are also slippery enough that dancers often rub rosin on them to increase the friction slightly. Special flooring is also used both for shock absorption and to further decrease friction between shoe and floor. Modern dance is usually performed barefooted, and the friction between foot and floor generally leads initially to blisters, followed by callus formation. Aerobic dance is the only form in which the shoes may have some degree of traction on the floor. Yet there are no ACL injuries reported in that activity either. Additional factors must play a role in protecting the ACL.

Center of Gravity and Proprioception

Video analyses of athletes at the moment of ACL tear have noted that the athlete's center of gravity is often posterior to the knee (Teitz 2001; Hutchinson, Williams, and Ireland 2002). Dancers and skaters are thought to have excellent proprioceptive sense and balance, although this has never been scientifically proven. Although there may be some natural selection of proprioceptively gifted athletes to remain in dance and skating, we don't find ACL injuries in young children who try these activities and then drop them because of insufficient skill.

Dancers start and land all jumps on the ball of the foot and in plié (bent knee). Skaters also tend to land on bent knee. These knee and foot positions tend to force the center of gravity forward. Moreover, skaters usually land jumps skating backward, which requires cocontraction of the quadriceps and hamstring muscles (Yu and Smith 2002). In addition, they do not land on a fixed foot but rather on a slippery surface. The ACL injuries described by Yu and Smith (2002) were sustained during incomplete triple jumps.

Choreography

Perhaps the key unique feature of dance and most forms of skating compared with other sports is that with the exceptions of in-line skating and ice hockey, all skating and all dance forms are choreographed. A sequence of movements is known and practiced. These athletes do not have to react suddenly to the unanticipated movements of an opposing athlete. When injuries occur, they tend to occur from an incompletely executed movement or from faulty choreography. The latter was noted by Garrick (personal communication, 2004) in two male dancers who were injured doing exactly the same jump in the show "Billy the Kid."

Additional Considerations

Two other differences between dance and skating and other sports are the lack of a specific sport season and the gradual progression of skills. Although all serious athletes practice many hours per day and many days per week, athletes in most field or gym sports have an off-season. This is not the case for serious dancers or skaters, who continue year-round. Although this schedule contributes to the prevalence of overuse injuries in dancers and skaters, traumatic injuries are less common.

With regard to skill progression, skaters and dancers progress slowly from relatively simple movements to more complex movements. Children playing soccer or basketball, on the other hand, do the same types of pivoting and jumping movements required for their sports as do adults. Dancers and skaters, on the other hand, take years to develop the ability to do jumps and are not required to do these jumps until they are thought to have adequate strength and balance.

What About Gymnasts?

According to the NCAA Injury Surveillance database, female gymnasts have the highest rate of ACL injuries of all athletes, male or female (Hutchinson and Ireland 1995). Yet gymnasts have many characteristics in common with dancers and skaters. Gymnasts do single-leg work and work on the ball of the foot during both the balance beam and floor exercise events. They seem proprioceptively gifted and their routines are choreographed. They also gradually advance their routines with regard to skills required and degree of difficulty. Gymnasts perform barefooted as do modern dancers.

In what ways do gymnasts differ from dancers and skaters? First, gymnasts do not emphasize lower limb external rotation. Second, although their tumbling routines, dismounts, and landings from flips are meant to occur on a bent knee, gymnasts are often landing from an aerial inverted position, and momentum may make it more difficult to get their center of gravity in front of their knees. They also must suddenly stop their forward momentum while tumbling and land on both legs. Third, they may be more innately ligamentously lax than dancers or skaters. Uhorchak and colleagues noted that ligamentous laxity was a risk factor in female athletes sustaining ACL injuries (Uhorchak et al. 2003).

Summary

Clearly the lack of ACL injuries in dancers and skaters is multifactorial. Recreational skaters and dancers don't practice intensely year-round, are not necessarily proprioceptively blessed, and may not have strong ACL antagonist muscles; yet they do not tear their ACLs. Nevertheless, the lack of ACL injuries in these athletes supports the concepts of strengthening hip, hamstring, and calf muscles to prevent ACL injuries. The fact that female dancers and skaters are not at increased risk for ACL injuries does not support the theories that lower limb anatomy, notch width, or hormonal changes may lead to ACL injuries in the female athlete.

Chapter 17

The Role of Biofeedback in Preventing Noncontact ACL Injuries

Julie R. Steele, PhD
Bridget J. Munro, PhD

Biofeedback involves measuring and quantifying an individual's bodily processes, which are usually subconscious, and then feeding this information back to the individual in a form that allows the individual to change or control those processes via practice and training. Often used to alter brain activity, blood pressure, chronic pain, muscle tension, heart rate, and other bodily functions that are normally beyond voluntary control, biofeedback can be provided in various ways, including visual, auditory, and tactile forms of feedback. For example, muscle biofeedback involves placing electrodes on the skin overlying muscles of interest and recording the electrical signal generated by these muscles. Feedback related to muscle activity, such as an audible tone or visual representation to indicate when muscle intensity has reached a desired level, can then be provided to the individual for a wide variety of applications, such as enhancing lower extremity function following stroke (Moreland, Thomson, and Fuoco 1998), eliciting strength gains during isometric exercises (Lucca and Recchiuti 1983), or during rehabilitation following knee surgery (Draper 1990; Draper and Ballard 1991).

The Role of Biofeedback in ACL Injury Prevention

A perpetual challenge confronting practitioners implementing ACL prevention programs is the ability to monitor the technique of athletes during training sessions and then to feed this information back to athletes in real time so they can modify their motion to minimize ACL injury risk. To address this challenge, sophisticated biofeedback devices have been developed to monitor aspects of performance, particularly muscle activity and joint motion. Despite a plethora of research pertaining to ACL injury prevention, only limited research has addressed whether biofeedback training can be used to alter the biomechanics of healthy athletes, as a method of reducing ACL injury risk. The purpose of this chapter is to provide an overview of the limited literature pertaining to the use of biofeedback devices during landing training programs that are designed to reduce the rate of noncontact ACL ruptures. The devices to be reviewed include biofeedback systems designed to retrain muscle recruitment as well as systems to increase knee joint motion during dynamic landings.

Biofeedback, Neuromuscular Activity, and ACL Injury Prevention

Correct recruitment of the lower limb muscles during abrupt deceleration tasks such as landing is an important factor for reducing loads on the ACL and subsequent risk of injury (Steele and Brown 1999). Although the ACL provides primary restraint to anterior tibial translation (Butler, Noyes, and Grood 1980), the hamstring muscles act as synergists to this ligament, recruited on demand when the ACL is excessively loaded to provide secondary restraint (Solomonow, Baratta, and D'Ambrosia 1989). The hamstring muscles therefore play an important role in reducing stress to the ACL and decreasing injury susceptibility. Kain and colleagues (1988) suggested that a muscle recruitment strategy whereby the hamstring muscles contract prior to the quadriceps muscles, thereby initiating a posterior tibial drawer and negating the quadriceps-initiated anterior tibial drawer, offered optimal protection to the ACL. However, during abrupt decelerative landings, there is insufficient time for this sequencing of muscle activity to occur reflexively, and therefore it must be preprogrammed (Andriacchi 1990). DeMont and colleagues (1999) suggested that players who had better neural programming experienced better joint protection through muscle stabilization and a subsequent decrease in ACL injury susceptibility. Likewise, Shultz and Perrin (1999b) suggested that efficient neuromuscular control was essential to ensure knee joint stability and protection during dynamic activity.

The importance of optimal hamstring-quadriceps muscle synchrony to protect the ACL was reinforced by Steele and Brown (1999), who examined the compensatory mechanisms developed by 11 functional, chronic, isolated-ACL-deficient patients during a task known to excessively stress the ACL, namely abrupt dynamic landings. Compared to their matched controls, these chronic ACL-deficient athletes showed significantly altered muscular coordination during landing. The ACL-deficient patients delayed activation of their hamstring muscles so that peak hamstring activity better coincided with the high tibiofemoral shear forces generated during the deceleration task.

As landing occurred with the knee near full extension, the more synchronous activation of the hamstring muscles with the peak tibiofemoral shear forces was thought to assist in stabilizing the knee via increasing tibiofemoral joint compression and, to a lesser extent, posterior tibial drawer when the knee would be most vulnerable to anterior subluxation. Steele and Brown (1999) speculated that these compensatory strategies used by the functional ACL-deficient patients to protect their knees against giving-way episodes were acquired through a learned motor program. If this speculation is correct, the question arises whether healthy athletes can be trained to learn alternative muscle recruitment strategies to protect their knees from noncontact ACL rupture. Can athletes be trained using biofeedback devices to recruit their hamstring and quadriceps muscles in a prescribed pattern? Will this lessen the forces that their knee is subjected to at landing and reduce the incidence of noncontact ACL ruptures?

The Need for Biofeedback Training to Alter Muscular Recruitment Patterns

Acknowledging the importance of correct muscle recruitment strategies, Cowling and colleagues (2003) investigated whether simply asking players to change the way they recruited their hamstring muscles, without specific muscle biofeedback retraining, was sufficient to enable them to alter their lower limb muscle activation patterns during dynamic landings. Twenty-four skilled, uninjured female netball players (mean age = 21.9 ± 4.8 years) were required to accelerate forward for approximately three paces, leap from their nondominant leg, and land on their dominant (test) limb in single-limb stance with their foot centrally located on a force platform while they caught a chest-high pass. This task was performed for 10 trials under four test conditions: (1) normal landing, (2) repeat normal landing, (3) landing after an instruction to increase knee flexion (knee instruction), and (4) landing after an instruction to recruit the hamstring muscles earlier (muscle instruction). Abrupt landing was chosen as the experimental task as it is a typical netball skill that has been shown to result in ACL rupture (Steele 1986). The ground reaction forces generated at landing and the activity of four muscles that control knee motion (rectus femoris, vastus lateralis, biceps femoris, and semimembranosus) were sampled (1000 Hz) using a force platform and an electromyographic (EMG) system, respectively. These data were then analyzed for each subject's dominant limb to provide an indication of the effect of simple verbal instructions on performing the deceleration task.

Analysis of the results indicated no significant differences in any of the temporal variables analyzed for the hamstring muscles among the four test conditions (see figure 17.1). However, the players activated the rectus femoris muscle earlier relative to initial foot–ground contact during the muscle instruction condition (110 ± 53 msec) compared to the other three conditions (normal landing = 83 ± 33 msec; repeat landing = 77 ± 27 msec; knee instruction = 72 ± 34 msec; $p < 0.05$; Cowling, Steele, and McNair 2003).

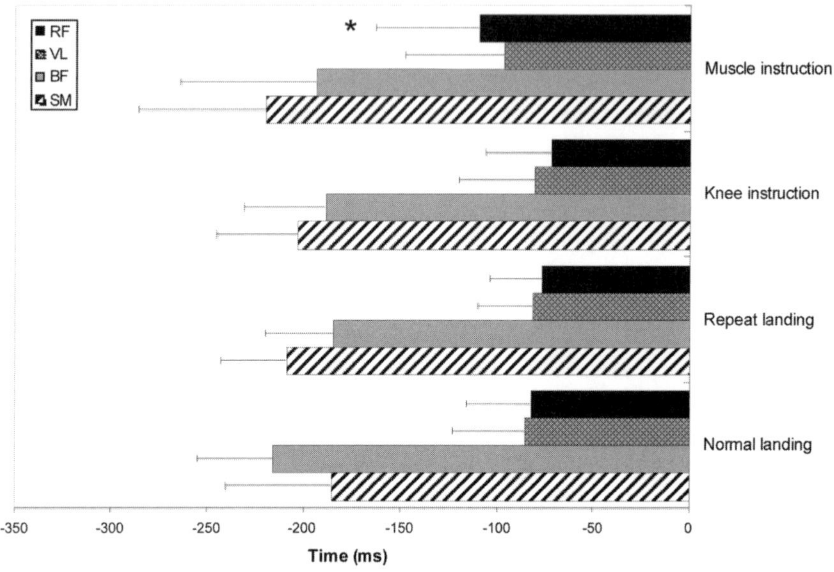

FIGURE 17.1 Average hamstring and quadriceps muscle onset time (msec) relative to initial foot–ground contact (IC; time = 0) displayed by 12 netball players during four landing conditions: normal landing, repeat normal landing, knee instruction, and muscle instruction. The asterisk denotes a significant ($p < 0.05$) between-condition difference in muscle onset for rectus femoris between the muscle instruction condition and all other conditions. A negative value indicates that a muscle was activated before IC.

As no significant differences were found in timing of the hamstring muscles among the four conditions, it was suggested that subjects were unable to selectively change the time at which they recruited their hamstring muscles when given only verbal instructions without prior muscle biofeedback training. Moreover, the simple muscle instruction actually resulted in earlier onset of the antagonistic quadriceps muscles prior to landing, thereby potentially imposing a greater risk of injury to the ACL during landing. The authors speculated that more extensive and specific muscle biofeedback training was required to enable skilled players to alter their hamstring-quadriceps muscle synchrony during a task as complex and as rapid as landing if safer landing practices were to be developed (Cowling, Steele, and McNair 2003).

Biofeedback and Neuromuscular Retraining

On the basis of their speculation, Cowling and Steele (2002) implemented a specialized muscle activation retraining program using muscle biofeedback in an attempt to determine whether players could be trained to modify their hamstring muscle recruitment patterns during a dynamic landing task to better protect their ACL. Retraining using muscle biofeedback has previously proven effective in clinical settings with patients such as children with cerebral palsy (Dursun, Durson, and Alican 2004) and hemiplegic patients (Colborne, Olney, and Griffin 1993) in improving their gait. It has also been used to facilitate hamstring relaxation during arthrometric assessment of knee laxity in patients having undergone unilateral ACL reconstruction (Feller, Hoser, and Webster 2000). However, despite the widespread use of muscle biofeedback in muscle rehabilitation and strengthening programs for patients (Feller, Hoser, and Webster 2000), it was unknown whether this method of muscle retraining could be used effectively in healthy noninjured populations to retrain lower limb muscles in order to better protect the knee during dynamic landings.

To address this question, Cowling and Steele (2002) recruited 28 healthy, skilled netball players to perform sets of the typical netball single-limb landings, described previously, during two test sessions that were scheduled six weeks apart: (1) before training and (2) posttraining. Sagittal plane motion, ground reaction forces, and muscle activity for the rectus femoris, vastus lateralis, biceps femoris, and semimembranosus of the landing limb were recorded for each landing trial using an optoelectronic motion analysis system (200 Hz), a force platform (1000 Hz), and a telemetered EMG system (1000 Hz), respectively. During the six-week interval between testing sessions, 14 of the players (experimental group) completed hamstring muscle biofeedback training for three 30 min sessions per week, while the additional 14 players (control group) performed the landing sessions with no intervention presented in the six-week interval.

This six-week training program focused on retraining the hamstring muscles and was designed to elicit earlier activation with respect to the quadriceps muscles and the time of landing (Kain et al. 1988). The players completed three 30 min individually supervised training sessions per week, with difficulty in the activities incremented over the six weeks. Six weeks was chosen as the length of the training program as previous ACL injury prevention training programs have successfully used a similar time frame and session duration (Caraffa et al. 1996; Hewett et al. 1999, 1996). The two representative hamstring muscles (biceps femoris and semimembranosus) were trained alternately using a commercially available EMG Retrainer (Chattanooga, TN) with audible feedback provided to each subject in relation to their muscle activity. The training sessions progressed from simple activities in which the players learned to contract their hamstring muscles while in static positions (lying prone, seated, standing) to more dynamic tasks (stepping, leaping, running to landing) with the end goal of replicating the test landing. The players were instructed to try to turn their hamstring muscles on earlier before landing, as this patterning has been suggested by Kain and colleagues (1988) to provide more time for these muscles to initiate a posterior tibial drawer before the onset of the antagonistic quadriceps muscles, and hence has been suggested to be protective of the ACL.

Interestingly, Cowling and Steele (2002) found that the training program was not effective in changing the hamstring muscle recruitment patterns displayed by the players after this intensive individualized six-week biofeedback training program. Although the training partially achieved the desired trend for earlier onset of the hamstring muscles, this trend was accompanied by unexpected changes in the quadriceps muscle group, as subjects also produced an earlier onset of these muscles. As a hamstring muscle biofeedback training program, the muscle training was deemed ineffective in selectively altering the timing of hamstring muscle recruitment with respect to landing. That is, in a concerted effort to successfully accomplish the training goals, the experimental players actually recruited their quadriceps earlier, which was speculated to be less, rather than more, protective to the ACL (Cowling and Steele 2002).

The results of Cowling and Steele (2002) could be interpreted to imply that the biofeedback training program was unsuccessful in retraining the muscle recruitment patterns displayed by healthy players performing this dynamic landing task. However, the hamstring muscle recruitment strategies displayed by individual players were affected by the training program in very different ways, despite each individual's having completed the same biofeedback training program (see figure 17.2). In fact, relative to the pretraining values, 8 of the 14 experimental subjects displayed significant changes in both their quadriceps

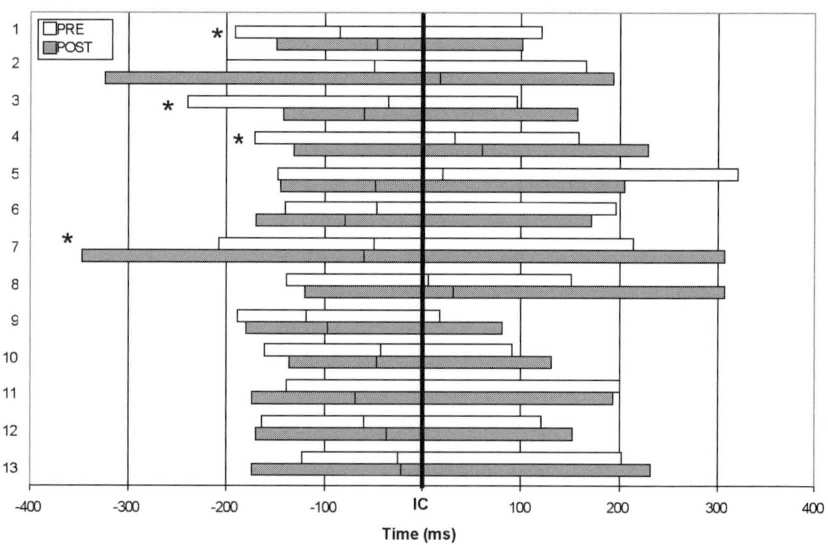

FIGURE 17.2 Average semimembranosus muscle activity (onset, peak, and offset times) relative to initial contact (IC; time = 0) displayed by each of the 13 subjects before (pre) and after (post) the six-week training program. The asterisk denotes a significant ($p < 0.05$) difference in the time from onset to initial contact before compared to after training. A negative value indicates that a muscle was activated before IC.

and hamstring muscle recruitment patterns following training, whereas four players displayed significant between-session differences in their quadriceps muscle recruitment patterns alone. In addition, one player altered only her hamstring muscle recruitment patterns after training, whereas another player displayed no significant differences in her quadriceps or hamstring muscle groups as a result of the training. These results suggested that healthy uninjured individuals do not display uniform adaptations to their lower limb muscle recruitment strategies following participation in muscle biofeedback training programs, somewhat confounding the role of group muscle biofeedback training programs as a strategy for ACL injury prevention. However, as only one study has addressed the use of muscle biofeedback training for ACL injury prevention, further research is recommended to examine the role of biofeedback as a tool to teach athletes to coordinate their lower limb muscle synchrony, without conscious control, so as to better protect the ACL from rupture. Other options, such as using biofeedback to retrain joint motion as an ACL injury prevention strategy, should also be considered.

Biofeedback, Knee Joint Motion, and ACL Injury Prevention

Many noncontact ACL injuries occur during landing from a jump with the knee close to full extension (Steele 1986; Boden et al. 2000; Olsen et al. 2004). During landing in this extended knee posture, contracting the quadriceps muscles, which are activated to prevent the lower limb from collapsing, unfortunately also increases ACL strain (Draganich and Vahey 1990; Torzilli, Deng, and Warren 1994). Furthermore, with the knee extended, the hamstring muscles are inefficient in providing sufficient posterior tibial drawer to counteract the quadriceps-induced anterior tibial translation, due to their inefficient line of action (Kain et al. 1988; Pandy and Shelburne 1997). For this reason, it is strongly advocated that individuals bend their knees when landing to enable the hamstring muscles to more effectively protect against high ACL strain. Flexing the knees throughout the landing action can also cushion the forces generated at foot–ground contact (McNair, Prapavessis, and Callender 2000; Prapavessis et al. 2003; Onate et al. 2005), thereby reducing the jarring effects of landing, as well as lowering an individual's center of gravity and in turn enhancing stability (Steele and Milburn 1987a, 1987b). Therefore, to reduce the potential for noncontact ACL injury, it is advocated that individuals land with a relatively high knee flexion angle combined with a large range or amplitude of joint motion over which to dissipate the energy in muscles (Mizrahi and Susak 1982a, 1982b).

Although Cowling and associates (2003) revealed that players were unable to selectively change the time at which they recruited lower limb muscles when given only verbal instructions, the results of their study suggested that the players were able to accurately respond to a simple command related to the kinematics of the movement, such as to bend the knee more on landing. McNair and colleagues (2000) had also previously established that athletes could be trained to alter their range of knee joint motion during a vertical drop jump, via simply being asked to do so, and showed that this increased knee flexion resulted in diminished ground reaction forces during landing. That is, subjects were able to modify their landing technique to reduce their risk of injury when simply asked to bend their knees more. More recently, Onate and colleagues (2005) confirmed that providing college-age recreational athletes with visual augmented feedback, in the form of videotapes depicting model jump-landing technique, not only increased maximum knee flexion angles and knee angular displacement displayed during a basketball jump-landing task, but also reduced the peak vertical forces generated during landing. Interestingly, the video augmented feedback was found to be more effective as a training tool when athletes were allowed to review their own landing technique in addition to, or instead of, reviewing an expert landing model only, which reinforces the need for individualized feedback.

Despite video augmented feedback, which appears promising as an instructional method to teach safe landing technique in ACL injury prevention programs (Onate et al. 2005), there is an inherent delay in athletes' reception of information about their performance after they complete each landing task. To ensure that all athletes are flexing their knees adequately when participating in landing training programs, it is imperative that each athlete receive immediate and individualized feedback about his or her knee joint motion during each and every landing via an appropriate biofeedback device.

Biofeedback Systems to Monitor Knee Joint Motion

Biofeedback devices that are currently commercially available to monitor joint motion in clinical and research settings (known as electrogoniometers) typically have rigid components that do not conform to the individual's body shape, thereby interfering with their natural motion during performance of a movement and possibly posing a safety hazard. Coaches, athletic trainers, and medical personnel have been typically forced to eyeball the performance of their athletes or patients and guess whether the correct motion, including knee flexion, is being used before providing verbal feedback to the individual to change movement patterns. Thus, although the benefits of landing training programs in reducing ACL injuries are readily acknowledged and implemented in sports such as Australian Rules Football (Seward et al. 1999), soccer, volleyball, and basketball (Caraffa et al. 1996; Hewett et al. 1999, 1996), participants in such programs traditionally have had no method to ensure that they are bending their knees sufficiently during training. However, recent advances in polymer science and textile technology have seen the emergence of electronic textiles, creating the opportunity to develop wearable textile sensors that offer novel biomonitoring options for use in ACL injury prevention programs (De Rossi,

Della Santa, and Mazzoldi 1999). These textile sensors, with strain gauge-like properties that have a wide dynamic range, are ideal for biomonitoring applications in that they can be worn without interfering with normal human motion. When connected to appropriate electronic circuitry, these textile sensors can also serve as unique wearable systems capable of providing biofeedback to the wearer with respect to joint motion.

Increasing Knee Flexion During Landing via Biofeedback

To ascertain whether immediate audible biofeedback provided by the flexible knee sleeve was effective in assisting athletes to learn to flex their knees more during dynamic landing movements, a pilot trial was completed involving 37 subjects (age 23.6 ± 4.0 years), all of whom were involved in sports requiring landings and had no history of knee joint disease or trauma. Before and after a six-week training program, each subject performed a series of abrupt decelerative landing movements, similar to those described previously, whereby they landed with their dominant foot centrally located on a force platform while catching a football. During each testing session the three-dimensional kinematic data (200 Hz) characterizing landing technique and ground reaction force data (1000 Hz) were collected using standard biomechanical procedures. At the completion of initial testing, the athletes, who were matched for age, height, body mass, injury history, and playing ability, were divided into three groups:

- Athletes who participated in a landing training program and who received audible feedback from the flexible knee sleeve during this training (knee sleeve-trained group)
- Athletes who participated in a landing training program wearing the flexible knee sleeve but did not receive any audible feedback during training, as the device was not connected (placebo-trained group)
- Athletes who did not participate in the landing training program (control group)

Athletes in the knee sleeve-trained and placebo-trained groups then participated in the six-week landing training program to learn correct landing mechanics, completing three 30 min training sessions per week.

Comparison of each subject's pre- and posttraining landing technique showed that after training, the control and placebo-trained groups displayed, on average, less knee flexion at the time of initial foot–ground contact during landing (control = –11%; placebo = –23%), at the time they generated the peak resultant force (control = –8%; placebo = –4%), and when the maximum knee flexion angle occurred (control = –4%; placebo = –6%). In contrast, after training, the knee sleeve-trained subjects displayed the desired increases in knee flexion at initial foot–ground contact (+14%), peak resultant force (+1%), and maximum knee flexion angle (+7%). In fact, although not statistically significant, the increase in maximum knee flexion angle from pre- to posttraining displayed by the knee sleeve-trained group was on average 8°, an increase that was considered functionally relevant. Interestingly, although both the placebo- and knee sleeve-trained groups participated in the same intensive six-week landing training program, only those subjects who received the immediate audible feedback during the training achieved the positive changes in their knee flexion angle. As the subject numbers and statistical power in this pilot investigation were low, further investigation is warranted to confirm whether participating in a landing training program using audible biofeedback teaches athletes to bend their knees more during landing or decelerating.

The Role of Biofeedback in Preventing ACL Reinjury

Apart from the preventive landing training biofeedback applications just described, biofeedback systems can also be incorporated into rehabilitation programs following ACL reconstructive surgery to ensure that patients perform their rehabilitation exercises properly and in turn reduce the chance of reinjuring their ACL. That is, as the primary goals of postoperative ACL reconstructive surgery are to regain full knee range of motion and to recover muscle strength and control (Draper 1990), biofeedback can help patients learn how to move their knee through a desirable range of motion or to recruit their lower limb musculature more effectively during typical rehabilitation exercises. This, in turn, should promote the recovery of knee range of motion and muscle function. For example, Draper (1990) found that the addition of biofeedback to muscle strengthening exercises facilitated the rate of recovery of quadriceps femoris muscle function following ACL reconstruction. Furthermore, a 12-week training program involving EMG biofeedback during thigh muscle exercises, balance exercises, and gait training has been shown to decrease muscle inhibition, increase maximal isometric knee flexion and extension torques, and increase walking speed in an individual with chronic knee instability due to bilateral ACL injury (Maitland, Ajemian, and Suter 1999). Biofeedback systems may therefore increase the effectiveness of rehabilitation for ACL-reconstructed patients, perhaps simultaneously promoting the recovery of knee muscle strength and neuromuscular control and reducing the noticeable asymmetric loss of knee flexion and extension (Millet, Wickiewicz, and Warren 2001).

Future Directions for Biofeedback and ACL Injury Prevention

One of the challenges confronting those wishing to monitor human performance for ACL injury prevention, whether it be neuromuscular control or knee joint motion, is the ability to design truly wearable biofeedback systems. That is, biofeedback systems designed to be as "unobtrusive as clothing" (Engin et al. 2005, p. 174), although capable of sustained real-time data processing during dynamic forms of activity, need to be developed if biofeedback is to be a feasible option for ACL injury prevention programs. Once such devices become commercially available, it is imperative that future research studies focus on ascertaining optimal biofeedback training programs to promote safe landing technique, particularly in those sports known to give rise to high rates of noncontact ACL injury. However, irrespective of the many challenges to be faced with biofeedback training techniques in relation to ACL injury prevention, the primary question that must be answered is whether changes in human performance, such as increases in knee joint flexion or altered neuromuscular patterns, can in fact translate to a reduction of noncontact ACL injuries in the field.

Part IV

Hormonal and Anatomic Risk Factors and Preventive Bracing for ACL Injuries

Sandra J. Shultz, PhD, ATC, CSCS

Chapter 18: Ligament Biology and Its Relationship to Injury Forces

This chapter introduces a multifactorial model that identifies relationships among factors that determine susceptibility to injury. The model is useful for identifying gaps in our understanding of ACL biology and for defining parameters that may contribute uniquely to the sex disparity in injury rate. In particular, the model highlights the potential effects of sex-specific regulation on the remodeling and adaptation of connective tissues in response to use. Consistent with this model, recent studies have identified sex-derived differences in ligament injury, biomechanics, and expression of genes encoding ligament remodeling components.

Key Points

- Proposed causes of sex differences in ACL injury range from extrinsic factors such as footwear and training to intrinsic factors such as anatomy, neuromuscular control of the leg, ligament biomechanics, and hormonal effects. Although seemingly distinct, these factors are in fact interdependent: Anatomy influences choice of footwear, and coaching can influence neuromuscular control of the leg. Likewise, sex hormones affect anatomical, neuromuscular, and other intrinsic differences between the sexes.

- Of the numerous factors that influence susceptibility to ACL injury, they must ultimately affect either the mechanical load placed on the ligament or the value of the ligament's intrinsic load at failure.
- Extrinsic factors exert their effects on ACL injury by affecting the applied external load. The extent to which this external load is transmitted to the ACL is dependent in part on anatomy and neuromuscular control, both of which are influenced by sex and their associated hormones. Changes in sex hormones begin to diverge during puberty and are responsible for a variety of musculoskeletal differences between sex, including changes in fat distribution, musculoskeletal strength, growth, and shape.
- The ACL's geometry (size or shape), macromolecular composition, and ultrastructure (internal organization) all determine the intrinsic properties of the ligament, thus the magnitude of the load the ligament can withstand before failure. Tissue remodeling and sex hormones are two important determinants of the ACL's geometry.

Chapter 19: Hormonal Influences on Ligament Biology

It is well known that males and females differ dramatically both in the type and level of circulating sex hormones. Because of these differences and the higher incidence of anterior cruciate ligament (ACL) tears in females, research over the past decade has begun to examine the complex relationship between sex hormones and ACL injury through three primary avenues of study. Sex hormones have been examined for their influence on the structure and metabolism of the ligament using basic science studies and for their effects on knee joint laxity and stiffness using clinical studies. Epidemiological studies have attempted to investigate the relationship between menstrual cycle phase and ACL injury incidence. This chapter critically reviews the evidence in each area of study relative to both endogenous and exogenous hormones.

Key Points

- Physiologic levels of estradiol and progesterone appear to have some influence on collagen metabolism, particularly in the first three days following increased exposure. However, the mechanical properties of the ACL after prolonged exposure to physiological concentrations of estrogen have not been demonstrated. Studies examining acute changes in mechanical properties of the ACL following acute cyclic changes in sex hormones across a normal menstrual cycle are needed.

- Females have greater knee laxity than males. While some females experience cyclic increases in knee laxity across the menstrual cycle, others do not. This appears to be mediated in part by their absolute nadir and peak estrogen and progesterone concentrations. A relationship between relaxin levels and joint laxity has not been demonstrated in either pregnant or nonpregnant females.
- Epidemiological studies have not yet conclusively demonstrated whether there is a time in the menstrual cycle when the greatest numbers of injuries occur. While the majority of evidence suggests that more injuries occur near the beginning and end of the follicular phase, the exact hormone milieu that may mediate injury occurrence is unknown.
- Although a significant percentage of high school and collegiate female athletes use oral contraceptives, studies examining the influence of oral contraceptive use on joint laxity and injury risk are limited and inconclusive. Given the various preparations on the market, future studies examining the relationship between birth control hormones, joint laxity, and ACL injury risk should consider the type and concentrations of the hormones delivered, and the studies should confirm bioavailable concentrations of both exogenous and endogenous hormones.
- Females vary substantially in their hormone profiles in regard to cycle length (both follicular and luteal phases), hormone phasing (i.e., timing of changes in one hormone relative to another), day of ovulation, and absolute changes in hormone levels across the cycle. These variations highlight the limitations of using a specific day or range of days to represent the same time in the cycle for all females. Further, these individual variations in cycle characteristics may result in some females' experiencing greater effects of sex hormones on ligament biology compared to others.

Chapter 20: Anatomical Factors in ACL Injury Risk

Anatomical characteristics are often cited as one of four risk factor classifications (environmental, anatomic, hormonal, and neuromuscular or biomechanical) that have been proposed to explain the increased risk of anterior cruciate ligament (ACL) injury in females. While much has been learned about gender differences in neuromuscular and biomechanical function in recent years, the influence of anatomical factors on neuromuscular and biomechanical function and ACL risk remains elusive. This chapter reviews what is known about gender differences in anatomical factors and their potential relationships with dynamic knee joint function and noncontact ACL injury.

Key Points

- A smaller femoral intercondylar notch width has been associated with a greater risk of ACL injury in a variety of athletic populations, including high school, college, military, and European club sports. The biomechanical implications of a smaller notch width relative to ACL injury risk remain unclear.

- Females have greater generalized joint laxity (GJL), and the difference is consistent across ages. While prospective and retrospective studies support a relationship between generalized joint laxity and ACL injury risk, the mechanism by which increased GJL leads to increased risk of ACL injury is unknown.
- Knee laxity is greater in females than males, and increased knee laxity has been found in combination with other anatomical factors to be significant predictors of ACL injury status. Limited evidence suggests greater knee laxity has the potential to alter joint mechanics and muscle activation strategies during weight bearing.
- The extent to which sex differences in postural alignment impair neuromuscular and biomechanical function and may contribute to the increased risk of ACL injury in females remains largely theoretical at this time. Clinical observations suggest that females have greater anterior pelvic tilt, hip anteversion, knee valgus, and recurvatum, yet large-scale, appropriately powered studies to validate these clinical observations are lacking.
- Based on retrospective, matched control studies, the alignment characteristic most consistently linked to ACL injury risk is foot pronation. The literature comparing foot pronation in males and females does not support a sex difference, suggesting this alignment factor alone does not explain the greater risk of ACL injury in females.
- Because of the interdependency between independent alignment factors, postural alignment of the entire lower extremity kinetic chain (from the pelvis to the foot) should be considered when examining the relationship between anatomic alignment, dynamic knee function, and the potential for ACL injury risk.

Chapter 21: Intrinsic and Extrinsic Forces Associated With ACL Injury

This chapter reviews what is currently known about the effectiveness of knee bracing in preventing injury to the ACL and reinjury of ACL grafts. The mechanisms behind how braces influence ACL biomechanics are examined, and clinical studies that have focused on the efficacy of prophylactic and functional knee braces in preventing ACL injuries are reviewed. This review reveals that very little is known about the effectiveness of prophylactic braces in preventing ACL injuries or the effectiveness of functional knee braces in preventing injury of healing ligaments and ACL grafts.

Key Points

- Brace performance is determined by at least four characteristics: brace design, the brace–limb interface, the forces produced on the leg by the brace strap tensions, and the magnitude of contraction of the leg musculature as well as the compressive joint load produced by body weight.
- When the aforementioned factors are controlled, bracing has been shown to significantly reduce ACL strain values for anterior-directed shear loading of the tibia with the subject in nonweight-bearing and weight-bearing postures and with internal–external torques applied to the non-weight-bearing knee.
- In the ACL-deficient knee, functional knee braces reduce abnormal AP laxity of the knee during nonweight-bearing and weight-bearing activities. However, they do not reduce abnormal increases in anterior displacement of the tibia relative to the femur as the knee transitions from nonweight-bearing to weight-bearing conditions.
- Prospective, randomized, controlled studies examining the effectiveness of braces in preventing ACL injury, ACL graft injury, and injury in the ACL-deficient knee are very limited and therefore inconclusive.
- There is a need for large-scale, long-term studies addressing the effect of bracing on the prevention of knee ligament injury and graft injury. Ideally these studies should be conducted across a variety of sports and should consider the interactions with intrinsic factors such as anatomical alignment and neuromuscular function.

Chapter 18

Ligament Biology and Its Relationship to Injury Forces

James R. Slauterbeck, MD
John R. Hickox, MS
Daniel M. Hardy, PhD

Twenty years have passed since the first report of increased ACL injury rate in female athletes (Ford et al. 2005). Numerous subsequent studies have confirmed this initial observation, and it is now clear that ACL injury is 3 to 10 times more common in females than in males (Arendt, Bershadsky, and Agel 2002; Bahr and Krosshaug 2005; Hewett et al. 1999; Myklebust et al. 1998). Despite an abundance of theories about why females are more susceptible to this injury, to date no definitive causal link has been found between sex and ACL rupture.

Defining the causes of female susceptibility to ACL rupture has proved difficult for several reasons. First and perhaps foremost is the complexity and uniqueness of the human knee itself. The knee is an extraordinary biomechanical device that, in humans, is specially adapted to our bipedal gait. Humans are the only bipedal mammal. Consequently, studies of nonhuman models, though informative and valuable, are nonetheless subject to criticism until their relevance to the human knee is established. Second, and similarly, the sex disparity in ACL injury is not only an anatomical question but also a reproductive biology question, and reproductive processes vary dramatically among species. Thus humans' unique reproductive endocrinology further complicates the interpretation of results from studies in nonhuman models. Finally, although various explanations have been proposed for the increased injury rate in females, few have been tested because many of them are interrelated and therefore not very amenable to isolation and study.

Relationships Among ACL Injury Factors

Proposed causes of sex differences in ACL injury range from extrinsic factors such as footwear and training to intrinsic factors such as anatomy (LaPrade and Burnett 1994; Lund-Hanssen et al. 1994; Souryal, Moore, and Evans 1988; Souryal and Freeman 1993; Tillman et al. 2002; Uhorchak et al. 2003), neuromuscular control of the leg (Ford et al. 2005), ligament biomechanics (Chandrashekar et al. 2006; Chandrashekar et al. 2005), and hormonal effects (Slauterbeck et al. 2002; Slauterbeck and Hardy 2001; Wojtys et al. 2002). These seemingly distinct, competing hypotheses are in fact interdependent. For example, anatomy influences choice of footwear, and coaching can influence neuromuscular control of the leg. Likewise, sex hormones affect anatomic, neuromuscular, and other intrinsic differences between the sexes.

What are the relationships between and among these interdependent factors, and how do their collective influences translate into an effect on ACL injury? To address this question, we constructed a model (figure 18.1) that places the various factors in a hierarchy and identifies pathways by which they contribute to ACL injury. According to this model, the numerous factors that influence susceptibility to ACL injury all must ultimately affect either the mechanical load placed on the ligament or the value of the ligament's intrinsic "load at failure." When the applied load exceeds the ligament's failure load, ACL injury occurs.

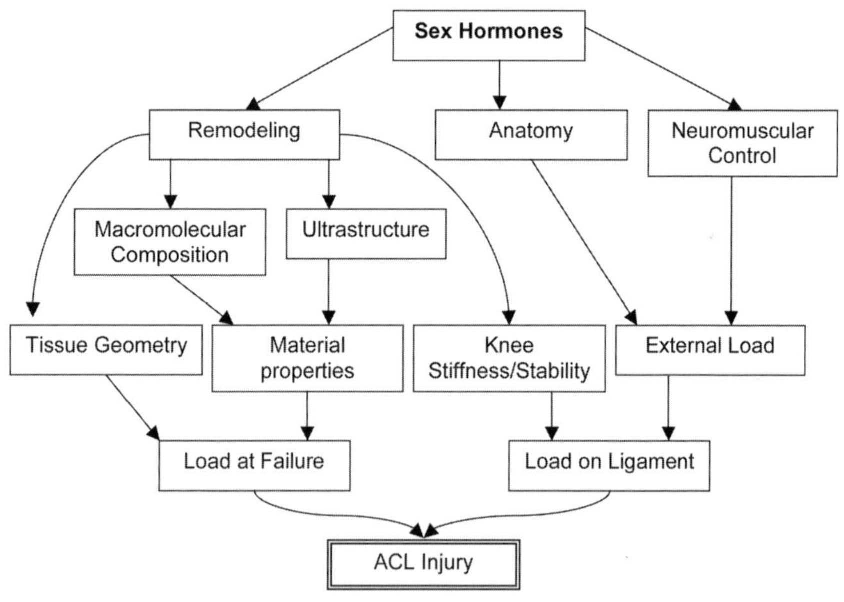

FIGURE 18.1 Relationship of potential factors affecting rate of ACL injury.

In this view of ACL injury, the biomechanical load on the ACL is determined in part by the applied external load on the knee. The portion of this applied external load that is transmitted to the ACL is in turn dependent upon various "intrinsic" factors (discussed later). Factors previously described as "extrinsic" all exert their effects on ACL injury by affecting the applied external load. Applied external load is also determined in large measure by neuromuscular control of the leg (hamstring vs. quadriceps firing patterns, jumping and landing strategies, or balancing strategies). For example, athletes exhibiting poor neuromuscular control (medial knee collapse) may increase the applied load to the knee because of the position (valgus) or internal torque placed on the leg during a landing event (Hewett et al. 1996; Markolf et al. 1997). Applied external load is also substantially affected by differences in collective anatomic structure (femoral length, tibial length). A longer tibia, for example, may place greater load on the knee because the increased length will apply a greater torque to the knee for a given force applied to the foot. A lower extremity with greater valgus may place a greater moment to the knee because both internal tibial torques and valgus moments at the knee combined with anterior sheer forces to increase the load on the ACL (Markolf et al. 1995). Therefore, the magnitude of the loads ultimately transmitted to the ACL depends in part on the external loads applied to the knee, which in turn depend on an individual's specific anatomy (femoral length, body mass index, lower extremity alignment) and neuromuscular control.

Knee stiffness and stability also affect how a load is transmitted to the ACL. If a given load is applied to a knee with less stiffness, a greater load is transmitted to the ACL. In humans, knee stiffness is lower in females than in males with muscular cocontraction (Wojtys, Ashton-Miller, and Huston 2002). Therefore, it is likely that for a given load to the knee, a greater proportion will be applied directly to the ACL in females as compared to males.

The second major determinant of ACL injury is the ligament's intrinsic load at failure. The ACL's geometry (size or shape), macromolecular composition, and ultrastructure (internal organization) all determine the magnitude of the load that the ligament can withstand before failure. In humans, the female ACL is smaller than that in males (Chandrashekar et al. 2005). With respect to load at failure, an ACL of smaller size and similar composition will fail at lower loads compared to an ACL of larger size. Conversely, an ACL of inferior internal composition or structure (material properties), compared to one of similar size with superior internal composition or structure, will fail at lower stresses (Chandrashekar et al. 2005). The size and material properties of the ACL are dependent on how effectively the ligament remodels in response to loads placed on it, and are important determinants of susceptibility to injury.

Effects of Tissue Remodeling

Tissue remodeling is the process whereby old or damaged structures are degraded and replaced with newly synthesized molecules (Dahlberg 1994; DiGirolamo

1996; Edwards 1996a; Everts 1996; Gaire 1994). This process has the potential to affect several aspects of ACL injury susceptibility (see figure 18.1). First, tissue remodeling determines the size, shape, and internal composition of the ACL. Any difference or change in structural or geometric quality of the ACL alters the ligament's intrinsic susceptibility to failure. Second, tissue remodeling can affect knee stiffness, defined as resistance to anterior tibia translation, by modifying the soft tissues about the knee. Third, a major remodeling event in humans occurs during puberty when sex hormones directly affect the size and shape and structure of the human body. Differences in width, ligament laxity, knee laxity, femur and tibia length, and neuromuscular control during puberty will collectively affect how loads are placed upon the ACL. Thus, remodeling may alter not only the load at which an ACL will fail, but also the magnitude of the applied load.

Tissue remodeling occurs continuously in both normal and injured tissues. The balance between the degradative and biosynthetic arms of this process is determined by the rate at which new structural components are synthesized, and by the relative activities of matrix metalloproteinases (MMPs) and tissue inhibitors of metalloproteinases (TIMPs) (Dahlberg 1994; DiGirolamo 1996; Everts 1996; Gaire 1994). Matrix metalloproteinases are endoproteinases that are responsible for matrix breakdown (Gaire 1994), and TIMP proteins block the hydrolytic activities of MMPs (Edwards 1996b; Mankin, Mow, and Buckwalter 1994). Together, TIMPs and MMPs function as molecules that dictate the rate of matrix breakdown during tissue remodeling. In general, the activity of MMPs is greater than that of TIMPs in the breakdown component of tissue remodeling (Edwards 1996a; Kozaci 1997; Pinals 1996; Salamonsen and Woolley 1996). Conversely, repair is favored when TIMP activity increases relative to MMPs. Thus, whether a noninjured tissue gets larger, gets smaller, or stays the same size is determined in part by expression of genes encoding structural proteins, enzymes that degrade them, and inhibitors of those enzymes. Likewise, whether an injured tissue is adequately repaired is also determined in part by expression of these genes.

Recent studies have characterized expression of genes that encode tissue remodeling components in the human ACL. Matrix metalloproteinases are expressed by many cell types, including macrophages, neutrophils, fibroblasts, trophoblasts, endometrial cells, epithelial cells, and various tumor cells; these enzymes are also present in connective tissues (e.g., cartilage) and in synovial fluid (Lohmander 1994; Matrisian 1994; Meikle 1994). Nine MMPs and all four known TIMPs are expressed in healthy human ACL tissue (Foos et al. 2001). The ACL, medial collateral ligament, and patellar tendon from rabbits also express collagenase (a tissue breakdown enzyme) activity after six days in tissue culture (Harper and Amiel 1988). Immediately after injury, ACLs exhibit increased protease (enzymes that break down proteins) activity that decreases with time during recovery (Amiel 1989; Chandrashekar et al. 2006; Lohmander 1994). Some of the increased MMP activity in injured ACL derives from inflammation, but some if not most may originate in the ligament itself (Amiel 1989). Collectively these studies show that MMP and TIMP genes are expressed in normal, healthy ACLs and that their expression changes dynamically after injury.

Tissue remodeling is evident in the injured ACL and in the tissues used for ACL reconstruction. For example, in sheep ACL subjected to thermal injury, the ligament's size increases and its internal composition changes as the injured tissue is repopulated with new cells (Jackson et al. 1991). Additionally, after a tendon is used to reconstruct the injured ACL, the tendon undergoes a remodeling process called "ligamentization" as it transforms into a ligament (Amiel 1989). Despite the essential roles of normal remodeling events in maintenance and repair of all tissues, including the ACL, their potential contribution to the sex disparity in ACL injury rate has not been fully evaluated.

Sex, Hormones, and ACL Injury

Sex and its associated hormones influence several determinants of human ACL function and injury, including effects on both the load on the ligament and its intrinsic load at failure (see figure 18.1). No sex difference in ACL injury prior to puberty has been reported. After puberty, however, ACL injury rates accelerate in females but not in males (Arendt 1994; Hewett et al. 1999). Concomitantly, neuromuscular strategies controlling landing and jumping diverge during puberty. After puberty, males continue to land with their knees wide apart, and females land in valgus (Hewett, Myer, and Ford 2004). This valgus moment around the knee is associated with ACL injury (Hewett et al. 2005b). Anatomically, sex hormones are responsible for the musculoskeletal changes occurring during puberty, including changes in fat distribution and musculoskeletal strength, growth, and shape. Some of these anatomic differences between males and females are considered risk factors for ACL injury (Ireland 2002; Uhorchak et al. 2003). Such sex-dependent changes in human anatomy and neuromuscular control influence ACL injury rate through their effect on the load on the ligament (see figure 18.1).

Various studies have further implicated sex hormones in the sex disparity in ACL injury. Anterior cruciate ligament injuries are not uniformly distributed through the human menstrual cycle (Arendt, Bershadsky, and Agel 2002; Myklebust et al. 1998; Slauterbeck et al. 2002; Wojtys et al. 2002). Instead, clusters of injuries are observed at different points in the cycle, although the timing of peak injury rate seems to vary depending on the activity that produced the injury (e.g., basketball vs. skiing). In dogs, ACL injury is more prevalent in spayed females and neutered males than in their gonadally intact counterparts (Slauterbeck et al. 2004b). Estrogen decreases the failure load of the rabbit ACL (Slauterbeck et al. 1999) but not the sheep ACL (Seneviratne et al. 2004; Strickland et al. 2003), a discrepancy that may reflect species differences in the response to this sex hormone. Though these studies do not establish a definitive link between sex hormones and ACL injury, they are consistent with such a link.

Sex hormones exert their biological effects almost entirely by affecting the regulation of gene expression. Estrogen and progesterone regulate the transcription of several MMP and TIMP genes (Matrisian 1994; Rajabi 1991; Schneikert 1996; Wahl 1977). For example, expression of different MMPs in cycling human endometrium is dependent on the phase of the menstrual cycle (Matrisian 1994). Several endometrial MMPs degrade type I collagen, which is the collagen in the ACL (Aimes 1995; Krane 1996; Rajabi 1991; Woo, An, and Arnoczky 1994). Estrogen-dependent degradation of type I collagen results in dilation of the guinea pig cervix during birth (Rajabi 1991). Estrogen-dependent collagenase production and progesterone-dependent inhibition of collagenase have been observed in pig pubic ligaments (Wahl 1977). Specific to the ACL, receptors for estrogen, progesterone, and testosterone are present in the human ACL (Hamlet et al. 1997; Liu et al 1996; Sciore, Frank, and Hart 1998); and increasing the concentration of estrogen in an ACL tissue culture model has been shown to result in a decrease in procollagen production (Liu et al 1997). Collectively, these studies suggest that variation in steroid hormone levels during the menstrual cycle could affect expression of tissue remodeling genes in the ACL, including those for structural proteins, MMPs, or TIMPs, that could in turn affect the ligament's intrinsic load at failure.

Tissue remodeling genes are differentially expressed between the sexes. Both the range and average level of matrix metalloproteinase-3 (MMP3, proteases responsible for matrix breakdown) messenger ribonucleic acid (mRNA) expression in the human ACL were found to be higher in females compared to males (Hardy et al. 2002). The measured amount of MMP3 protein in human ACL correlated with expression of its mRNA (Hardy et al. 2002). Similarly, the ratios of MMP3 and matrix metalloproteinase-1 (MMP1) to collagen 1α1 gene expression were found to be higher in ACLs from women than in those from men (Slauterbeck et al. 2004a). These ratios can be viewed as measures of the relative rates of collagen synthesis and degradation. Therefore, at least three genes responsible for ligament remodeling are differentially expressed between the sexes, and their expression appears to favor ligament degradation in females as compared to males.

In summary, the model presented in figure 18.1 illustrates that ACL injury is determined by two variables—the mechanical load on the ligament and the ligament's intrinsic load at failure. All factors that contribute to ACL injury must do so by affecting one or both of these two basic variables. Some factors, such as sex hormones and tissue remodeling, have a multifaceted effect on both the load at ACL failure and the magnitude of the load on the ligament. The relationships defined by this model provide a useful framework for interpretation of results on risk factors for ACL injury, and may also generate new questions to be answered by future research in this area. Finally, the model also illustrates the potentially profound effects that sex hormones and tissue remodeling likely have on female susceptibility to these injuries.

Chapter 19

Hormonal Influences on Ligament Biology

Sandra J. Shultz, PhD, ATC, CSCS

It is well known that males and females differ dramatically in both the type and level of circulating sex hormones. Unlike males, females are exposed to rhythmic fluctuations in endogenous hormones, with the absolute concentrations of sex hormones and their ratio to one another varying considerably during the course of the menstrual cycle. Because of these differences and the higher incidence of ACL tears in females, research over the past decade has begun to address the complex relationship between sex hormones and ACL injury through three primary avenues of study. At the microscopic level, sex hormones have been examined for their influence on the structure and metabolism of the ligament through laboratory studies in cell culture as well as animals and human ligament tissues. At a macroscopic level, sex hormones have been investigated for their effects on knee joint laxity and stiffness; comparisons are drawn between males and females as well as within females across different phases of their menstrual cycle. Lastly, epidemiological studies have addressed the relationship between menstrual cycle phase and ACL injury incidence. This chapter critically reviews the evidence in each area of study regarding how sex hormones may play a role in noncontact ACL injury. The clinical relevance and limitations of these studies are examined, as are important directions for future research. To set a foundation for discussion of these studies, the chapter begins with a brief review of sex hormone profiles and how they vary across the menstrual cycle.

Sex Hormone Profiles: Not All Menstrual Cycles Are Created Equal

The menstrual cycle is typically described as a 28-day cycle, with cycle lengths ranging between 26 and 32 days considered "normal." Over the course of this

28-day cycle, the absolute levels of estrogen and progesterone and their ratio to each other are known to vary considerably. On the basis of these and other hormone concentration changes, the menstrual cycle is divided into two distinct phases, the follicular and luteal phases, which are separated by ovulation (figure 19.1). While ovulation is often considered a phase in itself (e.g., typically reported as occurring during days 10-14), in actuality it represents a point in time (i.e., 24-36 hr) that is marked by a surge in luteinizing hormone (LH).

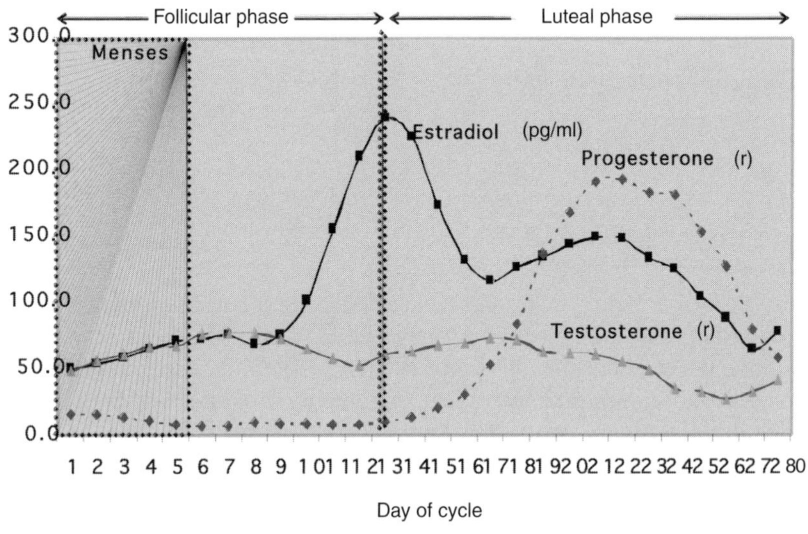

FIGURE 19.1 An exemplar graph showing the general phases of a 28-day menstrual cycle and the relative changes in estrogen, progesterone, and testosterone.

Typical Phases of the Menstrual Cycle

During the early follicular phase of the cycle (days 1-9), concentrations of both estrogen and progesterone are low. In the later half of the follicular phase (days 10-14) a rapid surge of estrogen (concentration increasing from ~100 to 800 pg/mL) occurs in the days prior to ovulation (~day 14), with progesterone remaining low (Guyton 1991; Larsen et al. 2003). Following ovulation, estrogen levels drop, but they stay somewhat elevated during the remainder of the cycle. The luteal phase (days 15-28) composes the later half of the cycle and is characterized by a second but smaller surge in estrogen (rise to ~400 pg/mL) and a considerable rise in progesterone levels (from 1 to 8 pg/mL) (Guyton 1991). As the cycle nears its end, hormone levels fall to their nadirs, stimulating menstruation. Therefore, estrogen levels are at their lowest concentration immediately before and during menses, while progesterone levels remain low from the days just prior to menses through ovulation.

Variations in Cycle Phase Characteristics

While the events just described are the "typical" events of a 28-day menstrual cycle, it is important to realize that in reality females vary substantially with regard to cycle length (both follicular and luteal phases), hormone phasing (i.e., timing of changes in one hormone relative to another), day of ovulation, and absolute changes in hormone levels across the cycle (Landgren, Unden, and Deczfalusy 1980; Nestour et al. 1993; Rossmanith, Schenkel, and Benz 1994; Smith et al. 1979). For example, in a study of 68 normal menstruating females, while the mean follicular and luteal phase lengths were 15 and 13 days, respectively, the actual phase length in these females ranged between 9 and 23 days for the follicular phase and 8 and 17 days for the luteal phase (Landgren, Unden, and Deczfalusy 1980). Although reports in the literature often suggest that the luteal phase is the most stable phase of the cycle, lasting 14 days, over 31% of the subjects had luteal phase lengths of less than 12 or more than 15 days. Moreover, approximately one-third of the subjects had peak LH and preovulatory estradiol levels either before day 12 or after day 19. These data suggest that ovulation, often identified by the surge in LH, frequently occurs outside the typical 10- to 14-day window.

In addition to cycle length, the actual concentration of hormones at various phases of the cycle can vary widely. Table 19.1 represents data from 22 females who were recruited based on self-reported normal and consistent menstrual cycles lasting from 28 to 32 days. These data demonstrate how variable the minimum and peak values are, as well as the variability of the day of the cycle on which these peaks and valleys occur. Although testosterone levels are not often studied in females, data from this table show that testosterone is also present in females and that the levels can vary substantially between females as well as within females across their cycle. Further, these levels appear to influence other cycle characteristics, as testosterone levels have been shown to be highly correlated with longer follicular phases and shorter luteal phases (Smith et al. 1979).

These findings highlight substantial individual variations in hormone profiles in normal menstruating females, and suggest that using a specific day or range of days to represent the same time in the cycle or hormone milieu for all women is likely inaccurate. Understanding this individual variability becomes important when one is critically reviewing methods and findings from studies that have examined ligament biology and ACL injury risk across the menstrual cycle.

Sex Hormone Effects on Collagen Structure and Metabolism

Sex-specific hormones have been investigated for their effects on a variety of collagen tissues, and the effect has been shown to be profound. When tissues are exposed to estrogen, this hormone has been found to increase both collagen synthesis (Dyer, Sodek, and Heersche 1980; Hassager et al. 1990; Ho and Weissberger 1992; Hosokawa et al. 1981) and absorption (Dyer, Sodek, and

TABLE 19.1 Variability in Menstrual Cycle Characteristics[a]

Cycle characteristic	Mean ± SD	Range
VARIATIONS BY CYCLE DAYS		
Total number of days in cycle	27.80 ± 2.40	24.00-36.00
Day of ovulation	13.90 ± 2.70	9.00-20.00
Day of 1st estradiol peak (near ovulation)	15.00 ± 3.80	8.00-25.00
Day of 2nd estradiol peak (luteal phase)	21.90 ± 3.10	15.00-27.00
Day of progesterone rise (>2 ng/mL)	17.40 ± 3.50	11.00-27.00
Day of progesterone peak	21.60 ± 3.10	15.00-27.00
VARIATIONS IN HORMONE CONCENTRATIONS		
Absolute minimum estradiol (pg/mL)	39.90 ± 11.80	23.30-57.50
Absolute peak estradiol (1st peak) (pg/mL)	203.00 ± 53.60	85.60-295.00
Relative change$_{(peak-min)}$ in estradiol (pg/mL)	163.10 ± 55.90	30.30-264.80
Absolute minimum progesterone (ng/mL)	0.61 ± 0.27	0.30-1.10
Absolute peak progesterone (ng/mL)	14.30 ± 5.80	3.60-26.80
Relative change$_{(peak-min)}$ in progesterone (ng/mL)	13.90 ± 5.30	3.90-25.70
Minimum testosterone (ng/mL)	22.50 ±10.50	10.00-48.00
Peak testosterone (ng/mL)	68.90 ± 16.70	37.00-115.00
Relative change in testosterone (ng/mL)	43.50 ± 16.80	17.00-95.00

[a] Subjects were 22 normal, menstruating females with self-reported consistent cycle lengths of 28 to 32 days over the past six months.

Adapted, by permission, from S.J. Shultz et al., 2004, "Relationship between sex hormones and anterior knee laxity across the menstrual cycle," *Med Sci Sports Exerc* 36(7): 1165-1174; data from S.J. Shultz et al., 2005, "Sex differences in knee joint laxity change across the female menstrual cycle," *J Sports Med Phys Fit* 45: 594-603.

Heersche 1980; Fischer 1973), indicating increased metabolic activity. Structural changes in tissue have also been observed in response to exposure to estrogen, that is, decreases in total collagen and protein content, and in fiber diameter and density (Abubaker, Hebda, and Gunsolley 1996; Dubey et al. 1998; Hama, Yamamuro, and Takeda 1976). These tissue responses appear to be enhanced with exposure to estrogen and progesterone together (Abubaker, Hebda, and Gunsolley 1996; Dubey et al. 1998), but are diminished when the tissue is exposed to either progesterone or testosterone alone (Abubaker, Hebda, and Gunsolley 1996; Hama, Yamamuro, and Takeda 1976; Shikata et al. 1979). While these findings are based on a variety of connective tissues and research models, the general consensus from the literature is that collagen structure and metabolism are greatly influenced by estrogen and progesterone.

These investigations, along with the identification of sex hormone receptors on the human ACL (Dragoo et al. 2003; Hamlet et al. 1997; Liu et al. 1996; Sciore et al. 1997), have led to considerable interest in sex hormones as a risk factor for ACL injury (Hamlet et al. 1997; Liu et al. 1996; Yu et al. 1997). Investigations in this area include both animal and human models and to date have primarily addressed the effects of estrogen on the metabolism and structure of the collagen tissue, thus the ultimate strength of the ligament.

Effect on Collagen Metabolism

The effect of estrogen on collagen metabolism of the ACL has been studied in both animal (Liu et al. 1997; Seneviratne et al. 2004) and human models (Yu et al. 1999, 2001). Yu and colleagues (1999, 2001) examined human ACL tissue in cell culture to prospectively evaluate the effects of both physiologic and supraphysiologic levels of 17β-estradiol (range 2.9 pg/mL-2500 pg/mL) and progesterone on cell proliferation and collagen synthesis in vitro. These studies revealed two relevant findings. First, they showed as estradiol levels progressively increased, fibroblast proliferation and type 1 procollagen synthesis progressively decreased then eventually leveled off at supraphysiologic levels of estradiol. Increasing levels of progesterone attenuated this inhibitory effect; and when estradiol levels were controlled, increasing progesterone levels actually resulted in dose-dependent increases in fibroblast proliferation and type 1 procollagen synthesis. The second relevant finding is that these hormone effects were transient, with the most pronounced effects observed in the initial days after hormone exposure (days 1 and 3) and with effects beginning to attenuate within seven days of exposure. Collectively, these results suggest that large, transient changes in progesterone and estrogen concentrations across the menstrual cycle may influence ACL metabolism and collagen synthesis in an interactive dose- and time-dependent manner.

Results from animal models, on the other hand, are conflicting. Liu and colleagues (1997) prospectively examined female rabbit ACLs in cell culture after two weeks of exposure to physiologic and supraphysiologic concentrations of estradiol (0 [control], 2.9, 25, 250, 2500, and 25,000 pg/mL). A decrease in collagen synthesis and fibroblast proliferation was noted with increasing concentrations of estradiol, starting with 25 pg/mL, compared to values in a control group with no exposure to estradiol. Conversely, Seneviratne and colleagues (2004) prospectively examined sheep ACL fibroblasts in cell culture four and six days after they had been subjected to somewhat similar incremental doses of estradiol (2.2 [control], 5, 15, 25, 250, and 2500 pg/mL), and found no difference in fibroblast proliferation and collagen synthesis at any concentration level.

Because of the limited and conflicting studies in this area, it is difficult to draw meaningful conclusions at this time. Differences in the study designs, including the length of estradiol exposure and the control group used, make it somewhat difficult to directly compare results between studies. Whereas Liu and colleagues (1997) used a control group that received no estradiol and examined changes after two weeks of exposure, Seneviratne and colleagues (2004) used a control group receiving 2.2 pg/mL and examined changes four and six days following exposure. Yu and colleagues (1999) also compared their data to those for a control group that received no estradiol, and this was the only study to look at transient changes that occurred within days of exposure. More work is needed for a full understanding of both the concentration and time dependency effects of estrogen exposure, as well as of other sex hormones, on ACL tissue.

Effect on Mechanical Properties

Studies of estrogen's effects on the mechanical properties of the ACL have been limited to animal models, including rabbit (Slauterbeck et al. 1999), sheep (Strickland et al. 2003), and monkey (Wentorf et al. In press). Using a prospective, matched-control design, Slauterbeck and colleagues (1999) examined the ultimate failure load on the ACL in ovariectomized rabbits with and without 30 days of exposure to estradiol concentrations consistent with pregnancy levels. While biomechanical testing revealed that the estrogen-treated ACLs failed at a 10% lower load compared to control ACLs, these results were limited to supraphysiologic levels of estradiol exposure.

Studies addressing this relationship at more physiological levels have not demonstrated this effect (Strickland et al. 2003; Wentorf et al. In press). Strickland and colleagues (2003) examined the biomechanical properties of 6 ram and 38 ewe knee ligaments, six months following random assignment of the ewes to sham operation, ovariectomy, and ovariectomy plus estradiol implant, as well as low-dose and high-dose raloxifene (estrogen receptor agonist) treatment groups. In this case, estradiol was administered at concentrations near 2 pg/mL, which was deemed similar to the concentration experienced during the normal luteal phase of the ewe estrous cycle. While the ultimate stress of the ram ligaments was greater than the ewe ligaments, the authors observed no difference in ligament strength (maximum force, stiffness, energy to failure) between groups. Similar findings were reported by Wentorf and colleagues (In press), who examined the mechanical properties of the ACLs and patellar tendons obtained from cynomolgus monkeys two years after the animals had been divided into sham-operated and ovariectomized groups. These investigators found no difference in any of the mechanical or material properties tested, including failure load, stiffness, elongation at failure, ultimate stress or strain, or energy at failure. A strength of this latter study is it involved monkeys, whose estrogen levels and cyclic variations of the menstrual cycle closely mirror those of humans (Goodman et al. 1977).

While these studies suggest that mechanical properties of the ACL may not be altered after prolonged exposure to different physiological concentrations of estrogen, more work is needed in this area. Future studies should deal with sex hormones other than estrogen (either in combination or isolation), as estrogen alone may not be responsible for changes in ligament properties (Wentorf et al. In press). Further, no studies were found that addressed acute changes in mechanical properties with acute cyclic changes in sex hormones across a normal menstrual cycle. Given the transient hormone effects on collagen metabolism described by Yu and colleagues (1999), and the cyclic variations that occur in sex hormones across the female menstrual cycle, looking at both acute and chronic effects would seem prudent. Finally, more studies using human and ape models are recommended. While data from various animal studies have improved our understanding of the effects of estradiol on mechanical properties of the ligament, their clinical relevance to the human ACL has been questioned since nonprimates have estrous cycles rather than menstrual cycles and therefore experience very different hormone profiles (Griffin et al. In press-a).

Sex Hormones and Knee Joint Laxity and Stiffness

Basic science studies demonstrating hormone effects on collagen structure and metabolism have prompted clinical research on the effects of sex hormone concentration changes on knee joint laxity and stiffness (Beynnon et al. 2005; Deie et al. 2002; Heitz 1999; Karageanes, Blackburn, and Vangelos 2000; Romani et al. 2003; Shultz et al. 2004b, 2005b). The majority of these studies have measured females at isolated points of their menstrual cycle, typically based on day of the cycle. Also, in all except one study (Karageanes, Blackburn, and Vangelos 2000), hormone concentrations were obtained at the time of knee joint testing. Only two studies included males as a comparison group (Beynnon et al. 2005; Shultz et al. 2005b). Before a review of the work in this area, a brief discussion on measurement of knee laxity and stiffness is warranted.

Knee Joint Laxity Versus Stiffness

Knee joint laxity and stiffness represent two clinical measures of knee joint behavior, most often measured with the KT-1000 or KT-2000 knee arthrometers (MedMetric Corp, San Diego, CA). While knee joint laxity characterizes the amount of joint displacement at a given force, knee joint stiffness characterizes the linear slope of the line between changes in force and changes in displacement across a given force range (figure 19.2). As will be noted in the studies discussed next, laxity and displacement have been defined at various ranges of the force–displacement curve. Another important distinction is that measures of knee joint laxity and stiffness are not direct measures of ACL laxity and stiffness. Because the force is applied externally to the knee joint to displace the tibia on the femur, laxity and stiffness more accurately represent a combination of joint (ligament and capsular) and musculotendinous (active and passive) restraints. Although research has demonstrated that the ACL is the predominant structure that restrains anterior translation of the tibia relative to the femur (Beard et al. 1993; Brask, Lueke, and Soderberg 1984; Butler, Noyes, and Good 1980), the exact contribution of the ACL cannot be determined with these clinical tests. Hence this discussion uses the terms "knee joint laxity" and "knee joint stiffness" throughout.

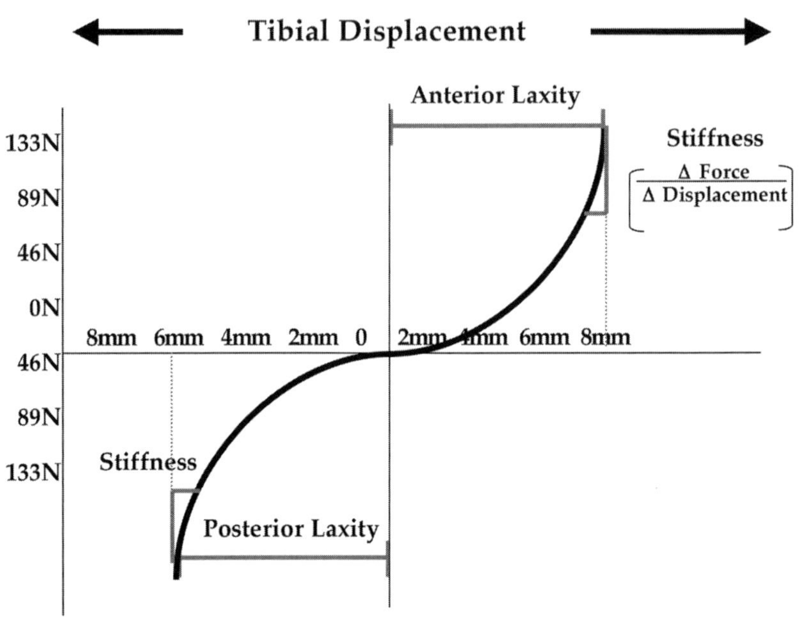

FIGURE 19.2 Measurement of knee joint laxity and terminal stiffness along the force–displacement curve with anterior- and posterior-directed loads on the tibia relative to the femur.

Sex Hormones and Knee Joint Laxity

Through use of a standard knee arthrometer to apply anterior-directed loads of 89 N and 134 N to displace the tibia relative to the femur, significant increases in anterior knee laxity have been found during the periovulatory and luteal phases compared to menses (i.e., the early follicular phase) (Deie et al. 2002; Heitz 1999). Deie and colleagues (2002) found significant increases in knee laxity in the ovulatory phase at 89 N of anterior force, and in the luteal phase at both 89 N and 134 N of anterior force, when compared to menses. These authors reported that cycle phase was based on basal body temperature and weekly serum estradiol and progesterone levels but did not report the criteria for defining cycle phases. Heitz (1999) also found significant differences in the periovulatory and luteal phases compared to menses, measuring knee laxity (133 N) and serum levels of estrogen and progesterone on days 1 (phase 1), 10 to 13 (phase 2), and 20 to 23 (phase 3) in seven normal menstruating females. In both studies, multiple measures were taken across the menstrual cycle, and data were pooled within the defined phases.

In contrast, Shultz and colleagues (2005b) obtained daily measures of serum hormone concentrations and knee laxity through one complete menstrual cycle and compared these values to those for males who were measured once per week for four weeks. Cycle phase was based on actual serum hormone concentrations rather than days of the cycle; menses was defined as the first five days following the onset of menstrual bleeding; the periovulatory phase was defined as the first five days following a 2 standard deviation increase in menstrual-level estradiol levels; early luteal phase was defined as the first five days once progesterone levels exceeded 2 ng/mL; and the late luteal phase was defined as the first five days after progesterone levels peaked. The findings revealed that females had increased knee laxity values on day 5 of the initial estradiol rise near ovulation compared to day 3 of menses, and on days 1 to 3 of the early luteal phase compared to all days of menses and day 1 near ovulation. Consequently sex differences in knee laxity were cycle dependent, with differences being greatest in the first three days of the early luteal phase (~1.5 mm) and least during the days of menses.

Other work has not demonstrated these cyclic changes in knee laxity (Beynnon et al. 2005; Karageanes, Blackburn, and Vangelos 2000; Van Lunen et al. 2003). One study (Karageanes, Blackburn, and Vangelos 2000) relied purely on subject recall versus actual hormone concentrations to confirm cycle phase. Two other studies confirmed cycle phase by measuring serum hormone concentrations on the day of testing, but the testing was limited to a single day to represent a particular phase of the menstrual cycle for all females (Beynnon et al. 2005; Van Lunen et al. 2003). Beynnon and colleagues (2005) compared 17 males and 17 females on anterior-posterior knee laxity at a single time point during each of days 1 to 3 (early follicular), 11 to 13 (late follicular), 20 to 22 (mid luteal), 27 to 28 (late luteal), and days 1 to 3 of the subsequent cycle, with all days corresponding to a 28-day cycle. While they found that females had significantly greater knee laxity compared to males, they observed no differences in knee laxity within females across phases of the cycle. Similarly, Van Lunen and colleagues (2003) found no difference in knee laxity (133 N) between the first day of menses, a day near ovulation (within 10 to 34 hr of a positive ovulation test), and a day in the luteal phase (day 23). Given the variability in the timing of cyclic events as previously described, it is questionable whether a single test day (e.g., day 23, or a day between days 11 and 13) will adequately capture the same hormone milieu for all women within a given phase.

Relationship Between Sex Hormones and Cyclic Changes in Knee Laxity

From the studies showing cyclic increases in knee laxity (Deie et al. 2002; Heitz 1999; Shultz et al. 2005b), what remained unknown was whether the cyclic increases in knee laxity observed in the early luteal phase were a delayed response to rising estradiol levels at ovulation versus a rise in both estradiol and progesterone levels with the onset of the early luteal phase. To address this question, Shultz and colleagues (2004b) examined the relationship between hormone concentration changes and knee laxity changes with and without the possibility of a time lag between these changes (range 0-8 days). On average, knee laxity changes were observed approximately three to four days following changes in sex hormone concentrations. When this time delay was accounted for, changes in estradiol, progesterone, and testosterone explained on average 63.3 ± 7.7% of the change in knee laxity across the cycle. However, when this time delay was not accounted for, the three hormones explained only 26% of the variance in knee laxity.

Important observations from this work (Shultz et al. 2004b, 2005b) are that not all females have greater knee laxity than males, and not all women experience marked changes in knee laxity across their menstrual cycle (range 1.5-5.3 mm). In an effort to better understand the hormone characteristics that mediate these variable responses in knee laxity, the data were further analyzed to determine if absolute hormone concentrations could predict the amount of cyclic increase experienced from menses to the early luteal phase (Shultz et al. 2006a). Findings revealed that minimum estrogen and progesterone levels during menses (early follicular phase) appeared to play a critical role in predicting cyclic increases in knee laxity in response to rising estrogen levels. In particular, females who had higher minimum progesterone levels and lower minimum estrogen levels during the menstrual phase experienced greater increases in knee laxity once estrogen and testosterone levels peaked near ovulation. These findings again highlight the substantial individual variations in hormone profiles and knee laxity changes in normal menstruating females, further exposing the potential inaccuracy of use of a specific day or range of days to represent the same time in the cycle for all women. Hence, it may be important for future studies to identify this individual variability, as some women may experience greater effects of sex hormones on ligament biology than others, potentially exposing them to a greater risk of injury.

Sex Hormones and Knee Joint Stiffness

The effects of sex hormones on knee joint stiffness have been investigated less frequently. In studies on this issue, differences in knee joint stiffness between sexes (Shultz et al. 2005b), or within females across their menstrual cycle (Deie et al. 2002; Romani et al. 2003; Shultz et al. 2005b), have not been observed. While Romani and colleagues (2003) found a significant correlation between anterior knee stiffness and estradiol levels near ovulation, their results revealed no mean difference from one measurement time point to the next. These results are consistent with basic science studies demonstrating no change in mechanical properties in sheep and monkey ACLs with estradiol exposure (Strickland et al. 2003; Wentorf et al. In press). While more work is needed in this area, the limited findings suggest that hormone-mediated increases in knee laxity are not associated with significant alterations in the mechanical behavior of capsuloligament structures.

Pregnancy, Relaxin, and Knee Laxity

During pregnancy, significant increases in joint laxity have been observed (Blecher and Richmond 1998; Charlton, Coslett-Charlton, and Ciccotti 2001;

Dumas and Reid 1997; Schauberger et al. 1996). The fact that the hormone relaxin is present at higher concentrations during pregnancy, and thus may contribute to changes in ligament integrity, has led to investigations of the relationship between serum relaxin hormone levels and ACL biology. Using cell cultures, Dragoo and colleagues (2003) demonstrated binding of relaxin to the female ACL, suggesting the presence of relaxin receptors on the female ACL but not the male ACL. However, no studies to date have demonstrated a relationship between relaxin levels and joint laxity in either pregnant women (Schauberger et al. 1996) or nonpregnant female athletes (Arnold et al. 2002). In fact, one study showed incremental increases in mean knee joint laxity from the first to third trimesters, while relaxin levels incrementally decreased (Schauberger et al. 1996). Although it has been suggested that alterations in tissue remodeling may lag behind significant changes in relaxin concentrations (Dragoo et al. 2003), time delay effects relative to this hormone have not been examined. Alternatively, it is possible that estrogen and progesterone are the primary mediators of laxity changes during pregnancy, as it is known that these levels steadily increase from 6 to 42 weeks (Tulchinsky et al. 1972). While a relationship between estradiol and knee laxity during pregnancy was suggested in one study (Charlton, Coslett-Charlton, and Ciccotti 1999), no correlations were reported. Future time series, case control studies are needed to determine the potential interactive relationships between the various hormones and changes in knee laxity.

Menstrual Cycle and ACL Injury

Given the known effects of sex hormones on peripheral tissues as previously described, other research has focused on ACL injury incidence and whether variations in hormone concentrations across the menstrual cycle influence the likelihood of occurrence of injury. The difficulty with these studies has to do with the ability to accurately capture the phase of the menstrual cycle when injury occurs. As noted in the previous section, this determination is not a simple matter.

Relationship Between Cycle Phase and ACL Injury

A variety of study designs have been used to examine the relationship between menstrual cycle phase and ACL injury risk. Some studies showed a greater number of noncontact ACL injuries than expected during the perimenstrual (Myklebust et al. 2003, 1998; Slauterbeck et al. 2002) or ovulatory (Wojtys et al. 2002) days of the cycle, while two other studies generally identified the follicular phase as the phase of higher risk for noncontact ACL injury (Arendt, Bershadsky, and Agel 2002; Beynnon et al. 2006).

Cycle Phase Based on Self-Report Questionnaires Initial work in this area used retrospective recall of menstrual cycle status at the time of injury via telephone interviews and questionnaires. Following an ACL injury, Myklebust and colleagues (1998) contacted ACL-injured female team handball players via personal or telephone interview, and on the basis of the respondents' self-reported menstrual cycle history and a 28-day cycle, classified injuries as occurring in the menstrual (days 1-7), follicular (days 8-14), early luteal (days 15-21), and late luteal (days 22-28) phases. Of the 23 females injured, only 17 provided menstrual histories; 8 of these were using oral contraceptives while 9 were menstruating normally. In these 17 females, 29% of the injuries occurred in the menstrual phase and 53% occurred in the late luteal phase. Unfortunately, the authors did not separate out the data for normal menstruating females versus those on oral contraceptives. Results were somewhat different in a subsequent study using the same methods and population (Myklebust et al. 2003). For a total of 69 injuries recorded, reliable menstrual data were obtained on 46 of the subjects; 28 used oral contraceptives and 18 were normally menstruating. In both groups, there were significant differences in injury rates by phase, with 50% of injuries occurring during the menstrual phase. In females who were menstruating normally and those using oral contraceptives, respectively, 22% and 29% of the injuries occurred in the follicular phase, 6% and 14% in the early luteal phase, and 22% and 7% in the late luteal phase.

Similarly, Wojtys and colleagues (1998) obtained menstrual history data from 28 ACL-injured females within three months of injury to define the subjects' menstrual cycle phase at the time of injury. Only subjects who had regular menstrual cycles (less than three-day variation in cycle length from month to month) were included. Three phases of the cycle were defined: follicular (days 1-9), ovulatory (days 10-14), and luteal (day 15 to end of cycle). Using these criteria, the authors found a nonsignificant trend ($p = 0.09$) toward a greater prevalence of injury in the ovulatory phase (29% observed, 18% expected) and a lower than expected prevalence in the follicular phase (13% observed, 32% expected) (Wojtys 2000; Wojtys et al. 1998). A study of female collegiate basketball players by Arendt and colleagues (2002) presented contrasting findings. Menstrual cycle history was captured in 58 normal menstruating players (cycle length 28 days, number of cycles 10-12 per year) and 28 oral contraceptive users who sustained a noncontact ACL injury. The follicular phase was generally identified as a higher-risk phase compared to the luteal phase.

The limitation of these studies is that they did not measure actual serum hormone concentrations to confirm cycle phase. Although Wojtys and colleagues (2002) subsequently found that the questionnaire yielded consistent responses from one administration to the next, they noted that the accuracy of this method was not validated against actual hormone concentrations. Further, the aforementioned results are based on the assumption of a 28-day cycle, with relatively fixed cycle lengths. Still, these findings represent important first steps in examining the relationship between cycle phase and ACL injury risk, as they have been instrumental in generating considerable interest and subsequent studies in this area.

Cycle Phase Confirmed by Serum Hormone Concentrations Given the limitations of self-report questionnaires, an effort has been made in subsequent studies to document serum hormone concentrations at the time of injury to confirm cycle phase. In a follow-up study, Wojtys and colleagues (2002) used a case series design to measure urine hormone levels (estradiol, progesterone, and LH) in 69 females (51 normal menstruating, 14 on oral contraceptives) within 24 hr of the time of injury. An added strength of this study is that the investigators also measured LH to further delineate whether females were in their ovulatory or luteal phase. While again more injuries were identified around the ovulatory phase (high estrogen levels), fewer injuries were identified in the luteal phase in women not taking oral contraceptives. Of interest, Wojtys and colleagues also compared the results from identification of cycle phase based on subject recall alone with those based on confirmation of actual urine hormone concentrations. They found substantial discrepancies between the two methods, particularly for the follicular and ovulatory phases. These results confirm the questionable validity of using subject recall to define cycle phase and the need to accurately document the hormone milieu at the time of the injury.

Employing a similar case series approach, Slauterbeck and colleagues (2002) used subject questionnaires and saliva-based estradiol and progesterone levels within 72 hr of injury to document cycle phase in 37 ACL-injured females. Within this cohort, 21 females provided both saliva samples and menstrual histories, while 10 females provided only saliva samples and 6 provided only menstrual histories. For the 21 who provided both saliva samples and menstrual histories, the authors used hormone concentrations of estradiol and progesterone to confirm self-reported cycle phase (the criteria for doing so were not reported, however). Moderate correlations were found between estrogen (0.73) and progesterone (0.72) concentrations derived from saliva samples and those obtained from serum. From these data, the authors identified a higher frequency of ACL injury on the day immediately before and on days 1 and 2 immediately after the onset of menses, and a lower probability of sustaining injury during days 25 to 28 and days 7 to 8 based on a 28-day cycle. The limitations of this study are that hormone concentrations were obtained as long as 72 hr after injury, when levels may have differed dramatically from those at the time of injury. This is of particular concern for the days near ovulation when estradiol increases fourfold, as well as in the early and late luteal phase when both progesterone and estrogen are steadily increasing and decreasing, respectively.

A limitation of studies using the case series design is that they do not include a control group; thus it is assumed that all participants have equal cycle lengths and are equally likely to participate on each day of their menstrual cycle (Beynnon et al. 2006). Hence, Beynnon and colleagues (2006) examined the likelihood of occurrence of an ACL injury by cycle phase using a case control study of 91 alpine skiers (46 injured, 45 uninjured). Using a self-report questionnaire and serum progesterone concentrations obtained immediately after the injury (within 2 hr), the authors divided the menstrual cycle into preovulatory (serum concentrations of progesterone less than 2.0 ng/mL) and postovulatory (serum concentrations of progesterone equal to or greater than 2.0 ng/mL) phases. With cycle phase based on actual serum hormone data, they determined that the odds of occurrence of an ACL injury were significantly elevated in the preovulatory compared to the postovulatory phase of the menstrual cycle (odds ratio = 3.22), with 74% of the injured skiers being in the preovulatory phase and only 56% of the control skiers in the preovulatory phase. With cycle phase based only on subject questionnaires, the odds of occurrence of an ACL injury in the preovulatory versus postovulatory phase were not significant.

Limitations Due to Variability in Cycle Characteristics

If sex hormones play a role in ACL injury risk, why is it that some females are more predisposed to ACL injury than others? One possible explanation may be the individual variations in menstrual cycle characteristics among females. This variability violates the assumption that all females who have "normal" and consistent cycle lengths from month to month will have common phase lengths within a given cycle length and will have similar magnitude and timing of hormone concentrations. The variability further reinforces the inaccuracy of predicting cycle phase based solely on the athlete's recall (Beynnon et al. 2006; Wojtys et al. 2002), and suggests that a single hormone measure may be limited in its ability to accurately identify the participant's day in the cycle or to characterize the hormone milieu in the days preceding injury.

While the ultimate study design would be one that prospectively measured hormone concentrations each day of the cycle until injury occurred, ACL injuries do not occur frequently enough to make this study design practical. Although this justifies the use of a case control design (Beynnon et al. 2006), the limitations lie in the assumptions that a "normal" ovulatory menstrual cycle has occurred and that the hormone levels taken at the time of injury will accurately reflect the phase in the cycle. Because these studies are by necessity retrospective, confirmation of ovulation cannot be documented in these reports. This may result in inaccuracies in phase identification, as anovulatory cycles can result in substantially altered progesterone levels (Israel et al. 1972; Shepard and Senturia 1977). Moreover, because samples are taken after the injury has occurred, it is not possible to measure the hormone milieu that preceded the injury. This may be of greatest concern during the early follicular phase, when estrogen and progesterone levels drop significantly at the time of menses, and in the late follicular phase, when estrogen and progesterone rise substantially in the days surrounding ovulation. Given reports that have identified greater numbers of injuries both at the onset and at the end of the follicular phase, understanding the timing and magnitude of hormone variations prior to the ACL injury may be particularly relevant.

A final concern is the potential variability in cycle characteristics from one month to the next and the effect of this variability on ACL injury risk. While variations in cycle characteristics within a given female from one month to the next are not as great, some variations do exist (Lenton et al. 1983). This is particularly true in physically active females, in whom menstrual disturbances (i.e., oligomenorrhea, amenorrhea) are more common than in less active females (Otis et al. 1997; Shangold and Mirkin 1988). Hence the decision by authors to exclude subjects who do not have consistent, regular cycles (Arendt, Bershadsky, and Agel 2002; Beynnon et al. 2006; Wojtys et al. 2002) limits the ability to generalize findings to all physically active females. While this inclusion criterion was necessary to accurately identify cycle phase based on questionnaire and a single hormone measurement, its potential to bias the sample and study findings should be recognized and considered in future study designs.

If sex hormones are truly a risk factor for ACL injury, it may very well be that the individual differences in the absolute magnitude and relative timing of sex hormone profiles across the menstrual cycle may in part explain why some women sustain ACL injuries while others do not. Hence, there is a need to develop methods that will allow researchers to reasonably capture these individual differences in hormone profiles so that we may further clarify the relationship between sex hormones and ACL injury in future prospective studies. For example, work is ongoing to develop an algorithm that characterizes female hormone responders versus nonresponders (those who will experience cyclic changes in knee laxity vs. those who do not) based on nadir and peak hormone concentrations obtained at key points of the cycle (Shultz et al. 2006a). It may also be advisable to examine, in addition to the hormone milieu at the time of injury, the hormone characteristics in a subsequent cycle, as this may offer additional information to further clarify the hormone milieu that may have been present in the days preceding the injury. However, the reliability of these methods must first be established.

Summary

On the basis of the published research to date, members of the 2005 Hunt Valley II conference determined that there was yet no clear consensus as to the hormonal level or the specific time in the menstrual cycle in which noncontact ACL injury is more likely to occur. However, studies conducted over the past seven years have led to important advances in our understanding of the relationship between cycle phase and ACL injury risk, and have prompted us to think more about the role of hormones as an ACL injury risk factor. In the studies defining cycle phase based on actual hormone concentrations, results appear to consistently implicate the follicular phase as the higher-risk phase, as no study has yet to identify a greater risk of injury in the luteal phase. To build on this early work, study designs that can better capture the unique characteristics of each female's menstrual cycle are needed. It is also important to consider the time dependency effects of sex hormones on collagen metabolism (Yu et al. 1999) and knee laxity (Shultz et al. 2004b). Hence future studies should consider ways to document or predict hormone concentrations in the days preceding the injury (rather than on the day of injury), as these levels may be equally important for accurately characterizing the hormone milieu leading up to the injury event.

Birth Control Hormones, Ligament Biology, and ACL Injury

Reports from the United States have indicated a prevalence of oral contraceptive use ranging from 8% to 14% in the adolescent population (Miller et al. 1999; Paulus, Saint-Remy, and Jeanjean 2000) and 26.7% in the collegiate athlete population (Beals and Manore 2002). In a recent study of 3150 NCAA basketball and soccer athletes, 28% of the basketball players and over 42% of the soccer players reported using contraceptive hormones (Agel, Bershadsky, and Arendt 2006). But while it is known that a significant percentage of physically active females take contraceptive hormones, very little is known about the effects of these hormones on ligament biology and ACL injury risk.

Bioactivity of Oral Contraceptives

The ability of sex hormones to access their target tissues (e.g., ligament), and thus become biologically active, is dependent on the extent to which they are freely circulating in the blood. Contraceptive hormones deliver synthetic ethinyl estradiol and progesterone at levels often much higher than those observed during the normal menstrual cycle. These exogenous hormones effectively reduce the bioavailability of circulating endogenous hormones by two mechanisms. First, they inhibit ovarian maturation and synthesis of estradiol by interfering with the hypothalamus-pituitary-ovarian axis and suppressing the release of follicle stimulating hormone (FSH) and LH (Clark et al. 2001; Coney and DelConte 1999). Secondly, the presence of synthetic ethinyl estradiol causes a two- to threefold increase in the levels of sex hormone binding globulin (SHBG), which effectively binds the hormones and dramatically reduces their free fraction concentration, making them less available for biological action (Henzyl 2001; London et al. 1992; Wreje et al. 2000).

Regardless of the specific compounds and doses used in the various contraceptive preparations that are common today, the actions just outlined typically result in profound suppression of endogenous progesterone (<1 ng/mL) and estradiol (<20 pg/mL) concentrations to early follicular levels, and in a 30% to 70% reduction in free testosterone levels depending on the progesterone compound used (Aden, Jung-Hoffman, and Kuhl 1998; Casazza et al. 2002; Coney and DelConte 1999; Hammond et al. 2003; Rabe, Nitsche, and Runnebaum 1997; Wiegratz et al. 2003; Wreje et al. 2000). In studies of women receiving either monophasic or triphasic 28-day oral contraceptives that deliver synthetic hormones for 21 days and a placebo for seven days (allowing menstruation), estradiol levels remained below 20 pg/mL during hormone delivery weeks and remained well below 50 pg/mL (14-39 pg/mL) during the hormone-free week (Aden, Jung-Hoffman, and Kuhl 1998; Casazza et al. 2002; Creinin et al. 2002; Rabe, Nitsche, and Runnebaum 1997). Thus, contraceptive hormones appear to provide consistent cycle control that may effectively manipulate biologically available endogenous hormone levels. Studying physically active females who use these preparations may help us gain a better understanding of the hormone phasing and concentrations that may affect knee laxity and ACL injury risk.

Birth Control Hormones and Knee Laxity

Research examining the effects of contraceptive hormones on knee laxity is quite limited. In fact, a review of the literature revealed only two studies that addressed the effects of oral contraceptive use on knee joint laxity. In a study of collegiate female athletes, Martineau and colleagues (2004) compared 42 athletes using low-dose oral contraceptive preparations (OCP) to 36 nonusers on measures of anterior knee laxity (at 67 N and 89 N) and ligament compliance (between 89 N and 67 N) using a KT-1000 knee arthrometer. They found that OCP users had significantly less knee laxity (~1 mm) than nonusers. In contrast, Pokorny and colleagues (2000) compared 30 low-dose OCP users and 25 nonusers on anterior knee laxity and digit joint motion and found no significant differences between groups. Knee laxity was measured with the KT-1000 at 89 N and 134 N, and the mean value of the two measures was used for analysis. Both studies used a criterion of three months for OCP use versus nonuse for group assignment, and both excluded subjects with irregular cycles. The primary difference between the two studies is that Pokorny and colleagues (2000) did not measure subjects during the menstrual week, since OCP users were not on contraceptive hormones during those days. Unfortunately, neither study reported serum hormone levels, so it is impossible to compare hormone profiles in the OCP user groups and nonuser groups across the two studies. Of interest, Pokorny and colleagues (2000) observed more variability in knee laxity in nonusers compared to OCP users who were tested at different days of the menstrual cycle.

Future prospective case control study designs are needed to clarify the relationship between endogenous versus exogenous hormone concentrations and knee laxity. Comparisons should include OCP users and nonusers as well as a male comparison group in order to clarify differences between groups, as well as the stability of knee laxity values within each group across time. Documentation of hormone concentrations (both exogenous and endogenous) is imperative not only to accurately define cycle phase, but also to account for differences in bioavailable concentrations.

Birth Control Hormones and ACL Injury

Because females on oral contraceptives are thought to have lower and more stable bioavailable concentrations of endogenous hormones across the cycle, investigators have examined whether OCP users may be at reduced risk for traumatic knee injury compared to normal menstruating females. Of the studies previously reported that addressed the association between ACL injury and cycle phase, four included females who used oral contraceptives (Arendt, Bershadsky, and Agel 2002; Myklebust et al. 1998; Slauterbeck et al. 2002; Wojtys et al. 2002). Of these four studies, three presented separate findings for oral contraceptive users (Arendt, Bershadsky, and Agel 2002; Slauterbeck et al. 2002; Wojtys et al. 2002), and two documented actual hormone concentrations to identify cycle phase (Slauterbeck et al. 2002; Wojtys et al. 2002).

Of the 65 ACL-injured females who met the inclusion criteria in the study by Wojtys and colleagues (2002), 14 were OCP users. While no association was found between cycle phase (secondary to a small sample size), a trend toward more injuries in the ovulatory phase and fewer in the follicular phase was reported. Conversely, six of the 37 ACL-injured females in the study by Slauterbeck and colleagues (2002) were OCP users, with five of the six sustaining an ACL injury in the early follicular phase. Similar findings were reported by Arendt and colleagues (2002), who showed that OCP users (N = 25) were at higher risk in the follicular phase compared to the luteal phase, with a shift to more injuries at the beginning of the cycle. However, a follow-up study revealed no periodicity in the OCP group (Agel, Bershadsky, and Arendt 2006). In each of these studies, the association between ACL injury and cycle phase appeared to be relatively similar when OCP users were compared to normal menstruating females.

While one might be tempted to conclude that the prevalence of ACL injury is lower in females using OCP, because each study reported fewer OCP users than nonusers in its ACL-injured population, no conclusion can be drawn in this regard without knowledge of the proportion of OCP users versus nonusers in the total population from which the sample was obtained. In what appears to be the largest study to date of OCP users, contraceptive hormones do not seem to have a protective effect on ankle or knee injury. Agel and colleagues (2006) examined ankle and ACL injury risk over two seasons in a cohort of 3150 NCAA Division I collegiate basketball and soccer players. In this sample, 28% of the total basketball players and 42% of the total soccer players who enrolled in the study used contraceptive hormones. There were a total of 45 noncontact ACL injuries and 116 noncontact ankle sprains. Comparison of injury rates (per 1000 exposures) between athletes using contraceptive hormones and those not using contraceptive hormones revealed no difference in ankle sprains or noncontact ACL injury rates. While the authors also reported no difference in periodicity in injury rates across the cycle in athletes using contraceptive hormones, the analyses of these data were based on a smaller subset of the data (eight ACL and 18 ankle injuries), as only those athletes who reported 28 days or less between onset of menses and time of injury were included.

Variability in Contraceptive Hormone Preparations

While it is well established that contraceptive hormones effectively reduce endogenous hormones to their nadirs, what remains unclear is the bioactivity of the contraceptive hormones. Studies on pre- and postmenopausal females who use birth control and hormone replacement therapy, respectively, have shown that exogenous hormones have the same biological effects as endogenous hormones on both reproductive (uterus, breast) and nonreproductive (bone, hypothalamus, pituitary) tissues (Larsen et al. 2003). This would suggest that exogenous hormones may also influence ligament biology, and that low-dose versus high-dose oral contraceptive preparations may have differential effects on these tissues given the large difference in hormone concentrations they deliver. Unfortunately, current assay techniques allow detection of only the drug itself or its metabolized by-products, so it is difficult to determine biologically active concentrations. However, pharmokinetic parameters for common contraceptive preparations, as well as one report showing that 64% of synthetic ethinyl estradiol is metabolized in the first 24 hr to biologically inactive estrogen sulphates (Wild, Rudland, and Black 1991), suggest that bioavailable exogenous concentrations are substantially lower than endogenous concentrations found in the early follicular to midfollicular phase of normal menstruating females. This reduced bioavailability is further supported by findings of reduced collagen turnover in those taking contraceptive hormones compared to normal menstruating females (Wreje et al. 2000).

Although these findings suggest that exogenous concentrations have a negligible effect on ligament biology, more research is needed for an understanding of the differences in bioavailable hormone concentrations in OCP users versus nonusers, and of the extent to which this relationship might differ from one hormone preparation to the next. For example, some preparations maintain constant levels for 21 days (monophasic) while others provide incremental changes in concentrations from one week to the next (triphasic). Preparations also differ in the absolute concentration of hormones delivered, as well as the type of hormones delivered (i.e., estrogen only, progesterone only, and combination of estrogen and progesterone). Future studies on the relationship between OCP use, joint laxity, and ACL injury risk may need to further stratify the data by type and concentration of hormones delivered and confirm bioavailable concentrations through actual serum sampling. Although the recent study by Agel and colleagues (2006) documents the type of contraceptive hormone used by NCAA Division I female athletes (monophasic, triphasic, or other), the authors determined that sample sizes were not sufficient to compare injury rates among athletes using the various hormone preparations.

Summary

While sex hormones constitute a promising area of study relative to ACL injury, it is clear that much remains unknown regarding the effects of sex hormones on ligament biology and injury risk. Although sex hormones appear to have a profound effect on collagen and have been shown to mediate cyclic increases in knee laxity as measured by knee arthrometer testing across the cycle, further research is needed to determine the neuromuscular and biomechanical implications of these biological changes and, ultimately, their relationship to injury risk (see chapter 21 for further discussion on this topic). Moreover, universal agreement is still lacking on whether there is a time in the menstrual cycle when the greatest numbers of injuries occur. While the preponderance of evidence to date suggests that more injuries occur in early and late follicular phase, the exact hormone milieu that may mediate injury occurrence remains relatively unknown.

To further clarify the relationship between sex hormones, ligament biology, and ACL risk, it is imperative that future researchers consider and appreciate the inherent individual variability in cycle characteristics between females. Paramount to this understanding is the need to study all females at risk for injury, including those who are on oral contraceptives and those who experience irregular cycles from one month to the next (e.g., amenorrheic, oligomenorrheic). This will require accurate documentation of each female's hormone milieu at the time of testing or injury (and perhaps on the days preceding testing or injury) via obtaining actual hormone concentrations through reliable means (e.g., serum, urine, saliva). Finally, when examining data across phases of the menstrual cycle, researchers are strongly encouraged to align data based on actual hormone concentrations instead of using a particular day or ranges of days in the menstrual cycle to represent a particular phase.

Chapter 20

Anatomical Factors in ACL Injury Risk

Sandra J. Shultz, PhD, ATC, CSCS
Anh-Dung Nguyen, MS Ed, ATC
Bruce D. Beynnon, PhD

The ACL is the most vulnerable to injury during activities that require sudden deceleration or change of direction with the foot planted (Boden et al. 2000; Olsen et al. 2004). One mechanism often described is a "functional valgus collapse" of the knee (Ireland 1999; Olsen et al. 2004), characterized by valgus and external rotation of the tibia relative to the femur, as the knee transitions from nonweight bearing to weight bearing (Olsen et al. 2004). Expert consensus in 1999 suggested that sex differences in neuromuscular and biomechanical function are the most compelling reasons more females are injured by these mechanisms (Griffin et al. 2000). However, we have yet to fully understand the underlying causes for these sex differences in neuromuscular and biomechanical function or their specific relationship to injury risk.

Lower extremity anatomy and posture differ markedly between males and females. However, the extent to which these sex differences in anatomy and posture contribute to sex differences in neuromuscular and biomechanical function of the knee joint, or independently contribute to ACL injury risk, remains poorly understood. In fact, expert consensus in 1999 concluded that the data were insufficient to relate lower extremity anatomical alignment to ACL injury risk and that more research was needed (Griffin et al. 2000). Unfortunately, our understanding of this relationship has progressed little over the past six years. The reason may be that anatomical factors are often overlooked in injury prevention programs because they are considered structural in nature

The authors wish to thank David H. Perrin, PhD, ATC, for his critical review and feedback on the chapter.

and therefore not modifiable through training. While that may be true of some factors, others are modifiable or can be compensated for through the use of orthotics, bracing, and functional training. Moreover, if we are to accurately identify those at greatest risk for injury and target our intervention strategies accordingly, it is imperative that we gain a better understanding of the potential underlying causes for dynamic knee joint dysfunction and injury risk. To that end, this chapter explores anatomical factors that are known to differ between males and females and examines how they may influence dynamic function and injury risk.

Notch Size and Width

A smaller femoral intercondylar notch width has been associated with a greater risk of ACL injury in a variety of athletic populations, including those in high school, college, the military, and European club sports. In a study of high school athletes, Souryal and Freeman (1993) reported that athletes with a small intercondylar notch width index (the ratio of the width of the anterior outlet of the intercondylar femoral notch to the total condylar width at the level of the popliteal groove) were at significantly increased risk for sustaining an ACL injury. Research on collegiate athletes showed similar findings (LaPrade and Burnett 1994). Uhorchak and colleagues (2003) performed a study of military academy cadets and reported that several risk factors predisposed them to noncontact ACL injury. Significant risk factors included a small femoral notch width, generalized joint laxity, and, in women, higher than normal body mass index and KT-2000 arthrometer measurements of anterior-posterior knee laxity that were 1 standard deviation or more above the mean. Lund-Hanssen and colleagues (1994) studied female European team handball athletes and reported that an increased risk of ACL injury was associated with a decreased femoral notch width. Female handball athletes with a femoral notch width of 17 mm or less were six times more susceptible to ACL injury than athletes with larger femoral notch widths. As well, Ireland and colleagues (2001) reported that individuals with smaller femoral notch width were at increased risk of suffering an ACL injury compared to those with larger notch widths. In contrast, Lombardo and colleagues (2005) studied professional male basketball athletes and reported that intercondylar femoral notch width could not be used to identify an athlete at risk for an ACL tear.

The biomechanical implications of a smaller notch width relative to ACL injury risk remain unclear. It has been suggested that an imbalance between the size of the ACL and the notch width may be the predisposing factor for injury. Proportionally, a smaller notch may lead to abnormal loading of the ACL, while a smaller ACL may have a lower ultimate failure strength to withstand loads applied to the knee (Souryal, Moore, and Evans 1988; Uhorchak et al. 2003). While females appear to have smaller ACLs than males, consistent with their smaller stature (Anderson et al. 2001; Rizzo, Holler, and Bassett 2001; Staeubli et al. 1999), sex differences in femoral notch width (Anderson et al. 2001; Chandrashekar et al. 2005; Charlton et al. 2002; Shelbourne, Davis, and Klootwyk 1998) and the relationship between notch size and ACL size (Chandrashekar et al. 2005; Charlton et al. 2002) are inconclusive.

Generalized Joint Laxity

Generalized joint laxity (GJL) is most often measured using the Beighton score described by Carter and Wilkinson (1964) and later modified by Beighton and colleagues (1969, 1973). The score reflects an overall measure of joint hypermobility (between 0 and 9) based on bilateral examination of fifth finger extension beyond 90°, opposition of the thumb to the forearm, elbow hyperextension beyond 10°, knee hyperextension beyond 10°, and forward flexion of the trunk so that the palms of the hands rest on the floor. Differences in GJL have been reported in comparisons of sex, age, ethnicity, and limb dominance. Females have greater GJL laxity compared to males, and the difference is consistent across ages (Beighton, Solomon, and Soskolne 1973; Jansson et al. 2004). Generalized joint laxity is greatest in infancy and declines as age increases in both males and females (with the greatest decline during childhood), but the decline in females tends to be slower than in males (Birrell et al. 1994). One report suggests that the greatest difference between sexes occurs around the age of 15, coincident with hormonal changes during puberty (Jansson et al. 2004).

Relationship to Injury Risk

Several investigations have addressed the relationship between GJL and lower extremity injury in general (Acasuso-Diaz, Collantes-Esteves, and Sanchez-Guijo 1993; Nicholas 1970), or GJL and all knee ligament injuries (Decoster et al. 1999; Grana and Moretz 1978) considered as a group; however, very little is known about the relationship between GJL and ACL injury. The most comprehensive study currently available on the topic was reported by Uhorchak and colleagues (2003), who performed a prospective study of the relationship between intrinsic risk factors and ACL injury in athletes attending the U.S. Military Academy. The Beighton test was used to evaluate GJL, and subjects with excessive laxity bilaterally in at least three joints were considered to have increased GJL. When male and female athletes were considered as a group, those with increased GJL had a 2.8 times increased risk of suffering an ACL injury. Males with increased GJL had a relative risk value of 3.1, while females had a relative risk value of 2.7.

A retrospective, matched-control study by Ramesh and colleagues (2005) also supports a relationship between GJL and ACL injury. The authors assessed the degree of genu recurvatum of the uninjured knee and GJL in 169 ACL-injured patients prior to reconstructive surgery, and compared these values to those for

65 age- and gender-matched control subjects. Generalized joint laxity was measured using the Beighton score, and a score greater than 6 defined hypermobility. The results revealed a significantly greater proportion of subjects with GJL in the ACL-injured group (42.6%) compared to the control group (21.5%).

Genu recurvatum (figure 20.1), one of the five measures that compose the Beighton score for GJL, has also been assessed independently relative to ACL injury risk. In the work of Ramesh and colleagues (2005), the proportion of subjects with genu recurvatum was 78.7% in the ACL-injured group and 37% in the control group. Loudon and colleagues (1996) also found genu recurvatum to be a significant predictor of ACL injury status, in combination with foot pronation.

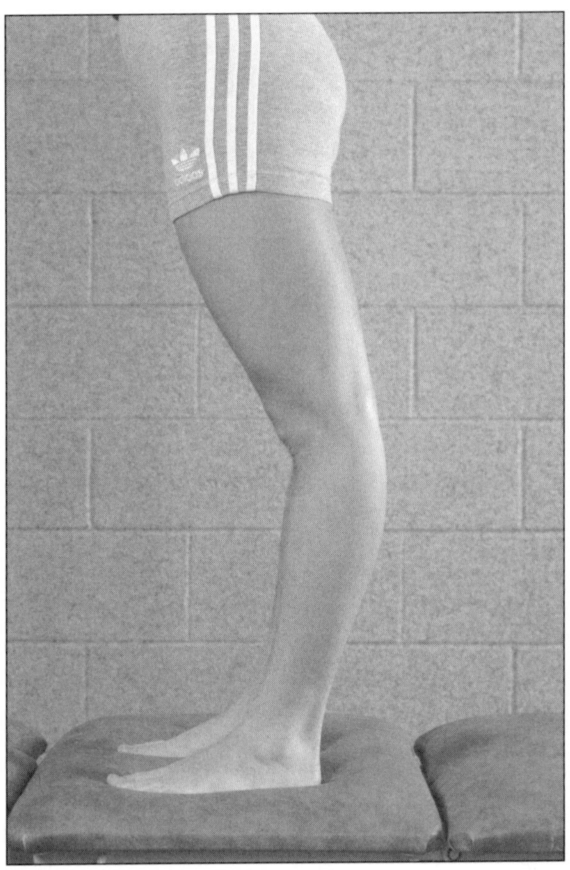

FIGURE 20.1 Genu recurvatum (knee hyperextension) greater than 10° is considered to reflect hypermobility.

Reprinted, by permission, from S.J. Shultz, P. Houglum, and D.H. Perrin, 2005 *Examination of musculoskeletal injuries*, 2nd ed. (Champaign, IL: Human Kinetics), 466.

Neuromuscular and Biomechanical Implications

Currently we do not fully understand the mechanism by which increased GJL leads to increased risk of ACL injury. In part, this is because the relationships between GJL, neuromuscular function, and the biomechanical response of the knee during at-risk activities such as landing from a jump or performing a plant and pivot maneuver have not been fully established and understood. It is important for us to point out that GJL does not consider the knee in isolation and does not provide an evaluation of joint biomechanics with multiple degrees of freedom (the situation that occurs when an ACL is torn). For example, it may be that the anterior-posterior and varus-valgus load displacement responses of the knee considered in combination with the internal-external torque rotation response of the joint is more predictive of ACL injury than GJL. Evidence for such a hypothesis is provided by the recent report by Hewett and colleagues (2005b) indicating that females with increased knee abduction angle when landing from a jump were at increased risk of suffering an ACL tear. While it remains unclear whether or not anatomic alignment of the lower extremity, neuromuscular function, and the biomechanical behavior of the ligaments that span the knee contribute to injury in isolation or combination, this certainly warrants future study for a complete understanding of ACL injury mechanisms.

Anterior Knee Laxity

Knee laxity has often been cited as a potential ACL injury risk factor, and it is generally agreed that females have greater knee laxity than males (Grana and Moretz 1978; Larsson, Baum, and Mudholkar 1987; Rosene and Fogarty 1999; Rozzi et al. 1999; Shultz et al. 2005b). Further, marked cyclic increases in knee laxity have been observed in some females from menses to the early luteal phase of their menstrual cycle (Deie et al. 2002; Heitz 1999; Shultz et al. 2005b). Thus it is somewhat surprising how little research has directly addressed knee laxity as an independent ACL injury risk factor.

Relationship to Injury Risk

A comprehensive review of the literature identified only two studies (one prospective, one retrospective) that included anterior knee laxity among a group of variables to predict ACL injury risk.

The most compelling data in this regard were reported by Uhorchak and colleagues (2003), who prospectively followed 1200 U.S. Military Academy cadets during their four-year tenure at the academy. Of the 14 variables measured on each participant, GJL (in both males and females) and anterior knee laxity values that exceeded 1 standard deviation (SD) of the mean (in females) were both considered significant predictors of ACL injury risk. When all subjects were considered, a model including narrow femoral notch width, higher than average body mass index (BMI), GJL, and anterior knee laxity (134 N with the KT-2000 knee arthrometer) values greater than 1 SD above the mean was determined to be the most predictive of ACL injury risk. However, this model explained only 28% of the variance in ACL-injured subjects and correctly predicted only 17% of those who injured their ACL. When females were considered alone, a model that included femoral notch width, BMI, and GJL or anterior knee laxity was able to correctly predict nearly 75% of those who sustained a noncontact ACL injury and 98% of those who were not injured. The contribution of anterior knee laxity to the prediction model for women was particularly compelling given that the relative risk of ACL injury increased considerably when anterior knee laxity (greater than 1 SD above the mean) was combined with either a narrow femoral notch (risk ratio 16.8) or higher BMI values (37.7). The relative risk for each variable alone, while significant, was much lower (knee laxity = 2.7, BMI = 3.5, and femoral notch = 4.0). In fact, all ACL-injured females had a combination of a narrow femoral notch, a BMI greater than 1 SD above the mean, and either GJL or anterior knee laxity greater than 1 SD above the mean.

The findings from this prospective study implicating anterior knee laxity as a contributory risk factor are further supported by a retrospective study showing that increased knee laxity and navicular drop values correctly predicted ACL injury status in 88% of the females and in 71% of all cases (both males and females) (Woodford-Rogers, Cyphert, and Denegar 1994). The major limitation of these studies is that very few ACL-injured subjects were included. For example, Uhorchak and colleagues (2003) followed 1200 cadets over four years, and this generated eight women with ACL disruptions. Therefore, it is important to confirm these findings in a larger cohort of athletes that generates a larger number of ACL-injured women.

Neuromuscular and Biomechanical Implications

The specific mechanism or mechanisms by which anterior knee joint laxity (as measured nonweight bearing) may modify ACL risk are currently unknown. However, it is well known that the ACL acts as a primary static stabilizer of the knee, providing the majority of restraint to anterior translation of the tibia relative to the femur in both nonweight-bearing and weight-bearing postures (Beard et al. 1993; Beynnon et al. 2002; Brask, Lueke, and Soderberg 1984; Butler, Noyes, and Grood 1980; Hsieh and Walker 1976; Lofvenberg et al. 1995; Smith, Livesay, and Woo 1993). Mechanoreceptors present in the human ACL (Schultz et al. 1984; Zimney, Schutte, and Dabezies 1986) also enable the ligament to provide sensory feedback about changes in ligament length and tension, thereby modifying neuromuscular strategies (Barrack, Lund, and Skinner 1994; Fujita et al. 2000; Johannson, Sjolander, and Sojka 1990; Sojka et al. 1989; Solomonow et al. 1987). Based on the role of the ACL as both a primary ligament restraint and dynamic sensory modality, potential mechanisms include reduced proprioceptive sensitivity to joint displacements and loads (Rozzi et al. 1999; Shultz, Carcia, and Perrin 2004) and altered biomechanics during weight bearing (Shultz et al. 2006b). Hormonal effects also represent a potential mechanism given the noted relationships between sex hormones and knee joint laxity (Deie et al. 2002; Heitz 1999; Shultz et al. 2004b), ligament tensile strength (Slauterbeck et al. 1999), and injury risk (Beynnon et al. 2006; Slauterbeck and Hardy 2001; Wojtys et al. 2002) (see chapter 20).

Altered Biomechanics During Weight Bearing One of the more common ACL injury mechanisms is described as occurring just after foot strike, with the knee near full extension. During the transition from nonweight bearing to weight bearing, research indicates that there is a natural anterior shift of the tibia relative to the femur when the knee is near full extension (Beynnon et al. 2002; Fleming et al. 2001; Torzilli, Deng, and Warren 1994). Studies of ACL-intact versus ACL-deficient knees have shown that this anterior shift of the tibia relative to the femur is restrained by the ACL in the normal knee (Fleming et al. 2001; Torzilli, Deng, and Warren, 1994). These findings, combined with evidence that tibiofemoral contact is located more posterior on the tibia in the ACL-deficient knee (Scarvell et al. 2005), indicate that the ACL plays an important role in maintaining normal tibiofemoral joint position and biomechanics upon initial ground contact during activities such as landing from a jump or in the foot strike phase of gait. Hence, it is possible that increased knee laxity may allow greater anterior displacement of the tibia relative to the femur upon weight acceptance of the limb and potentially disrupt the normal alignment of joint surfaces. These biomechanical alterations would be of greatest concern during rapid deceleration maneuvers that are accompanied by large quadriceps forces, which have the potential to further accentuate anterior displacement of the tibia relative to the femur and thus increase ACL strain values (DeMorat et al. 2004; Torzilli, Deng, and Warren, 1994).

Shultz and colleagues (2006b) initially explored the relationship between non-weight-bearing anterior knee laxity (using the KT-2000 knee arthrometer) and the magnitude of anterior translation of the tibia relative to the femur produced during the transition from nonweight-bearing to weight-bearing conditions (using the Vermont Knee Laxity Device). Examination of 20 subjects revealed that subjects with greater anterior knee laxity also had greater anterior tibial translation, with a 1 mm increase in anterior knee laxity predicting an approximate 0.5 mm increase in anterior tibial translation. However, this study did not account for other relevant factors that may also influence the amount of anterior tibial translation with an applied compressive load to the joint, namely joint geometry (i.e., the slope of the tibial plateau) and muscle coactivation levels.

Research has clearly established the contribution of the hamstrings, both singularly and in coactivation with the quadriceps, in regulating joint stiffness and ACL protection by preventing or decreasing anterior and rotary displacement of the tibia relative to the femur (Hirokawa et al. 1991; Renstrom et al. 1986). Further, the slope of the tibial plateau in the sagittal plane has been found to vary widely in the human knee (0-20° with a mean ± SD of 10 ± 3°) (Dejour and Bonnin 1994; Jiang, Yip, and Liu 1994), and research suggests that a 10°

increase in anterior to posterior tibial slope can increase anterior tibial translation by as much as 6 mm upon weight acceptance (single-leg stance) (Dejour and Bonnin 1994). Accounting for these factors in future studies will further our understanding of the relationship between anterior knee laxity (measured clinically) and knee joint biomechanics during weight bearing. Additionally, this initial study did not examine gender differences, and it is unknown if the relationship between anterior tibial translation produced during the transition from nonweight bearing to weight bearing and anterior knee laxity is similar for males and females.

Reduced Proprioception and Altered Neuromuscular Responses The cruciate ligaments have a sensory role in joint stabilization, providing proprioceptive feedback in response to relatively small tensile loads (5-40 N) by heightening gamma motor neuron activation and muscle spindle sensitivity (Johannson, Sjolander, and Sojka 1990; Sojka et al. 1989). The sensory role of the ACL has been demonstrated in the ACL-deficient knee, with these subjects showing reduced proprioception (Mizuta et al. 1992; Roberts, Andersson, and Friden 2004), increased reflex delays with sudden anterior tibial translations (Beard et al. 1993; Wojtys and Huston 1994), and altered neuromuscular control strategies during cutting (Branch, Hunter, and Donath 1989) and landing maneuvers (Gauffin and Tropp 1992; McNair and Marshall 1994) when compared to subjects with uninjured knees. Further, in a cohort of ACL-injured subjects, a greater decrease in knee joint proprioception (threshold to detection of passive motion) was observed in those who had greater joint laxity (as measured by the Lachman exam) (Roberts, Andersson, and Friden 2004). Given these findings, the question arises whether increased knee laxity (in an otherwise healthy knee) may allow greater joint displacement and loads before a proprioceptive threshold is reached, thus potentially delaying sensory feedback and protective neuromuscular responses. To date, few studies have addressed the neuromuscular consequences of increased knee joint laxity in healthy knees.

Rozzi and colleagues (1999) measured knee joint laxity (KT-1000 at 133 N), joint kinesthesia (threshold to detection of passive knee motion), single-leg balance (stability index), time to peak torque of the knee flexors and extensors measured isokinetically at 180°/sec, and muscle activity in response to a landing task (surface electromyography; EMG) in healthy male and female collegiate basketball and soccer athletes (N = 34). Compared to males, females had greater knee laxity (mean difference of ~1.25 mm), increased threshold to detect knee extension motion, and increased peak amplitude of the lateral hamstring muscle when landing from a jump. The authors proposed that the greater joint laxity in females may have rendered the knee less sensitive to joint motion and that increased hamstring activity was an active strategy to stabilize the knee in the presence of reduced passive (capsule-ligamentous) stability. While direct correlations between knee joint laxity and neuromuscular variables were not reported in their study, other work (Shultz, Carcia, and Perrin 2004) supports this hypothesis.

Shultz, Carcia, and Perrin (2004) compared neuromuscular responses (preactivity, reflex time and amplitude) produced during a single-leg weight-bearing perturbation in females with above-average knee laxity versus those with below-average knee laxity. Females with above-average knee laxity had increased lateral hamstring amplitude throughout the perturbation (pre and post), yet significantly longer reflex delays in the hamstring muscles in response to the perturbation. Other studies, while not directly measuring anterior knee laxity, also indicate proprioceptive and neuromuscular changes in subjects with increased knee laxity. Loudon (2000) compared females with high (>5°) and low (<5°) genu recurvatum on weight-bearing knee joint reproduction at 10°, 30°, and 60°. Genu recurvatum was positively correlated with absolute angular error, with the high recurvatum group demonstrating greater reproduction errors at all angles. Further static and cyclic loading of the knee (resulting in creep and temporary increases in anterior knee joint laxity) has been shown to alter neuromuscular responses of the quadriceps and hamstrings (Chu et al. 2003; Sbriccoli et al. 2005).

While these studies suggest that increased knee laxity has the potential to alter knee joint proprioception and neuromuscular activation strategies, more studies are needed. Rozzi and colleagues (1999) examined sex differences in knee laxity and neuromuscular variables, making inferences regarding the relationship between these variables since they were all greater in females than in males. Conversely, Shultz, Carcia, and Perrin (2004) examined the effects of knee joint laxity on neuromuscular responses, but did not include males. Therefore, it is unknown whether similar neuromuscular patterns would be observed in both males and females who have similar knee laxity values. Further, given the dynamic nature of these tasks (landing, perturbations), studies incorporating both neuromuscular and biomechanical analyses are needed to fully interpret the clinical implications of the hamstring EMG responses observed in females with above-average knee laxity during weight-bearing activities (Rozzi et al. 1999; Shultz, Carcia, and Perrin 2004). Whether these altered responses represent proprioceptive deficits in response to joint loading (e.g., delayed hamstring responses), or are simply successful compensatory strategies to control altered knee biomechanics during weight bearing (e.g., increased lateral hamstring activation to restrain anterior translation and internal tibial rotation in the lax knee), will have significant bearing on our approach to injury prevention.

Hormonal Influences As discussed in the previous chapter, knee laxity is affected by sex hormone concentrations, which have also been studied as an independent ACL injury risk factor (see chapter 20). To date, these variables have not been studied in combination as they relate to dynamic knee joint function and ACL injury risk. If continued research in this area concludes that increased knee laxity adversely influences neuromuscular and biomechanical control of the knee during weight bearing, it is plausible that cyclic increases in knee laxity during a female's menstrual cycle may further compromise the dynamic biomechanical response of the knee in those who already have comparatively greater baseline knee laxity values compared to males. In other words, females may experience reduced neuromuscular and biomechanical control of the knee in the days following significant changes in hormone concentrations (e.g., postovulatory/early luteal days of the cycle), supporting epidemiological evidence that ACL injury is cycle dependent (Beynnon et al. 2006; Slauterbeck et al. 2002; Wojtys et al. 2002).

Relationship With Varus-Valgus and Internal-External Knee Laxity Anterior-posterior knee laxity has been used as the primary measure of knee joint laxity because it can be readily determined in most clinical settings. While this laxity measure represents only sagittal plane joint biomechanics, there is some evidence that healthy young adult females who have greater anterior knee laxity compared to males also have greater varus-valgus and internal-external rotational knee laxity (Markolf, Graff-Radford, and Amstutz 1978; Sharma et al. 1999b). It is conceivable therefore that increased anterior knee laxity may actually be correlated with increased knee laxity in multiple planes. Consequently joint biomechanics may also be altered in the frontal plane with increased varus-valgus laxity and, when increased anterior knee laxity is also present, in the transverse plane as well. To date, varus-valgus laxity has been primarily studied as a risk factor for osteoarthritis (not ACL injury risk). Research is therefore needed to determine if females who have greater absolute and cyclic increases in anterior knee laxity also have greater absolute and cyclic increases in varus-valgus and internal-external rotational laxity of the knee. Research is also needed to understand the neuromuscular and biomechanical consequences of multidirectional knee laxity on weight bearing knee joint function and ACL injury risk.

Summary

Females generally have greater anterior knee laxity than males, and can experience marked increases in anterior knee laxity when they are in the early luteal phase of their menstrual cycle. Increased anterior knee laxity has been identified as a relevant factor in predicting female athletes at increased risk of suffering an ACL injury (Uhorchak et al. 2003), and limited evidence suggests that greater knee laxity has the potential to alter joint mechanics and muscle activation strategies during weight bearing. Should increased anterior knee laxity result in increased anterior tibial translation upon weight acceptance and reduced hamstring reflex sensitivity in response to joint loading, this may in part explain observations of preferential quadriceps activity (Huston and Wojtys 1996; Malinzak et al. 2001; Shultz et al. 2001) and greater anterior shear forces and decreased muscular stiffness (Granata, Padua, and Wilson 2002; Padua et al. 2002; Wojtys, Ashton-Miller, and Huston 2002) in females compared to males during functional tasks, all of which have the potential to increase ACL strain values (Fleming et al. 2001; Markolf et al. 1995). Further, the potential for increased anterior knee laxity to be related to increased varus-valgus and internal-external rotational knee laxity may in part explain the increased functional valgus collapse (Ford, Myer, and

Hewett 2003; Hewett, Myer, and Ford 2004; Zeller et al. 2003) and valgus-varus moments observed in females compared to males (Chappell et al. 2002; Hewett et al. 1996; Malinzak et al. 2001; McLean et al. 1999).

Anatomical Alignment

Anatomical alignment of the pelvis and lower extremity is often implicated as an ACL injury risk factor; however, no anatomical alignment variable has been reliably associated with increased risk of ACL injury (Griffin et al. In press-a). Clinical measures that are commonly used to describe lower extremity alignment and that have received attention as potential ACL injury risk factors include pelvic angle, femur-to-tibial length ratio, hip anteversion, quadriceps angle, tibiofemoral angle, genu recurvatum, tibial torsion, and foot pronation. The challenge with this body of literature is that the majority of studies have involved individual or a select group of alignment factors and their relationship to ACL injury risk, without an appreciation of the interdependence of other potential anatomical alignment abnormalities that may be present along the lower kinetic chain. This may in part explain why it has been difficult to reliably identify relationships between anatomic alignment factors and ACL injury risk.

Gender Differences in Lower Extremity Posture

While females are cited as having greater anterior pelvic tilt, femoral anteversion, tibiofemoral angle, quadriceps angle, tibial torsion, and foot pronation (Griffin et al. 2000; Hutchinson and Ireland 1995), many of these differences appear to be based on clinician observation, as few empirical data are available to support this notion. A comprehensive review of literature on normative data for anatomical measures revealed only one study reporting sex comparisons for pelvic tilt (greater in females than in males) (Hertel, Dorfman, and Braham 2004), and conflicting findings regarding sex differences in femoral anteversion (Braten, Terjesen, and Rossvoll 1992; Prasad et al. 1996) and tibiofemoral angle (Cooke et al. 1997; Hsu et al. 1990; Tang, Zhu, and Chiu 2000). While the literature consistently demonstrates greater quadriceps angles in females (Aglietti, Insall, and Cerulli 1983; Guerra, Arnold, and Gajdosik 1994; Hertel, Dorfman, and Braham 2004; Horton and Hall 1989; Hsu et al. 1990; Woodland and Francis 1992), the prevailing thought that the larger Q angles in females are a result of greater pelvic width has not been demonstrated (Guerra, Arnold, and Gajdosik 1994; Horton and Hall 1989; Kernozek and Greer 1993). Limited studies support a sex difference in genu recurvatum (Trimble et al. 2002), but not in tibial torsion (Pasciak, Stoll, and Hefti 1996; Staheli et al. 1985) or foot pronation as measured by navicular drop (Beckett et al. 1992; Hertel, Dorfman, and Braham 2004; Moul 1998; Trimble et al. 2002) and rearfoot angle (Astrom and Arvidson 1995; Sobel et al. 1999). The limitation with many of these gender comparison studies is that in most cases, individual alignment variables are examined and a relatively small sample is involved. Further, the measurement technique for a particular alignment factor can vary among studies. Currently, there are no published large databases that provide normative data and sex differences in a comprehensive selection of anatomic alignment variables obtained from the same individuals. This is important if we are to accurately define sex differences in lower extremity alignment and posture.

Relationship to Injury Risk

Although a standing posture of greater anterior pelvic tilt, internal femoral rotation, knee hyperextension, knee valgus, and foot pronation (figure 20.2) is thought to be associated with lower extremity dysfunction and biomechanical

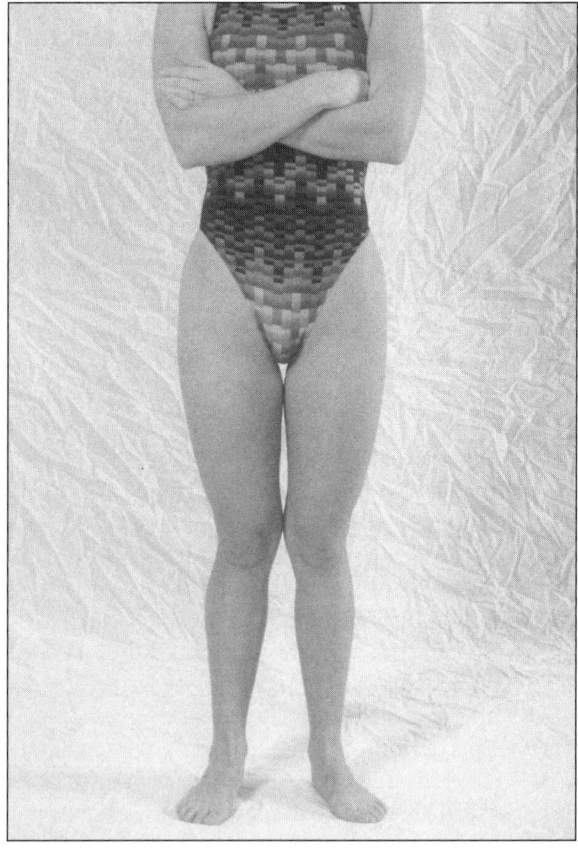

FIGURE 20.2 A standing posture of anterior pelvic tilt, internal femoral rotation, knee valgus, knee hyperextension, and foot pronation.

Reprinted, by permission, from P. Houglum, 2005, *Therapeutic exercise for musculoskeletal injuries*, 2nd ed. (Champaign, IL: Human Kinetics), 333.

abnormalities (Hruska 1998; Hutchinson and Ireland 1995; Loudon, Jenkins, and Loudon 1996), it is unknown if this posture increases the risk of ACL injury. Table 20.1 lists published studies of lower extremity alignment variables and their relationship to the likelihood of ACL injury. These retrospective studies differ considerably in the variables examined, with only one study including a comprehensive list of postural factors. From these data, the alignment characteristic most consistently linked to ACL injury risk is foot pronation (Beckett et al. 1992; Hertel, Dorfman, and Braham 2004; Loudon, Jenkins, and Loudon 1996; Woodford-Rogers, Cyphert, and Denegar 1994). Interestingly, the literature comparing navicular drop values in males and females has consistently shown no gender difference (Beckett et al. 1992; Hertel, Dorfman, and Braham 2004; Moul 1998; Trimble et al. 2002), suggesting that this alignment factor alone does not explain the greater risk of ACL injury in females. In fact, navicular drop has been found to be a predictor of ACL injury risk in combination with pelvic tilt (Hertel, Dorfman, and Braham 2004), genu recurvatum (Loudon, Jenkins, and Loudon 1996), and knee laxity (Woodford-Rogers, Cyphert, and Denegar 1994)—variables that do differ between sexes. As the predictive ability of each variable is specific only to the variables entered in the model, there is a need for large, prospective, multifactorial studies that examine posture characteristics of the entire lower extremity chain. Only when we take a comprehensive approach and account for all relevant postural variables (admittedly a very difficult task) will we be able to determine the relationship between lower extremity posture and the risk of occurrence of an ACL injury.

Neuromuscular and Biomechanical Implications

One of the more common mechanisms of ACL injury has been described as a "functional valgus collapse" of the knee (Ireland 1999; Olsen et al. 2004). This is characterized by valgus and either internal or external rotation of the tibia relative to the femur as the lower limb transitions from nonweight bearing to full weight bearing (figure 20.3) (Olsen et al. 2004). Females are often found to land and cut with greater knee valgus angles (Ford, Myer, and Hewett 2003; Hewett, Myer, and Ford 2004; Zeller et al. 2003) and greater valgus-varus moments (Chappell et al. 2002; Hewett et al. 1996; Malinzak et al. 2001; McLean et al. 1999) compared to males. These motions were identified in a recent prospective controlled cohort study of 205 adolescent female soccer, basketball, and volleyball players as predictive of ACL injury risk (Hewett et al. 2005b) and are known to strain the ACL during weight bearing (Fleming et al. 2001). However, the reason more females are prone to these at-risk knee positions remains unknown. While neuromuscular (strength) deficits are thought to contribute to lack of knee control in the frontal plane (Hewett et al. 2005b, 1996), research suggests that postural malalignments may also have the potential to significantly alter biomechanical function, internal-external rotation, and laxity of the knee joint (Bates et al. 1979; Beckett et al. 1992; Coplan 1989; Cornwall and McPoil 1995; Hruska 1998; Ilahi and Kohl 1998; Krivickas

TABLE 20.1 Studies Examining Lower Extremity Alignment Variables for Their Ability to Predict ACL Injury Status

Reference	Study type	Sample[a]	Variables examined	Statistical analysis	Predictors	Variance explained
Beckett et al. 1992	Retrospective case control	50 ACL-I (11F, 39M); 20 ACL-NI (18F, 32M)	Navicular drop	2 × 2 ANOVA (group, side)	Navicular drop > in ACL-I group (P = 0.001)	Not reported
Woodford-Rogers et al. 1994	Retrospective case control	22 ACL-I (14M, 8F); 22 ACL-NI (14M, 8F)	Navicular drop, knee laxity, rearfoot angle	Discriminate analysis	Navicular drop, knee laxity	All = 20% (71% correctly classified); males = 22% (71% correctly classified); females = 60% (88% correctly classified)
Loudon et al. 1996	Retrospective case control	20 F ACL-I; 20 F ACL-NI	Pelvic angle, hip anteversion, knee recurvatum, quadriceps angle, hamstring length, navicular drop, rearfoot angle	Logistic regression (univariate and multivariate)	Pelvic angle[a], recurvatum, navicular drop, rearfoot angle; [a]Univariate predictor only	Not reported
Hertel et al. 2004	Retrospective case control	20 ACL-I (10M, 10F); 20 ACL-NI (10M, 10F)	Pelvic angle, quadriceps angle, navicular drop, hip rotation range, true and apparent leg length	Stepwise, logistic regression	Navicular drop, pelvic angle	42% (correctly predicted 74% ACL-I and 76% ACL-NI)

[a]F = female; M = male; I = injured; NI = noninjured.

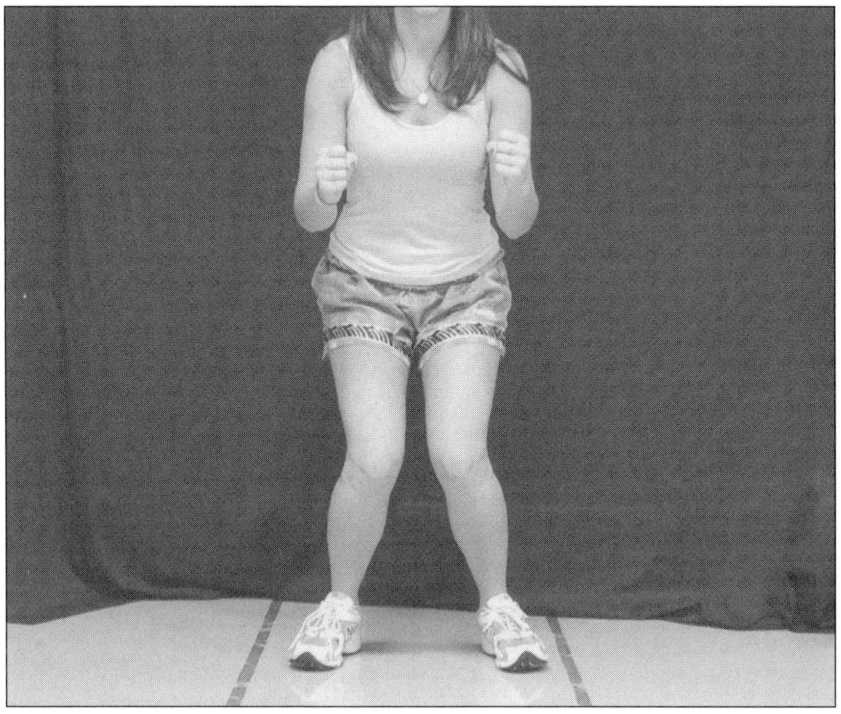

FIGURE 20.3 Functional valgus collapse characterized by internal femoral rotation, knee valgus, and external tibial rotation.
Photo courtesy of A. Nguyen.

1997; Loudon, Jenkins, and Loudon 1996). These changes may further influence proprioceptive orientation or feedback from the hip and knee, or both (Hruska 1998; Loudon, Jenkins, and Loudon 1996), as well as the mechanical efficiency and relative contribution of a muscle to control knee motion. Therefore, it is conceivable that neuromuscular control of the knee and the corresponding loads that are transmitted across this joint may be substantially different in athletes who possess lower extremity malalignments. Understanding how postural factors may influence dynamic control and biomechanical function of the knee may explain some of the sex differences that have been previously noted. Hence, the following sections address how various anatomic alignment variables may influence dynamic control of the knee and contribute to components of "functional valgus collapse."

Subtalar Pronation Subtalar joint pronation has been a variable of particular interest with respect to ACL injury because of the compensatory increase in internal tibial rotation on the foot that occurs with excessive pronation. Increased internal tibial rotation at the foot is thought to couple with increased internal tibial rotation at the knee (Beckett et al. 1992; Coplan 1989; Loudon, Jenkins, and Loudon 1996), which has been shown to increase ACL strain values during weight bearing (Fleming et al. 2001). Hence, excessive pronation may create increased ACL strain values during the stance phase of gait, particularly when the pelvis is externally rotating (Bates et al. 1979; Beckett et al. 1992; Cornwall and McPoil 1995; Cowan et al. 1996). While studies of normal gait and running have not demonstrated a significant increase of internal rotation of the tibia at the knee in subjects with excessive pronation (LaFortune et al. 1994; McClay and Manal 1997), a recent study has demonstrated this relationship during a single landing (Shimokochi et al. 2005).

As previously noted, subtalar pronation does not differ significantly between males and females, which suggests that subtalar pronation may be coupled with other alignment factors to increase biomechanical stresses at the knee. A secondary consequence of pronation and internal tibial rotation at the knee is the potential for increased internal femoral rotation and valgus angulation at the knee (Powers 2003). Hence, females who have a propensity for increased femoral rotation (e.g., excessive hip anteversion and excessive anterior pelvic tilt) may magnify the effects of subtalar pronation, further accentuating a valgus collapse of the knee.

Quadriceps Angle The quadriceps angle reflects a composite measure of pelvic angle, hip rotation, tibial rotation, patella position, and foot position (Hruska 1998; Ilahi and Kohl 1998; Powers 2003). It is defined clinically as the angle in the frontal plane that is formed by intersecting lines from the center of the patella to the anterior superior iliac spine (ASIS) and the center of the patella to the tibial tubercle (figure 20.4). Given the anatomical landmarks associated with this measure, the quadriceps angle can be greatly influenced by abnormal tibia and femur positions in the transverse and frontal planes. For example, when measured in a weight-bearing posture, the quadriceps angle may be increased with greater anterior pelvic tilt, which can change the orientation of the acetabulum and result in internal rotation of the femur (Hruska 1998). Quadriceps angle may also increase with greater hip anteversion and knee valgus (moving the patella more medially relative to the ASIS and tibial tubercle) and external tibial rotation (moving the tibial tubercle laterally) (Powers 2003). Depending on the relative contributions and interactions of these various malalignments, excessive quadriceps angle may reflect a measure that contributes to dynamic knee valgus and increased torsion on the knee during weight bearing. However, the fact that the quadriceps angle can be increased or decreased by changes in any one of these variables creates challenges for efforts to ascertain its relationship to at-risk knee motions and ACL injury risk. In order to clarify the effects of excessive quadriceps angle on neuromuscular and biomechanical function of the knee, it may be necessary to classify the quadriceps angle based on the relative contribution of soft tissue, structural, or functional abnormalities that define the measure (Powers

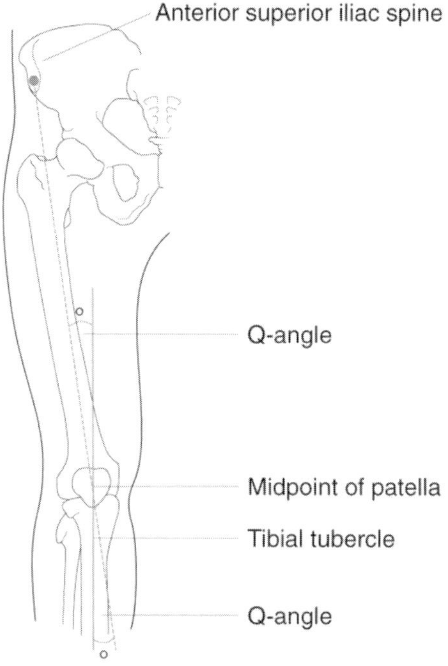

FIGURE 20.4 Measurement of the quadriceps angle.
Reprinted, by permission, from S.J. Shultz, P. Houglum, and D.H. Perrin, 2005, *Examination of musculoskeletal injuries,* 2nd ed. (Champaign, IL: Human Kinetics), 458.

2003). This further supports the need to consider alignment of the entire lower extremity rather than a single alignment variable.

Pelvic Angle As discussed in chapter 6 of this text, anterior pelvic tilt has been hypothesized to be a predictor of ACL injury because of its effect on lower extremity postural alignment. Clinically, excessive anterior tilt of the pelvis is thought to lead to an internal rotation and medial collapse of the extremities, specifically internal femoral rotation, genu valgus, genu recurvatum, and subtalar pronation (see figure 20.2) (Chaitow and DeLany 2000; Hruska 1998; Loudon, Jenkins, and Loudon 1996). In addition to preloading the ACL, this posture is thought to increase ligamentous laxity, place the hamstrings in a lengthened and weakened position, and alter proprioception and muscular activation (Coplan 1989; Hruska 1998; Kendall and McCreary 1983; Loudon, Jenkins, and Loudon 1996). Further, increased anterior pelvic tilt, along with the concomitant hip flexion and internal femoral rotation, may contribute to weakness and inefficiency of the gluteal muscles due to changes in the moment arms (Delp et al. 1999). Decreased function of these posterior-lateral hip muscles would further compromise control of hip adduction and internal femoral rotation, further accentuating "functional valgus collapse" of the knee. While two retrospective case control studies have identified a univariate relationship between ACL injury and excessive anterior pelvic tilt (Hertel, Dorfman, and Braham 2004; Loudon, Jenkins, and Loudon 1996), it is not clear whether pelvic tilt itself, versus the distal functional malalignments it creates (i.e., knee recurvatum, navicular drop, knee laxity [Beckett et al. 1992; Hertel, Dorfman, and Braham 2004; Loudon, Jenkins, and Loudon 1996; Uhorchak et al. 2003; Woodford-Rogers, Cyphert, and Denegar 1994]), is most predictive of ACL injury risk. While one study showed that pelvic tilt and navicular drop combined to predict injury risk (Hertel, Dorfman, and Braham 2004), the other showed that pelvic tilt was a predictor of risk only when examined independently, as it did not contribute to the multivariate model of injury risk based on genu recurvatum, rearfoot angle, and navicular drop (Loudon, Jenkins, and Loudon 1996).

Femoral Anteversion Femoral torsion is defined as the angle formed between the axis of the femoral neck and a transverse line through the femoral condyles (Crane 1959; Norkin and Levangie 1992). Femoral anteversion results from a forward projection of the femoral neck from the transcondylar plane and manifests clinically as internal femoral rotation and a toe-in gait (figure 20.5). As with increased anterior pelvic tilt, increased anteversion may contribute to the inefficiency of the gluteal muscles in controlling lower extremity motion. During static single-leg stance, a large abduction force is required to maintain

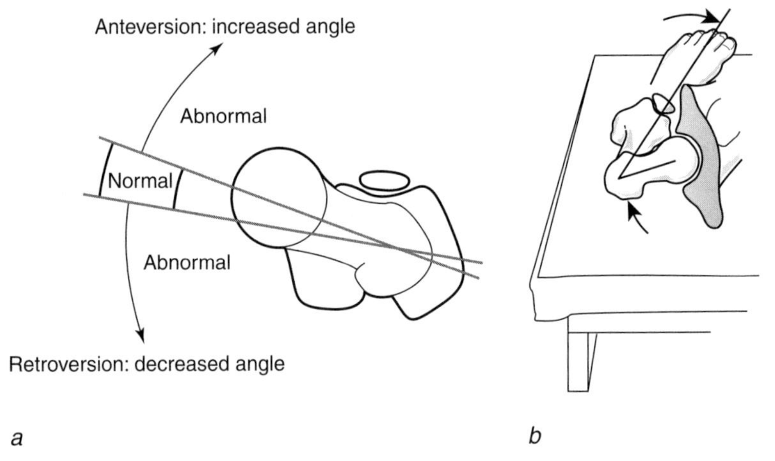

FIGURE 20.5 Hip anteversion is characterized by *(a)* an increased angulation of the femoral neck relative to the femoral condyles, resulting in *(b)* internal femoral rotation and a toe-in gait.

(a) Reprinted, by permission, from P. Houglum, 2005, *Therapeutic exercise for musculoskeletal injuries,* 2nd ed. (Champaign, IL: Human Kinetics), 332. *(b)* Reprinted, by permission, from S.J. Shultz, P. Houglum, and D.H. Perrin, 2005, *Examination of musculoskeletal injuries,* 2nd ed. (Champaign, IL: Human Kinetics), 488.

and stabilize a level pelvis. The reason is that the hip abductors have a relatively small internal moment arm and need to counteract a large adduction force produced by the body's weight and its larger external moment arm acting at the hip (Neumann 1989). Inability of hip abductors to produce the required force to counteract the adduction force produced by the body weight would result in adduction of the hip (contralateral pelvis dropping), a characteristic of "functional valgus collapse." In theory, increased femoral anteversion would decrease the internal moment arm of the gluteus medius, increasing the abduction force necessary to maintain stability of the pelvis. This theory is supported by work on muscle forces of the hip that used a simulated hip model in which an internally rotated femur, as is present with hip anteversion, required an increase in gluteus medius force to maintain a level pelvis compared to a neutral alignment of the femur (Merchant 1965). Further, decreased activation of the gluteus medius as measured by EMG amplitude has been demonstrated in those with increased relative femoral anteversion (Nyland et al. 2004). Hence, increased hip anteversion may lead to decreased frontal and transverse plane hip control as a result of decreased gluteus medius activation.

Summary

Females differ from males with regard to neuromuscular and biomechanical function of the knee because of a variety of factors that may include structural influences. However, the extent to which sex differences in postural alignment impair neuromuscular and biomechanical function and explain the increased risk of ACL injury in females remains largely theoretical at this point. Theory suggests that females have greater anterior pelvic tilt, hip anteversion, and knee valgus and recurvatum, yet there are no large-scale appropriately powered studies to validate this clinical observation. Moreover, while this posture has the potential to contribute to functional valgus collapse and increased loading about the knee during dynamic activity, empirical studies examining this relationship are quite limited. The interdependency that exists between independent alignment factors further complicates this relationship, as one segment or joint may profoundly influence the alignment of other segments or joints and ultimately the loads produced across the knee and ACL. Future studies should consider postural alignment of the entire lower extremity kinetic chain, from the pelvis to the foot, in order to determine the relationship between anatomic alignment, knee joint function, and ACL injury risk.

Conclusions

It is generally agreed that the risk for ACL injury is likely multifactorial. The focus of this chapter has been on anatomical factors that are known to differ between males and females and that have the potential to alter neuromuscular and biomechanical control of the knee, thus ACL injury risk. What becomes increasingly apparent in such a review is how little we still know about the role of anatomical factors. However, there is evidence suggesting that anatomical factors (i.e., notch width index, general and knee joint laxity, and postural alignment) may represent one component of this multifactorial problem. In order to determine which structural factors exert the greatest influence on neuromuscular and biomechanical function, large data sets are needed to examine all relevant intrinsic and extrinsic factors.

With increasing emphasis on ACL injury prevention programs, the anatomical correlates to ACL injury are often dismissed, as it is largely believed that anatomical factors are not modifiable. While it is true that factors such as notch width, hip anteversion, and tibial torsion are structural factors that cannot be modified, factors such as increased anterior pelvic angle are largely functional in nature and can be modified through flexibility and neuromuscular training. Hence, prevention strategies that improve core and gluteal muscle function, and thus functional alignment of the pelvis, have the potential to reduce the loads transmitted across the knee, improving hip control and dynamic control of knee alignment. Once we understand the relationship between anatomical factors and dynamic knee function, we can progress to studies that suggest how we can improve knee function in those who are found to be at increased risk of injury.

Chapter 21

Intrinsic and Extrinsic Forces Associated With ACL Injury

Can Functional Bracing Reduce the Risk of ACL Injury?

Bruce D. Beynnon, PhD
James R. Slauterbeck, MD

This chapter reviews what is currently known about the effectiveness of knee bracing in preventing injury to the ACL and reinjury of ACL grafts. We present the relevant literature on the mechanisms whereby braces influence ACL biomechanics. In addition, we review clinical studies focusing on the efficacy of prophylactic and functional knee braces in preventing ACL injuries, specifically those that provide the highest level of evidence: randomized, controlled trials. Our review revealed that very little is known about the effectiveness of prophylactic braces in preventing ACL injuries. As well, very little is known about the effectiveness of functional knee braces in preventing injury of healing ligaments and ACL grafts.

The Biomechanics of Knee Bracing

Knee braces have been used by the sports medicine community to treat instability of the knee due to an ACL disruption, to protect an ACL graft, and to prevent knee ligament injuries during sport. Both functional and prophylactic braces are designed with the objective of allowing normal joint kinematics while limiting unwanted displacements and rotations between the tibia and femur that might detrimentally strain a healing ligament or graft or produce intra-articular injury.

Subjective studies have shown that braces help most subjects with knee ligament injuries feel better and can even improve athletic performance in those with torn knee ligaments; however, many athletes report that knee bracing hinders their performance and that braces migrate and slide out of position on the leg during activity (Greene et al. 2000).

The Effect of Knee Braces on ACL Biomechanics

Indirect and direct techniques have been used to measure brace performance on knee and ligament biomechanics. Indirect measurement techniques (i.e., kinematic studies of the position of the tibia in relation to the femur) have shown that functional braces increase knee stiffness and reduce anterior-posterior displacement of the tibia relative to the femur, but only for low intersegmental shear loads. Direct measurement techniques have been performed by our group through instrumentation of the ACL of cadavers (Arms et al. 1987). This study showed that application of a functional brace resulted in an increase in ACL strain values with passive flexion-extension of the knee joint (i.e., the braces had a detrimental prestraining effect on the ACL), and suggested that bracing may be harmful for an injured ACL or a healing ACL graft.

This study motivated us to perform measurements of ACL strain in human subjects to determine if braces were harmful to the ACL, and that investigation revealed that bracing did not prestrain or harm the ACL (Beynnon et al. 1992). This finding was in direct contrast to those of our earlier cadaveric study and raised the question whether it is valid to use cadavers to study the effect of braces on ACL biomechanics. Further, we found that both custom and off-the-shelf brace designs significantly reduced ACL strain values for anterior-directed loads applied to the tibia (relative to the femur) up to the maximum anterior load of 140 N. Similarly, bracing significantly reduced ACL strain values in response to internal and external torques applied about the long axis of the tibia up to the maximum torque of 6 Nm. This is important because torque applied about the long axis of the tibia produces a substantial load on the ACL at the extremes of knee flexion and extension (Markolf et al. 1995) and can injure the ACL (Ryder et al. 1997). For both anterior loading and internal-external torques of the tibia, we determined that the protective strain-shielding effect of a functional brace on the ACL was dependent on the magnitude of applied load and torque. The protective effect of the brace on the ACL decreased as the magnitude of applied anterior load and internal-external torques increased.

From this investigation, we concluded that knee brace performance was determined by at least four different characteristics. The first is the brace design, composed of parameters such as the hinges, the uprights, and the strap versus shell attachment technique. The second is the brace–limb interface. This was thought to be of importance because the magnitude and sequence of contraction of the leg musculature alters the compliance of the soft tissue at the brace–leg interface, and therefore the capability of the brace to mechanically control the skeletal system, protect the ligaments, and prevent intra-articular injury. Third, we determined that it was important to monitor the forces produced on the leg by the brace strap tensions. Fourth, we found that the magnitude of contraction of the leg musculature, as well as the compressive joint load produced by body weight, affected ACL strain values and therefore were important to include.

We then progressed to an investigation in which we controlled the brace design and brace–limb interface variables by studying a single brace (the DonJoy Four Point Brace) while systematically examining the effect of the extrinsic forces produced by different brace strap tensions on ACL strain biomechanics. This was done in the presence of the intrinsic forces produced by leg musculature and body weight (Beynnon et al. 1997b). Bracing significantly reduced ACL strain values for anterior-directed shear loading of the tibia (to the limit of 140 N) with the subject in nonweight-bearing and weight-bearing postures. Similarly, functional bracing significantly reduced ACL strain values with internal-external torque applied to the tibia up to the limit of 6 Nm with the subject nonweight bearing. The posterior-directed load applied by the brace strap to the proximal tibia was adjusted between a low (22 N) and a high (45 N) setting (loading that we hypothesized would protect the ACL), but this did not modulate the effect of the brace on ACL strain values for the nonweight-bearing and weight-bearing conditions. Our most recent investigation of the same brace design confirmed that it can protect the ACL in response to anterior-posterior-directed shear loading with the knee nonweight bearing and weight bearing, as well as in response to internal torque applied to the nonweight-bearing knee (Fleming et al. 2000).

The Effect of Knee Braces on the Biomechanics of the ACL-Deficient Knee

Functional knee braces can reduce the abnormal anterior-posterior laxity of the ACL-deficient knee to within the limits of the normal knee during nonweight-bearing and weight-bearing activities (Beynnon et al. 2003). However, in the ACL-deficient knee, braces do not reduce the abnormal increased anterior displacement of the tibia relative to the femur that occurs as the knee transitions from nonweight-bearing to weight-bearing conditions (Beynnon et al. 2003, 2002).

The Effectiveness of Braces in Preventing ACL, ACL Graft, and ACL-Deficient Knee Injuries

In an effort to determine if bracing is effective in preventing ACL injury, ACL graft injury, or injury to the ACL-deficient knee, we considered the highest level of scientific evidence available in the literature. Anterior cruciate ligament injury or injury to the ACL-deficient knee is a relatively rare event, and therefore researchers focusing on the effectiveness of bracing in reducing these injuries must carefully study a large sample of athletes over a long time interval. Consequently, it is not surprising that only a few studies based on prospective, randomized, controlled study designs have been reported. A majority of the research has focused on the sport of American football, in which the injury mechanisms involve both direct and indirect contact.

The Effectiveness of Prophylactic Knee Braces in Preventing ACL Injuries

The use of prophylactic knee braces to prevent knee injuries has long been a contentious area of research. The best study to date of prophylactic knee braces and ACL injury remains a prospective, randomized study of 1396 cadets playing intramural tackle football at the U.S. Military Academy (Sitler et al. 1990). This study showed that prophylactic knee brace use did not significantly decrease the severity of ACL and MCL injuries. There was, however, a trend toward a reduced rate of less severe ACL and MCL injuries in athletes who used braces (Sitler et al. 1990). On the basis of the data published in that paper, we compute that the rate of ACL injury in the nonbraced cadets was 3.0 times higher (95%CI: 1.0-9.2) than in braced cadets. It should be noted that the number of ACL injuries was small. Only 16 ACL injuries occurred: four in the braced and 12 in the nonbraced condition. Other large epidemiologic studies conducted to date have focused on the effectiveness of prophylactic braces in reducing MCL injuries in the sport of football; however, these investigations have not dealt with the effect of bracing on the reduction of ACL injuries (Albright et al. 1994a, 1994b; Hewson, Mendini, and Wang 1986; Teitz et al. 1987). The efficacy of prophylactic knee braces in preventing ACL disruptions remains an unanswered question (Najibi and Albright 2005).

The Effectiveness of Functional Knee Braces in Preventing Injury to an ACL Graft

A prospective, randomized, multicenter study examined 100 cadets at the three largest U.S. military academies who underwent ACL reconstruction and were randomized to either functional brace use or no brace use (McDevitt et al. 2004). At one year postsurgery, the use of a functional brace appeared to have no effect on the incidence of graft injury; however, there were only five reinjuries (two in the braced and three in the nonbraced group).

The Effectiveness of Functional Knee Braces in Preventing Injury to an ACL-Deficient Knee

A prospective study of 180 ACL-deficient skiers, identified from screening of 9410 professional skiers, showed a higher risk of knee injury in skiers who did not wear a functional knee brace compared to those who wore functional knee braces (risk ratio of 6.4, based on a total of 12 injuries) (Kocher et al. 2003).

Conclusion

The evidence regarding the efficacy of prophylactic bracing in the prevention of ACL injuries, and the efficacy of functional bracing in the prevention of injury of ACL grafts, is mixed. Few methodologically rigorous randomized, controlled trials have been performed, and those that exist are limited by the small numbers of subjects with ACL injuries or reinjury. The biomechanical and epidemiologic literature on brace use (prophylactic and functional) is incomplete. In general, there is a need for studies addressing the effect of bracing on the prevention of knee ligament injury and graft injury. Such studies would also ideally consider the interaction of extrinsic factors such as sport and intrinsic factors such as anatomical alignment and neuromuscular function on the likelihood of occurrence of an ACL injury.

References

Abubaker, A.O., P.C. Hebda, and J.N. Gunsolley. 1996. Effects of sex hormones on protein and collagen content of the temporomandibular joint disc of the rat. *J Oral Max Surg* 54: 721-727.

Acasuso-Diaz, M., E. Collantes-Esteves, and P. Sanchez-Guijo. 1993. Joint hyperlaxity and musculoligamentous lesions: Study of a population of homogeneous age, sex and physical exertion. *Br J Rheumatol* 32: 120-122.

Aden, U., C. Jung-Hoffmann, and H. Kuhl. 1998. A randomized cross-over study on various hormonal parameters of two triphasic oral contraceptives. *Contraception* 58: 75-81.

Agel, J., L. Arendt, and B. Breshadsky. 2005. Anterior cruciate ligament injury in national collegiate athletic association basketball and soccer: A 13-year review. *Am J Sports Med* 33(4): 524-530.

Agel, J., B. Bershadsky, and E.A. Arendt. 2006. Hormonal therapy: ACL and ankle injury. *Med Sci Sports Exerc* 38(1):7-12.

Aglietti, P., J.N. Insall, and G. Cerulli. 1983. Patellar pain and incongruence, I: Measurements of incongruence. *Clin Orthop Rel Res* 176: 217-224.

Ahmed, A.M., and D.L. Burke. 1983. In-vitro measurements of static pressure distribution in synovial joints: I. Tibial surface of the knee. *Biomech Eng* 105: 216-225.

Aimes, R.T. 1995. Matrix metalloproteinase-2 is an interstitial collagenase. *J Biol Chem* 5872-5876.

Ala-Kokko, L., C.T. Baldwin, R.W. Moskowitz, et al. 1990. Single base mutation in the type II procollagen gene (COL2AI) as a cause of primary osteoarthritis associated with a mild chondrodysplasia. *Proc Natl Acad Sci USA* 87: 6565-6568.

Albright, J.P., J.W. Powell, W. Smith, A. Martindale, E. Crowley, J. Monroe, R. Miller, J. Connolly, B.A. Hill, D. Miller, D. Helwig, and J. Marshall. 1994a. Medial collateral ligament knee sprains in college football players: Brace wear preferences and injury risk. *Am J Sports Med* 22: 2-11.

Albright, J.P., J.W. Powell, W. Smith, A. Martindale, E. Crowley, J. Monroe, R. Miller, J. Connolly, B.A. Hill, D. Miller, D. Helwig, and J. Marshall. 1994b. Medial collateral ligament knee sprains in college football: Effectiveness of preventive braces. *Am J Sports Med* 22: 12-18.

Amiel, D. 1989. Injury of the ACL: The role of collagenase in ligament degeneration. *J Orthop Res* 7: 486-493.

Andersen, T.E., O. Larsen, A. Tenga, et al. 2003. Football incident analysis: A new video based method to describe injury mechanisms in professional football. *Br J Sports Med* 37: 226-232.

Anderson, A.F., D.C. Dome, S. Gautam, M.H. Awh, and G.W. Rennirt. 2001. Correlation of anthropometric measurements, strength, anterior cruciate ligament size, and intercondylar notch characteristics to sex differences in anterior cruciate ligament tear rates. *Am J Sports Med* 29(1): 58-66.

Andriacchi, T.P. 1990. Dynamics of pathological motion: Applied to the anterior cruciate deficient knee. *J Biomech* 23(Suppl. 1): 99-105.

Arendt, E.A. 1994. Orthopaedic issues for active and athletic women. *Clin Sports Med* 13: 483-503.

Arendt, E., J. Agel, and R. Dick. 1999. Anterior cruciate ligament injury patterns among collegiate men and women. *J Athl Train* 34: 86-92.

Arendt, E.A., B. Bershadsky, and J. Agel. 2002. Periodicity of noncontact anterior cruciate ligament injuries during the menstrual cycle. *J Gend Spec Med* 5(2): 19-26.

Arendt, E., and R. Dick. 1995. Knee injury patterns among men and women in collegiate basketball and soccer. NCAA data and review of literature. *Am J Sports Med* 23: 694-701.

Arms, S.W., D. Donnermeyer, P. Renström, M. Pope, R. Johnson, and S. Incavo. 1987. The effect of knee braces on anterior cruciate ligament strain. *Orthop Transl* 12: 245.

Arms, S.W., M.H. Pope, R.J. Johnson, R.A. Fischer, I. Arvidsson, and E. Eriksson. 1984. The biomechanics of anterior cruciate ligament rehabilitation and reconstruction. *Am J Sports Med* 12: 8-18.

Arnason, A., A. Tenga, L. Engebretsen, and R. Bahr. 2004. A prospective video-based analysis of injury situations in elite male football. Football incident analysis. *Am J Sports Med* 32(Sept. 6): 1459-1465.

Arner, E.C., and M.A. Pratta. 1989. Independent effects of interleukin-I on proteoglycan breakdown, proteoglycan synthesis, and prostaglandin E2 release from cartilage in organ culture. *Arthritis Rheum* 32: 288-297.

Arnoczky, S.P., M.K. Skyhar, and T.L. Wickiewicz. 1991. In J.B. McGinty (Ed.), *Basic science of the knee*. Operative Arthroscopy (pp. 155-192). New York: Raven Press

Arnoczky, S.P., and R.F. Warren. 1982. Microvasculature of the human meniscus. *Am J Sports Med* 10: 90-95.

Arnold, C., C. VanBell, V. Rogers, and T. Cooney. 2002. The relationship between serum relaxin and knee joint laxity in female athletes. *Orthopedics* 25(6): 669-673.

Arnold, J.A., T.P. Coker, L.M. Heaton, J.P. Park, and W.D. Harris. 1979. Natural history of anterior cruciate tears. *Am J Sports Med* 7: 305-313.

Astrom, M., and T. Arvidson. 1995. Alignment and joint motion in the normal foot. *J Orthop Sports Phys Ther* 22(5): 216-222.

Aune, A.K., P.W. Cawley, and A. Ekeland. 1997. Quadriceps muscle contraction protects the anterior cruciate ligament during anterior tibial translation. *Am J Sports Med* 25: 187-190.

Aune, A.K., P. Schaff, and L. Nordsletten. 1995. Contraction of knee flexors and extensors in skiing related to the backward fall mechanism of injury to the anterior cruciate ligament. *Scand J Med Sci Sports* 5: 165-169.

Bach, J.M., and M.L. Hull. 1998. Strain inhomogeneity in the anterior cruciate ligament under application of external and muscular loads. *J Biomech Eng* 120: 497-503.

Bahr, R., and I. Holme. 2003. Risk factors for sports injuries—a methodological approach. *Br J Sports Med* 37: 384-392.

Bahr, R., and T. Krosshaug. 2005. Understanding injury mechanisms: A key component of preventing injuries in sports. *Br J Sports Med* 39(6): 324-329.

Bahr, R., W. van Mechelen, and P. Kannus. 2002. Prevention of sports injuries. In: M. Kjær, M. Krogsgaard, P. Magnusson, L. Engebretsen, H. Roos, T. Takala, and S.L.Y. Woo (Eds.),

Textbook of sports medicine. Basic science and clinical aspects of sports injury and physical activity (pp. 299-314). Oxford: Blackwell Science.

Bally, A., and M. Del Pedro. 1990. Etude Sur les Lesions du genou a Ski. Rapport d'activite 1989-1990. Institute de mecanique appliquee et de construction des machines, Ecole polytechnique federale de Lausanne, pp. 9-33.

Baratta, R., M. Solomonow, et al. 1988. Muscular coactivation: The role of the antagonist musculature in maintaining knee stability. *Am J Sports Med* 16(2): 113-122.

Barber-Westin, S.D., M. Galloway, F.R. Noyes, G. Corbett, and C. Walsh. 2005. Assessment of lower limb neuromuscular control in prepubescent athletes. *Am J Sports Med* 33: 1853-1860.

Barone, M., V. Senner, and P. Schaff. 1999. ACL injury mechanism in alpine skiing: Analysis of an accidental ACL rupture. In R.J. Johnson (Ed.), *Skiing trauma and safety* (Vol. 12, pp. 63-81). ASTM STP 1345. Philadelphia: American Society for Testing and Materials.

Barrack, R.L., P.J. Lund, and H.B. Skinner. 1994. Knee joint proprioception revisited. *J Sport Rehab* 3: 18-42.

Barrack, R., H.B. Skinner, and S.L. Buckley. 1989. Proprioception in the anterior cruciate deficient knee. *Am J Sports Med* 17: 1-6.

Barrett, D.S. 1991. Proprioception and function after anterior cruciate reconstruction. *J Bone Joint Surg* 73B: 833-837.

Barrett, D.S., A.G. Cobb, and G. Bentley. 1991. Joint proprioception in normal, osteoarthritic and re-laced knees. *J Bone Joint Surg* 73B: 53-56.

Bates, B.T., L.R. Osternig, B. Mason, and L.S. James. 1979. Foot orthotic devices to modify selected aspects of lower extremity mechanics. *Am J Sports Med* 7(6): 338-342.

Beals, K.A., and M.L. Manore. 2002. Disorders of the female athlete triad among collegiate athletes. *Int J Sport Nutr Exerc Metab* 12: 281-292.

Beard, D.J., P.J. Kyberd, C.M. Fergusson, and C.A. Dodd. 1993. Proprioception after rupture of the anterior cruciate ligament: An objective indication for the need for surgery? *J Bone Joint Surg Br* 75-B: 311-315.

Beckett, M.E., D.L. Massie, K.D. Bowers, and D.A. Stoll. 1992. Incidence of hyperpronation in the ACL injured knee: A clinical perspective. *J Athl Train* 27(1): 58-60.

Beckman, S.M., and T.S. Buchanan. 1995. Ankle inversion injury and hypermobility: Effect on hip and ankle muscle electromyography onset latency. *Arch Phys Med Rehab* 76: 1138-1143.

Beighton, P., and F. Horan. 1969. Orthopaedic aspects of the Ehlers-Danlos syndrome. *J Bone Joint Surg Br* 51: 444-453.

Beighton, P., L. Solomon, and C.L. Soskolne. 1973. Articular mobility in an African population. *Ann Rheum Dis* 32: 413-418.

Belmont, P.J. Jr., S.B. Shawen, K.T. Mason, and S.J. Sladicka. 1999. Incidence and outcomes of anterior cruciate ligament reconstruction among U.S. Army aviators. *Aviat, Space, Environ Med* 70(4): 316-320.

Ben-Sira, D., A. Ayalon, and M. Tavi. 1995. The effect of different types of strength training on concentric strength in women. *J Strength Cond Res* 9: 143-148.

Berchuk, M., T.P. Andriacchi, B.R. Bach, et al. 1990. Gait adaptations by patients who have a deficient anterior cruciate ligament. *J Bone Joint Surg* 72A: 871-877.

Berns, G.S., M.L. Hull, and H.A. Patterson. 1992. Strain in the anteromedial bundle of the anterior cruciate ligament under combination loading. *J Orthop Res* 10: 167-176.

Besier, T.F., D.G. Lloyd, et al. 2001a. Anticipatory effects on knee joint loading during running and cutting maneuvers. *Med Sci Sports Exerc* 33(7): 1176-1181.

Besier, T.F., D.G. Lloyd, et al. 2001b. External loading of the knee joint during running and cutting maneuvers. *Med Sci Sports Exerc* 33(7): 1168-1175.

Besier, T.F., D.G. Lloyd, et al. 2003. Muscle activation strategies at the knee during running and cutting maneuvers. *Med Sci Sports Exerc* 35(1): 119-127.

Beynnon, B.D. 2003. Risk factors for knee ligament trauma. *J Orthop Sports Phys Ther* 33(8): A10-13.

Beynnon, B.D., I. Bernstein, A. Belisle, B. Brattbakk, P. Devanny, R. Risinger, and D. Durant. 2005. The effect of estradiol and progesterone on knee and ankle joint laxity. *Am J Sports Med* 33(9): 1298-1304.

Beynnon, B.D., and B.C. Fleming. 1998. Anterior cruciate ligament strain in-vivo: A review of previous work. *J Biomech* 31(6): 519-525.

Beynnon, B.D., B.C. Fleming, D.L. Churchill, and D. Brown. 2003. The effect of anterior cruciate ligament deficiency and functional bracing on translation of the tibia relative to the femur during nonweightbearing and weightbearing. *Am J Sports Med* 31(1): 99-105.

Beynnon, B.D., B.C. Fleming, R.J. Johnson, C.E. Nichols, P.A. Renstrum, and M.H. Pope. 1995. Anterior cruciate ligament strain behavior during rehabilitation exercises in vivo. *Am J Sports Med* 23: 24-34.

Beynnon, B.D., B.C. Fleming, R. Labovitch, and B. Parsons. 2002. Chronic anterior cruciate ligament deficiency is associated with increased anterior translation of the tibia during the transition from non-weightbearing to weightbearing. *J Orthop Res* 20: 332-337.

Beynnon, B.D., R.J. Johnson, et al. 1997a. The strain behavior of the anterior cruciate ligament during squatting and active flexion-extension: A comparison of open and closed kinetic chain exercise. *Am J Sports Med* 25(6): 823-829.

Beynnon, B.D., R.J. Johnson, S. Braun, M. Sargent, I. Bernstein, J.M. Skelly, and P.M. Vacek. 2006. The relationship between menstrual cycle phase and anterior cruciate ligament injury: A case-control study of recreational alpine skiers. *Am J Sports Med* 25(6):823-829.

Beynnon, B.D., R.J. Johnson, B.C. Fleming, G.D. Peura, P.A. Renström, C.E. Nichols, and M.H. Pope. 1997b. The effect of functional knee bracing on the anterior cruciate ligament in the weight-bearing and non-weight-bearing knee. *Am J Sports Med* 25: 353-359.

Beynnon, B.D., M.H. Pope, C.M. Wertheimer, R.J. Johnson, B.C. Fleming, L.D. Haugh, J.G. Howe, and C.E. Nichols. 1992. The effect of functional knee braces on anterior cruciate ligament strain in-vivo. *J Bone Joint Surg* 74A: 1298-1312.

Birrell, F.N., A.O. Adebajo, B.L. Hazleman, and A.J. Silman. 1994. High prevalence of joint laxity in West Africans. *Br J Rheumatol* 33(1): 56-59.

Biscevic, M., D. Tomic, V. Starc, and D. Smrke. 2005. Gender differences in knee kinematics and its possible consequences. *Croatia Med J* 46: 253-260.

Bjordal, J.M., F. Arnly, B. Hannestad, and F. Stand. 1997. Epidemiology of ACL injuries in soccer. *Am J Sports Med* 25: 341-345.

Blecher, A.M., and J.C. Richmond. 1998. Transient laxity of an anterior cruciate ligament-reconstructed knee related to pregnancy. *J Arthrosc Rel Surg* 14: 77-79.

Bobbert, M.F., and J.P. Vanzanwijk. 1999. Dynamics of force and muscle stimulation in human vertical jumping. *Med Sci Sports Exerc* 31(2): 303-310.

Boden, B.P., G.S. Dean, J.A. Feagin Jr., and W.E. Garrett Jr. 2000. Mechanisms of anterior cruciate ligament injury. *Orthopedics* 23: 573-578.

Borzekowski, D.L., and V.I. Rickert. 2000. Urban girls, internet use, and accessing health information. *J Pediatr Adolesc Gynecol* 13(2): 94-95.

Bowling, A. 1989. Injuries to dancers: Prevalence, treatment, and perceptions of causes. *Br Med J* 298: 731-734.

Boyer, B.T. 1990. A comparison of the effects of three strength training programs on women. *J Appl Sport Sci Res* 4: 88-94.

Branch, T.P., R. Hunter, and M. Donath. 1989. Dynamic EMG analysis of anterior cruciate deficient legs with and without bracing during cutting. *Am J Sports Med* 17(1): 35-41.

Brandt, K.D. 1985. Osteoarthritis: Clinical patterns and pathology. In: W.N. Kelley, E.D. Harris, and R.S. Sledge (Eds.), *Textbook of rheumatology* (2nd ed., pp. 1432-1448). Philadelphia: Saunders.

Brask, B., R.H. Lueke, and G.L. Soderberg. 1984. Electromyographic analysis of selected muscles during the lateral step-up exercise. *Phys Ther* 64(3): 324-329.

Braten, M., T. Terjesen, and I. Rossvoll. 1992. Femoral anteversion in normal adults. Ultrasound measurements in 50 men and 50 women. *Acta Orthop Scand* 63(1): 29-32.

Bray, R.C., and D.J. Dandy. 1989. Meniscal lesions and chronic anterior cruciate ligament deficiency. Meniscal tears occurring before and after reconstruction. *J Bone Joint Surg* 71B: 128-130.

Brock, R.M., and C.C. Striowski. 1986. Injuries in elite figure skaters. *Physician Sportsmed* 14: 111-115.

Bronner, S., and B. Brownstein. 1997. Profile of dance injuries in a Broadway show: A discussion of issues in dance medicine epidemiology. *J Orthop Sports Phys Ther* 26(2): 87-94.

Bronner, S., S. Ojofeitimi, and D. Rose. 2003. Injuries in a modern dance company. Effect of comprehensive management on injury incidence and time loss. *Am J Sports Med* 31(3): 365-373.

Bruce, W.J.M., M.J. Cross, and L. Pinczewski. 1989. Acute knee injuries in skiing. *J Bone Joint Surg* 71B: 159.

Buff, H.U., L.C. Jones, and D.S. Hungerford. 1988. Experimental determination of forces transmitted through the patella-femoral joint. *J Biomech* 21: 17-23.

Bullough, P.G., L. Munuera, J. Murphy, et al. 1970. The strength of menisci of the knee as it relates to their fine structure. *J Bone Joint Surg* 52(3): 564-567.

Butler, D.L., F.R. Noyes, and E.S. Grood. 1980. Ligamentous restraints to anterior-posterior drawer in the human knee. *J Bone Joint Surg Am* 62-A(2): 259-270.

Byhring, S., and K. Bo. 2002. Musculoskeletal injuries in the Norwegian National Ballet: A prospective cohort study. *Scand J Med Sci Sports* 12: 365-370.

Cahalan, T.D., M.E. Johnson, et al. 1989. Quantitative measures of hip strength in different age groups. *Clin Orthop Rel Res* 246: 136-145.

Cahill, B.R., and E.H. Griffith. 1978. Effect of preseason conditioning on the incidence and severity of high school football knee injuries. *Am J Sports Med* 6: 180-184.

Cameron, M.L., A. Buchgraber, H.H. Paessler, et al. 1994a. The natural history of the anterior cruciate ligament-deficient knee. *Am J Sports Med* 25: 750-754.

Cameron, M.L., H.H. Fu, H.H. Paessler, et al. 1994b. Synovial fluid cytokine concentrations as possible prognostic indicators in the ACL-deficient knee. *Knee Surg, Sports Traumatol, Arthrosc* 2: 38-44.

Caraffa, A., G. Cerulli, M. Projetti, G. Aisa, and A. Rizzo. 1996. Prevention of anterior cruciate ligament injuries in soccer: A prospective controlled study of proprioceptive training. *Knee Surg, Sports Traumatol, Arthrosc* 4: 19-21.

Carrivick, P.J., A.H. Lee, and K.K. Yau. 2002. Effectiveness of a workplace risk assessment team in reducing the rate, cost, and duration of occupational injury. *J Occup Environ Med* 44(2): 155-159.

Carson, W.G. Jr. 2004. Wakeboarding injuries. *Am J Sports Med* 32(1): 164-173.

Carter, C., and J. Wilkinson. 1964. Persistent joint laxity and congenital dislocation of the hip. *J Bone Joint Surg Br* 46: 40-45.

Carter, D.B., M.R. Beibert, and C.J. Dunn. 1990. Purification, cloning, expression and biological characterization of an interleukin-I receptor antagonist protein. *Nature* 344: 633-638.

Casazza, G.A., S.H. Suh, B.F. Miller, F.M. Navazio, and G.A. Brooks. 2002. Effects of oral contraceptives on peak exercise capacity. *J Appl Physiol* 93: 1698-1702.

Casscells, S.W. 1978. *Arthroscopic and cadaver knee investigations. Symposium on arthroscopy and arthrography of the knee*. American Academy of Orthopaedic Surgeons. St. Louis: Mosby, pp. 122-141.

Centers for Disease Control and Prevention. 2003. *Targeting arthritis: The nation's leading cause of disability.* Atlanta: U.S. Department of Health and Human Services.

Cerabona, F., M. Sherman, J. Bonamo, et al. 1998. Patterns of meniscal injury with acute anterior cruciate ligament tears. *Am J Sports Med* 16: 603-609.

Chaitow, L., and J.W. DeLany. 2000. The Pelvis. *Clinical application of neuromuscular techniques: The Lower Body* (Vol. 2, pp. 301-386). New York: Churchill Livingstone.

Chambat, P., O. Siegrist, P. Neyret, et al. 1997. ACL rupture mechanism during skiing [abstract no. 57]. Twelfth International Symposium on Ski Trauma and Safety, May 4-10, Whistler, Canada.

Chandrashekar, N., H. Mansouri, J. Slauterbeck, and J. Hashemi. 2006. Sex-based differences in the tensile properties of the human anterior cruciate ligament. *J Biomech*. 2006 Jan 4; [Epub ahead of print]

Chandrashekar, N., J. Slauterbeck, and J. Hashemi. 2005. Sex-based differences in the anthropometric characteristics of the anterior cruciate ligament and its relation to intercondylar notch geometry. *Am J Sports Med* 33(10): 1492-1498.

Chappell, J.D., D.C. Herman, B.S. Knight, D.T. Kirkendall, W.E. Garrett, and B. Yu. 2005. Effect of fatigue on knee kinetics and kinematics in stop-jump tasks. *Am J Sports Med* 33: 1022-1029.

Chappell, J.D., B. Yu, D.T. Kirkendall, and W.E. Garrett. 2002. A comparison of knee kinetics between male and female recreational athletes in stop-jump tasks. *Am J Sports Med* 30(2): 261-267.

Charlton, W.P.H., L.M. Coslett-Charlton, and M.G. Ciccotti. 1999. The effect of endogenous estrogen on the instrumented measurement of the anterior cruciate ligament. 25th Annual Meeting, American Orthopaedic Society for Sports Medicine, Traverse City, MI.

Charlton, W.P.H., L.M. Coslett-Charlton, and M.G. Ciccotti. 2001. Correlation of estradiol in pregnancy and anterior cruciate ligament laxity. *Clin Orthop Rel Res* 1(387): 165-170.

Charlton, W.P., T.A. St. John, M.G. Ciccotti, N. Harrison, and M. Schweitzer. 2002. Differences in femoral notch anatomy between men and women: A magnetic resonance imaging study. *Am J Sports Med* 30(3): 329-333.

Chiang, A.L., and C.D. Mote Jr. 1993. Translations and rotations across the knee under isometric quadriceps contraction. In: R.J. Johnson, C.D. Mote Jr., and J. Zelcer (Eds.), *Skiing trauma and safety* (pp. 62-74). Ninth International Symposium. ASTM STP 1182. Philadelphia: American Society for Testing and Materials.

Chilibeck, P.D., A.W. Calder, D.G. Sale, et al. 1998. A comparison of strength and muscle mass increases during resistance training in young women. *Eur J Appl Physiol Occup Physiol* 77: 170-175.

Chimera, N.J., K.A. Swanik, et al. 2004. Effects of plyometric training on muscle-activation strategies and performance in female athletes. *J Athl Train* 39(1): 24-31.

Chmelar, R.D., B.B. Shultz, R. Ruhling, et al. 1998. Isokinetic characteristics of the knee in female, professional and university, ballet and modern dancers. *J Orthop Sports Phys Ther* 9(12): 410-418.

Cholewicki J., and S.M. McGill. 1996. Mechanical stability of the in vivo lumbar spine: implications for injury and chronic low back pain. *Clin Biomech* (Bristol, Avon) 11(1):1-15.

Cholewicki J., and J.J. VanVliet. 2002. Relative contribution of trunk muscles to the stability of the lumbar spine during isometric exertions. *Clin Biomech* (Bristol, Avon) 17(2):99-105.

Chong, R.W., and J.L. Tan. 2004. Rising trend of anterior cruciate ligament injuries in females in a regional hospital. *Ann Acad Med Singapore* 33: 298-301.

Chu, D., R. LeBlanc, P. D'Ambrosia, R. D'Ambrosia, R.V. Baratta, and M. Solomonow. 2003. Neuromuscular disorder in response to anterior cruciate ligament creep. *Clin Biomech* 18: 222-230.

Clark, M.K., M. Sowers, B.T. Levy, and P. Tenhundfeld. 2001. Magnitude and variability of sequential estradiol and progesterone concentrations in women using depot medroxyprogesterone acetate for contraception. *Fertil Steril* 75(5): 871-877.

Coen, M.J., D.N.M. Caborn, and D.L. Johnson. 1996. The dimpling phenomenon: Articular cartilage injury overlying an occult osteochondral lesion at the time of anterior cruciate ligament reconstruction. *Arthroscopy* 12: 502-505.

Cohen, J. 1988. *Statistical power analysis for behavioral sciences*. Hillsdale, NJ: Erlbaum.

Colborne, G.R., S.J. Olney, and M.P. Griffin. 1993. Feedback of ankle joint angle and soleus electromyography in the rehabilitation of hemiplegic gait. *Arch Phys Med Rehab* 74: 1100-1106.

Colby, S., A. Francisco, B. Yu, D. Kirkendall, M. Finch, and W. Garrett. 2000. Electromyographic and kinematic analysis of cutting maneuvers. *Am J Sports Med* 28: 234-240.

Coleman, S., and S. Hansen. 1994. Reducing work-related back injuries. *Nurs Manage* 25(11): 58-61.

Coney, P., and A. DelConte. 1999. The effects of ovarian activity of a monophasic oral contraceptive with 100 μg levonorgestrel and 20 μg ethinyl estradiol. *Am J Obstr Gynecol* 181(5): S53-S58.

Cooke, I.D., A. Scudamore, J. Li, U. Wyss, T. Bryant, and P. Costigan. 1997. Axial lower-limb alignment: Comparison of knee geometry in normal volunteers and osteoarthritis patients. *Osteoarth Cartil* 5: 39-47.

Cooper, D.E., S.P. Arnoczky, and R.F. Warren. 1990. Arthroscopic meniscal repair. *Clin Sports Med* 9: 589-607.

Coplan, J.A. 1989. Rotational motion of the knee: A comparison of normal and pronating subjects. *J Orthop Sports Phys Ther* 10: 366-369.

Cornwall, M.W., and T.G. McPoil. 1995. Footwear and foot orthotic effectiveness research: A new approach. *J Orthop Sports Phys Ther* 21(6): 337-344.

Corrigan, J.P., W.F. Cashmen, and M.P. Brady. 1992. Proprioception in the cruciate deficient knee. *J Bone Joint Surg* 74B: 247-250.

Coventry, M.B. 1973. Osteotomy about the knee for degenerative and rheumatoid arthritis: Indications, operative technique and results. *J Bone Joint Surg* 55A: 23-48.

Cowan, D.N., B.H. Jones, P.N. Frykman, D.W. Polly, A. Harman, R.M. Rosenstein, and M.T. Rosenstein. 1996. Lower limb morphology and risk of overuse injury among male infantry trainees. *Med Sci Sports Exerc* 28(8): 945-952.

Cowling, E.J., and J.R. Steele. 2001. Is lower limb muscle synchrony during landing affected by landing? *J Electromyog Kinesiol* 11: 263-268.

Cowling, E.J., and J.R. Steele. 2002. *Hamstring muscle retraining: Is this a feasible option to decrease anterior cruciate ligament injury susceptibility?* Final Report to the NSW Sporting Injuries Committee, December, 24 pp.

Cowling, E.J., J.R. Steele, and P.J. McNair. 2003. Effect of verbal instructions on muscle activity and risk of injury to the anterior cruciate ligament during landing. *Br J Sports Med* 37: 126-130.

Crane, L. 1959. Femoral torsion and its relation to toeing-in and toeing-out. *J Bone Joint Surg Am* 41-A(3): 421-428.

Creinin, M.D., J.S. Lippman, S.E. Eder, A.J. Godwin, and W. Olson. 2002. The effect of extending the pill-free interval on follicular activity: Triphasic norgestimate/35μg ethinyl estradiol versus monophasic levonorgesterel/20μg ethinyl estradiol. *Contraception* 66: 147-152.

Crook, S., and M.L. Ireland. 2005. ACL injury prevention in female basketball players. In: T.L. Schuemann (Ed.), *Home study course: Rehabilitation concerns for the female athlete.* SPTS 2005: 2-12.

Cunningham, L.S., and J.L. Kelsey. 1984. Epidemiology of musculoskeletal impairments and associated disability. *Am J Pub Health* 74: 574-579.

Dahlberg, L. 1994. A longitudinal study of cartilage matrix metabolism in patients with cruciate ligament rupture-synovial fluid concentrations of aggrecan fragments, stromelysin-1 and tissue inhibitor of metalloproteinase-1. *Brit J Rheumatol* 33: 1107-1111.

Daniel, D.M., M.L. Stone, B.E. Dobson, et al. 1994. Fate of the ACL-injured patient. A prospective outcome study. *Am J Sports Med* 22: 632-644.

Davis, M.A., W.H. Ettinger, J.M. Neuhaus, et al. 1991. Knee osteoarthritis and physical functioning: Evidence from NHANES I epidemiologic follow-up study. *J Rheumatol* 18: 591-598.

Deacon, A., K. Bennell, Z.S. Kiss, K. Crossley, and P. Brukner. 1997. Osteoarthritis of the knee in retired, elite Australian Rules footballers. *Med J Aust* 166(4): 187-190.

Decker, M.J., M.R. Torry, D.J. Wyland, W.I. Sterett, and J.R. Steadman. 2003. Gender differences in lower extremity kinematics, kinetics, and energy absorption during landing. *Clin Biomech* 18: 662-669.

Decoster, L.C., J.N. Bernier, R.H. Lindsay, and J.C. Vailas. 1999. Generalized joint hypermobility and its relationship to injury patterns among NCAA lacrosse players. *J Athl Train* 34(2): 99-105.

DeHaven, K.E. 1980. The diagnosis of acute knee injuries with hemathrosis. *Am J Sports Med* 8: 9-14.

DeHaven, K.E. 1990. The role of the meniscus. In: J.W. Ewing (Ed.), *Articular cartilage and knee joint function. Basic science and arthroscopy* (pp. 103-115). New York: Raven Press.

Deibert, M.C., D.D. Aronsson, R.J. Johnson, C.F. Ettlinger, and J.E. Shealy. 1998. Skiing injuries in children, adolescents, and adults. *J Bone Joint Surg Am* 80(1): 25-32.

Deie, M., Y. Sakamaki, Y. Sumen, Y. Urabe, and Y. Ikuta. 2002. Anterior knee laxity in young women varies with their menstrual cycle. *Int Orthop* 26: 154-156.

Dejour, H., and M. Bonnin. 1994. Tibial translation after anterior cruciate ligament rupture. *J Bone Joint Surg Br* 76-B: 745-749.

Delfico, A.J., and W.E. Garrett. 1998. Mechanism of injury of the anterior cruciate ligament in soccer players. *Clin Sports Med* 17: 779-785.

de Loës, M., L.J. Dahlstedt, and R. Thomee. 2000. A 7-year study on risks and costs of knee injuries in male and female youth participants in 12 sports. *Scand J Med Science Sports* 10(2): 90-97.

Delp, S.L., W.E. Hess, D.S. Hungerford, and L.C. Jones. 1999. Variation of rotation moment arms with hip flexion. *J Biomech* 32(5): 493-501.

DeMaio, M., and K. McHale. 2003. Anterior cruciate ligament injuries in female athletes. In J.G. Garrick (Ed.), *Orthopedic knowledge update volume 3: Sports medicine.* Rosemont, IL: American Academy of Orthopaedic Surgeons.

DeMont, R.G., S.M. Lephart. 2004. Effect of sex on preactivation of the gastrocnemius and hamstring muscles. *Br J Sports Med* 38: 120-124.

DeMont, R.G., S.M. Lephart, J.L. Giraldo, C.B. Swanik, and F.H. Fu. 1999. Muscle preactivity of anterior cruciate ligament-deficient and -reconstructed females during functional activities. *J Athl Train* 34: 115-120.

DeMorat, G., P. Weinhold, T. Blackburn, S. Chudik, and W.E. Garrett. 2004. Aggressive quadriceps loading can induce noncontact anterior cruciate ligament injury. *Am J Sports Med* 32(2): 477-483.

De Rossi, D., A. Della Santa, and A. Mazzoldi. 1999. Dressware: Wearable hardware. *Mat Sci Eng* C(7): 31-35.

Devita, P., and W.A. Skelly. 1992. Effect of landing stiffness on joint kinetics and energetics in the lower extremity. *Med Sci Sports Exerc* 24: 108-115.

Diebert, M.C., D.D. Aronsson, R.J. Johnson, C.F. Ettlinger, and J.E. Shealy. 1998. Skiing injuries in children, adolescents, and adults. *J Bone Joint Surg* 80A(1): 25-32.

Dietz, V., J. Noth, et al. 1981. Interaction between pre-activity and stretch reflex in human triceps brachii during landing from forward falls. *J Physiol* 311: 113-125.

DiGirolamo, N. 1996. Increased matrix metalloproteinases in the aqueous humor of patients and experimental animals with uveitis. *Curr Eye Res* 15: 1060-1068.

Dikeman, J.S. 1998. Experimental simulation of mechanism of injury for non-contact, isolated anterior cruciate ligament ruptures. Master's thesis, North Carolina State University.

DiStefano, M., D.A. Padua, A. Van Doren, J.T. Blackburn, W.E. Prentice, and S.G. Karas. 2005. Gender Differences in Trunk and Hip Kinematics and Muscle Activation During a Cutting Task: A Comparison of Elite Soccer Athletes. Abstract presented at AOSSM annual meeting, Keystone CO.

Donohue, J.M., D. Buss, T.R. Oegema Jr., et al. 1983. The effects of indirect trauma on adult canine articular cartilage. *J Bone Joint Surg* 65A: 948-957.

Draganich, L.F., and J.W. Vahey. 1990. An in vitro study of anterior cruciate ligament strain induced by quadriceps and hamstring forces. *J Orthop Res* 8: 57-63.

Dragoo, J.L., R.S. Lee, P. Benhaim, G.A.M. Finerman, and S.L. Hame. 2003. Relaxin receptors in the human female anterior cruciate ligament. *Am J Sports Med* 31(4): 577-584.

Draper, V. 1990. Electromyographic biofeedback and recovery of quadriceps femoris muscle function following anterior cruciate ligament reconstruction. *Phys Ther* 70: 11-17.

Draper, V., and L. Ballard. 1991. Electrical stimulation versus electromyographic biofeedback in the recovery of quadriceps femoris muscle function following anterior cruciate ligament surgery. *Phys Ther* 71: 455-461; discussion 461-464.

Drawer, S., and C.W. Fuller. 2002. Evaluating the level of injury in English professional football using a risk based assessment process. *Br J Sports Med* 36: 446-451.

Dubey, R.K., D.G. Gillespie, E.K. Jackson, and P.J. Keller. 1998. 17B-Estradiol, its metabolites, and progesterone inhibit cardiac fibroblast growth. *Hypertension* 31(2): 522-528.

Dubravcic-Simunjak, S., M. Pecina, H. Kuipers, et al. 2003. The incidence of injuries in elite junior figure skaters. *Am J Sports Med* 31(4): 511-517.

Dumas, G.A., and J.G. Reid. 1997. Laxity of knee cruciate ligaments during pregnancy. *J Orthop Sports Phys Ther* 26: 2-6.

Dunn, T.G., S.E. Gillig, et al. 1986. The learning process in biofeedback: Is it feed-forward or feedback? *Biofeedback Self Reg* 11(2): 143-156.

Dürselen, L., L. Claes, and H. Kiefer. 1995. The influence of muscle forces and external loads on cruciate ligament strain. *Am J Sports Med* 23: 129-136.

Dursun, E., N. Dursun, and D. Alican. 2004. Effects of biofeedback treatment on gait in children with cerebral palsy. *Disabil Rehab* 26: 116-120.

Dyer, R., J. Sodek, and J.M. Heersche. 1980. The effect of 17 B-estradiol on collagen and noncollagenous protein synthesis in the uterus and some periodontal tissues. *Endocrinology* 107: 1014-1021.

Dyhre-Poulsen, P., E.B. Simonsen, et al. 1991. Dynamic control of muscle stiffness and H reflex modulation during hopping and jumping in man. *J Physiol* 437: 287-304.

Ebstrup, J.F., and F. Bojsen-Moller. 2000. Anterior cruciate ligament injury in indoor ball games. *Scand J Med Sci Sports* 10: 114-116.

Edwards, D.R. 1996a. Differential effects of transforming growth factor beta-1 on the expression of matrix metalloproteinases and tissue inhibitors of metalloproteinases in young and old human fibroblast. *Exp Gerontol* 31: 207-223.

Edwards, D.R. 1996b. The roles of tissue inhibitors of metalloproteinases in tissue remodeling and cell growth. *Int J Obes Rel Metab Disord* 20:Suppl. 3: 9-15.

Ekeland, A., and B.O. Thoresen. 1987. Isolated rupture of the anterior cruciate ligament by knee hyperflexion. In: C.D. Mote Jr. and R.J. Johnson (Eds.), *Skiing trauma and safety* (pp. 61-67). Sixth International Symposium. ASTM STP 938. Philadelphia: American Society for Testing and Materials.

Ekstrand, J., and J. Gillquist. 1983. Soccer injuries and their mechanisms: A prospective study. *Med Sci Sports Exerc* 15: 267-270.

Elmqvist, L.G., and R.J. Johnson. 1994. Prevention of cruciate ligament injuries. In: J.A. Feagin Jr. (Ed.) *The crucial ligaments* (2nd ed., pp. 495-505). New York: Churchill Livingstone.

Engebretsen, L., E. Arendt, and H.M. Fritts. 1993. Osteochondral lesions and cruciate ligament injuries. MRI in 18 knees. *Acta Orthop Scand* 64: 434-436.

Engin, M., A. Demirel, E.Z. Engin, and M. Fedakar. 2005. Recent developments and trends in biomedical sensors. *Measurement* 37: 173-188.

Engstrom, B., J.C. Johansson, and H. Tomkvist. 1991. Soccer injuries among elite female players. *Am J Sports Med* Jul-Aug 19(4): 372-375.

Ettlinger, C.F. 1986. Why all the knee injuries. *Skiing*, 70-78.

Ettlinger, C.F., R.J. Johnson, and J.E. Shealy. 1995. A method to help reduce the risk of serious knee sprains incurred in alpine skiing. *Am J Sports Med* 23(5): 531-537.

Ettlinger, C.F., R.J. Johnson, and J.E. Shealy. 2003. Where do we go from here? In: R.J. Johnson, M. Lamont, and J.E. Shealy (Eds.), *Skiing trauma and safety* (Vol. 14, pp. 53-64). ASTM STP 1440. West Conshohocken, PA: American Society for Testing and Materials.

Ettlinger, C.F., R.J. Johnson, and J.E. Shealy. 2005. Function and release characteristics of alpine ski equipment. Presented at the Sixteenth International Symposium on Ski Trauma and Skiing Safety, Arai Mountain, Niigata, Japan, April 17-23.

Evans, R.W., R.I. Evans, S. Caravajal, and S. Perry. 1996. A survey of injuries among Broadway performers. *Am J Pub Health* 86(1): 77-80.

Everts, V. 1996. Phagocytosis and intracellular digestion of collagen, its role in turnover and remodeling. *Histochem J* 28: 229-245.

Fagenbaum, R., and W.G. Darling. 2003. Jump landing strategies in male and female college athletes and the implications of such strategies for anterior cruciate ligament injury. *Am J Sports Med* 31: 233-240.

Fairbank, T.J. 1948. Knee joint changes after meniscectomy. *J Bone Joint Surg* 30B 664-670.

Faude, O., A. Junge, W. Kindermann, and J. Dvorak. 2005. Injuries in female soccer players: A prospective study in the German national league. *Am J Sports Med* 33(11): 1-7.

Feagin, J.A. Jr., and W.W. Curl. 1976. Isolated tear of the anterior cruciate ligament: 5-year follow-up study. *Am J Sports Med* 4: 95-100.

Feagin, J.A., K.L. Lambert, R.R. Cunningham, L.M. Anderson, J. Riegel, P.H. King, and L. VanGenderen. 1987. Consideration of the anterior cruciate ligament in skiing. *Clin Orthop Rel Res* 216: 13-18.

Feller, J., C. Hoser, and K. Webster. 2000. EMG biofeedback assisted KT-1000 evaluation of anterior tibial displacement. *Knee Surg, Sports Traumatol, Arthrosc* 8: 132-136.

Ferretti, A., F. Conteduca, A. De Carli, et al. 1991. Osteoarthritis of the knee after ACL reconstruction. *Int Orthop* 15: 367-371.

Ferretti, A., P. Papandrea, F. Conteduca, and P.P. Mariani. 1992. Knee ligament injuries in volleyball players. *Am J Sports Med* 20: 203-207.

Ferris, C.M., J.P. Abt, et al. 2004. Pelvis and hip neuromechanical characteristics predict knee biomechanics during a stop-jump task. *J Athl Train* 39(2): S-34.

Fischer, G.M. 1973. Comparison of collagen dynamics in different tissues under the influence of estradiol. *Endocrinology* 93: 1216-1218.

Fleck, S.J., and J.E. Falkel. 1986. Value of resistance training for the reduction of sports injuries. *Sports Med* 3: 61-68.

Fleming, B.C., P.A. Renstrom, B.D. Beynnon, B. Engstrom, and G. Peura. 2000. The influence of functional knee braces on the anterior cruciate ligament strain biomechanics in weight bearing and non-weight bearing knees. *Am J Sports Med* 28(6): 815-824.

Fleming, B.C., P.A. Renstrom, B.D. Beynnon, B. Engstrom, G.D. Peura, G.J. Badger, and R.J. Johnson. 2001. The effect of weightbearing and external loading on anterior cruciate ligament strain. *J Biomech* 34(3): 163-170.

Foos, M.J., J.R. Hickox, P.G. Mansour, J.R. Slauterbeck, and D.M. Hardy. 2001. Expression of matrix metalloprotease and tissue inhibitor of metalloprotease genes in the human anterior cruciate ligament. *J Orthop Res* 19: 642-649.

Ford, K.R., G.D. Myer, and T.E. Hewett. 2003. Valgus knee motion during landing in high school female and male basketball players. *Med Sci Sports Exerc* 35(10): 1745-1750.

Ford, K.R., G.D. Myer, H.E. Toms, and T.E. Hewett. 2005. Gender differences in the kinematics of unanticipated cutting in young athletes. *Med Sci Sports Exerc* 37: 124-129.

Fowler, P.J., and W.P. Regan. 1987. The patient with symptomatic chronic anterior cruciate ligament insufficiency: Results of minimal arthroscopic surgery and rehabilitation. *Am J Sports Med* 15: 321-325.

Freedman, K.B., M.T. Glasgow, S.G. Glasgow, and J. Bernstein. 1998. Anterior cruciate ligament injury and reconstruction among university students. *Clin Orthop Rel Res* 356: 208-212.

Freudiger, S., and N.F. Friederich. 2000. Critical load cases for knee ligaments at skiing—an engineering approach. In: R.J. Johnson, P. Zucco, and J.E. Shealy (Eds.), *Skiing trauma and safety* (Vol. 13, pp. 160-174). ASTM STP 1397. Philadelphia: American Society for Testing and Materials.

Fry, A.C., W.J. Kraemer, C.A. Weseman, et al. 1991. The effects of an off-season strength and conditioning program on starters and non-starters in women's intercollegiate volleyball. *J Appl Sport Sci Res* 5: 174-181.

Fujita, I., T. Nishikawa, H.E. Kambic, J.T. Andrish, and M.D. Grabiner. 2000. Characterization of hamstring reflexes during anterior cruciate ligament disruption: In vivo results from a goat model. *J Orthop Res* 18: 183-189.

Gaire, M. 1994. Structure and expression of the human gene for the matrix metalloproteinase matrilysin. *J Biol Chem* 269: 2032-2040.

Gardocki, R.J., R.G. Watkins, et al. 2002. Measurements of lumbopelvic lordosis using pelvic radius technique as it correlates with sagittal spinal balance and sacral translation. *Spine J* 2: 421-429.

Garrick, J.G. 1982. Figure skating injuries. *Med Sci Sports Exerc* 14: 141.

Garrick, J.G., D.M. Gillien, and P. Whiteside. 1986. The epidemiology of aerobic dance injuries. *Am J Sports Med* 14(1): 67-72.

Garrick, J.G., and R.K. Requa. 1993. Ballet injuries: An analysis of epidemiology and financial outcome. *Am J Sports Med* 21(4): 586-590.

Garrick, J.G., and R.K. Requa. 2001. ACL injuries in men and women—how common are they? In: L. Griffin (Ed.), *Prevention of noncontact ACL injuries* (chapter 1). Rosemont, IL: American Academy of Orthopedic Surgeons.

Gauffin, H., and H. Tropp. 1992. Altered movement and muscular-activation patterns during the one-legged jump in patients with an old anterior cruciate ligament rupture. *Am J Sports Med* 20(2): 182-192.

Gerberich, S.G., et al. 1987. Analysis of severe injuries associated with volleyball activities. *Physician Sportsmed* 6: 314-316.

Geyer, M., and C.J. Wirth. 1991. A new mechanism of injury of the anterior cruciate ligament. *Unfallchirurg* 94(2): 69-72.

Gilchrist, J., B. Mandelbaum, H.J. Silvers, et al. 2004a. ACL injury prevention in the Division I NCAA female soccer athlete. Presented at AOSSM Specialty Day.

Gilchrist, J.R., B.R. Mandelbaum, H. Melancon, et al. 2004b. A randomized controlled trial to prevent non-contact ACL injury in female collegiate soccer players. Presented at the American Orthopaedic Society for Sports Medicine, San Francisco.

Giove, T.P., S.J. Miller III, B.E. Kent, et al. 1983. Nonoperative treatment of the torn anterior cruciate ligament. *J Bone Joint Surg* 65A: 184-192.

Giza, E., K. Mithofer, L. Farrell, B. Zarins, and T. Gill. 2005. Injuries in women's professional soccer. *Br J Sports Med* 39(4): 212-216.

Gomez, E., J.C. DeLee, and W.C. Farney. 1996. Incidence of injury in Texas high school girls basketball. *Am J Sports Med* 24(5): 684-687.

Goodman, A.L., C.D. Descalzi, D.K. Johnson, and G.D. Hodgen. 1977. Composite pattern of circulating LH, FSH, estradiol, and progesterone during the menstrual cycle in cynomolgus monkeys. *Proc Soc Exper Biol Med* 155(4): 479-481.

Graf, B.K., D.A. Cook, A.A. DeSmet, et al. 1993. "Bone bruises" on magnetic resonance imaging evaluation of anterior cruciate ligament injuries. *Am J Sports Med* 21: 220-223.

Grana, W.A., and J.A. Moretz. 1978. Ligamentous laxity in secondary school athletes. *JAMA* 240: 1975-1976.

Granata, K.P., D.A. Padua, and S.E. Wilson. 2002. Gender differences in active musculoskeletal stiffness. Part II. Quantification of leg stiffness during functional hopping tasks. *J Electromyog Kinesiol* 12: 127-135.

Granata, K.P., S.E. Wilson, and D.A. Padua. 2002. Gender differences in active musculoskeletal stiffness. Part I. Quantification in controlled measurements of knee joint dynamics. *J Electromyog Kinesiol* 12: 119-126.

Gray, J., J.E. Taunton, D.C. McKenzie, D.B. Clement, J.P. McConkey, and R.G. Davidson. 1985. A survey of injuries to the anterior cruciate ligament of the knee in female basketball players. *Int J Sports Med* 6: 314-316.

Greene, D.L., K.R. Hamson, R.C. Bay, and C.D. Bryce. 2000. Effects of protective knee bracing on speed and agility. *Am J Sports Med* 28(4): 453-459.

Greenwood, R., and A. Hopkins. 1976. Landing from an unexpected fall and a voluntary step. *Brain* 99(2): 375-386.

Griffin, L.Y. 2000. The Henning Program. Rosemont: American Academy of Orthopaedic Surgeons; 2000.

Griffin, L.Y. 2001. The Henning program. In: L.Y. Griffin (Ed.), *Prevention of noncontact ACL injuries* (pp. 93-96). Rosemont, IL: American Academy of Orthopaedic Surgeons.

Griffin, L.Y., J. Agel, M.J. Albohm, E.A. Arendt, R.W. Dick, W.E. Garrett, J.G. Garrick, T.E. Hewett, L. Huston, M.L. Ireland, R.J. Johnson, W.B. Kibler, S. Lephart, J.L. Lewis, T.N. Lindenfeld, B.R. Mandelbaum, P. Marchak, C.C. Teitz, and E.M. Wojtys. 2000. Noncontact anterior cruciate ligament injuries: Risk factors and prevention strategies. *J Am Acad Orthop Surg* 8(3): 141-150.

Griffin, L.Y., M.J. Albohm, E.A. Arendt, E. Bahr, B.D. Beynnon, M. DeMaio, R.W. Dick, L. Engebretsen, W.E. Garrett, J. Gilchrist, J.A. Hannafin, T.E. Hewett, L.J. Huston, R.J. Johnson, S.M. Lephart, M.L. Ireland, B.R. Mandelbaum, B. Mann, P.H. Marks, S.W. Marshall, G. Myklebust, F.R. Noyes, C. Powers, C. Shields, S.J. Shultz, H. Silvers, J. Slauterbeck,

D. Taylor, C.C. Teitz, E.M. Wojtys, and B. Yu. In press-a. Update on ACL Prevention: Theoretical and practical guidelines. *Am J Sports Med.*

Griffin, L.Y., M.J. Albohm, E.A. Arendt, R. Bahr, B.D. Beynnon, M. DeMaio, R.W. Dick, L. Engebretsen, W.E. Garrett Jr., J.A. Hannafin, T.E. Hewett, L.J. Huston, M.L. Ireland, R.J. Johnson, S. Lephart, B.R. Mandelbaum, B. Mann, P.H. Marks, S.W. Marshall, G. Myklebust, F.R. Noyes, C. Powers, C. Shields Jr., S.J. Shultz, H. Silvers, J. Slauterbeck, D.C. Taylor, C.C. Teitz, E.M. Wojtys, and B. Yu. In press-b. Understanding and preventing non-contact ACL injuries: A review of the Hunt Valley II meeting, January 2005. *Am J Sports Med.*

Guerra, J.P., M.J. Arnold, and R.L. Gajdosik. 1994. Q angle: Effects of isometric quadriceps contraction and body position. *J Orthop Sports Phys Ther* 19(4): 200-204.

Guyton, A.C. 1991. Female physiology before pregnancy, and the female hormones. In: *Textbook of medical physiology* (pp. 899-914). Philadelphia: Saunders.

Gwinn, D., J. Wilckens, E. McDevitt, G. Ross, and T. Kao. 2000. The relative incidence of anterior cruciate ligament injury in men and women at the United States Naval Academy. *Am J Sports Med* 28: 98-102.

Haas, C.J., E.A. Schick, M.D. Tillman, J.W. Chow, D. Brunt, and J.H. Cauraugh. 2005. Knee biomechanics during landings: Comparison of pre- and postpubescent females. *Med Sci Sports Exerc* 37: 100-107.

Hagel, B.E., I.B. Pless, C. Goulet, R.W. Platt, and Y. Robitaille. 2005. Effectiveness of helmets in skiers and snowboarders: Case-control and case crossover study. *Br Med J* doi:10.1136/bmj.38314.480035.7C (published January 4, 2005).

Hagood, S., M. Solomonow, et al. 1990. The effect of joint velocity on the contribution of the antagonist musculature to knee stiffness and laxity. *Am J Sports Med* 18(2): 182-186.

Hama, H., T. Yamamuro, and T. Takeda. 1976. Experimental studies on connective tissue of the capsular ligament. Influences of aging and sex hormones. *Acta Orthop Scand* 47: 473-479.

Hame, S.L., D.A. Oakes, and K.L. Markolf. 2002. Injury to the anterior cruciate ligament during alpine skiing. *Am J Sports Med* 30(4): 537-540.

Hamilton, W.G., L.H. Hamilton, P. Marshall, and M. Molnar. 1992. A profile of the musculoskeletal characteristics of elite professional ballet dancers. *Am J Sports Med* 20(3): 267-273.

Hamlet, W.P., S.H. Liu, V. Panossian, and G.A. Finerman. 1997. Primary immunolocalization of androgen target cells in the human anterior cruciate ligament. *J Orthop Res* 15(5): 657-663.

Hammond, G.L., L.S. Abrams, G.W. Creasy, J. Natarajan, J.G. Allen, and P.K. Siiteri. 2003. Serum distribution of the major metabolites of norgestimate in relation to its pharmacological properties. *Contraception* 67: 93-99.

Hansen, M.S., B. Dieckmann, K. Jensen, and B.W. Jakobsen. 2000. The reliability of balance tests performed on the kinesthetic ability trainer (KAT 2000). *Knee Surg, Sports Traumatol, Arthrosc* 8: 180-185.

Hardacker, W.T., W.E. Garrett Jr., and F.H. Basset III. 1990. Evaluation of acute traumatic hemarthrosis of the knee joint. *South Med J* 83: 640-644.

Hardy, D.M., J.R. Hickox, S.M. Shepherd, R.A. Hirsch, M.P. Smith, and J.R. Slauterbeck. 2002. Gender differences in expression of MMP3 in human ACL. *Transactions of the annual meeting of the Orthopaedic Research Society* 27: 926.

Harmon, K.G., and R. Dick. 1998. The relationship of skill level to anterior cruciate ligament injury. *Clin J Sport Med* 8(4): 260-265.

Harner, C.D., L.E. Paulos, A.E. Greenwald, T.D. Rosenberg, and V.C. Cooley. 1994. Detailed analysis of patients with bilateral anterior cruciate ligament injuries. *Am J Sports Med* 22: 37-43.

Harper, J., and D. Amiel. 1988. Collagenase production by rabbit ligaments and tendon. *Conn Tissue Res* 17: 253-259.

Hart, D.A., C. Reno, C.B. Frank, and N.G. Shrive. 2000. Pregnancy affects cellular activity, but not tissue mechanical properties, in the healing rabbit medial collateral ligament. *J Orthop Res* 18: 462-471.

Hassager, C., L.T. Jensen, J. Podenphant, B.J. Riis, and C. Christiansen. 1990. Collagen synthesis in postmenopausal women during therapy with anabolic steroid or female sex hormones. *Metabolism* 39: 1167-1169.

Hawkins, R.J., G.W. Misamore, and T.R. Merrit. 1986. Follow up of the acute non-operated isolated anterior cruciate ligament tears. *Am J Sports Med* 14: 205-210.

Heidt, R.S., L.M. Sweeterman, R.L. Carlonas, J.A. Traub, and F.X. Tekulve. 2000. Avoidance of soccer injuries with preseason conditioning. *Am J Sports Med* 28(5): 659-662.

Heinegard, D., and A. Oldberg. 1989. Structure and biology of cartilage and bone matrix noncollagenous macromolecules. *FASEB* 3: 2042-2054.

Heise, G.D., M. Bohne, and E. Bressel. 2001. Muscle preactivation and leg stiffness in men and women during hopping. Abstract presented at the American Society of Biomechanics annual meeting, San Diego, CA.

Heitkamp, H.C., T. Horstmann, F. Mayer, et al. 2001. Gain in strength and muscular balance after balance training. *Int J Sports Med* 22: 285-290.

Heitz, N.A. 1999. Hormonal changes throughout the menstrual cycle and increased anterior cruciate ligament laxity in females. *J Athl Train* 343(2): 144-149.

Henning, C.E., and N.D. Griffis. 1990. Injury prevention of the anterior cruciate ligament [videotape]. Wichita, KS: Mid-America Center for Sports Medicine.

Henzyl, M.R. 2001. Norgestimate: From the laboratory to three clinical indications. *J Reprod Med* 46(7): 647-661.

Hertel, J.N., J.H. Dorfman, and R.A. Braham. 2004. Lower extremity malalignments and anterior cruciate ligament injury history. *J Sports Sci Med* 3: 220-225.

Hertling, D. and R. Kessler. 1996. *Management of common musculoskeletal disorders: Physical therapy principles and methods.* (pp. 512-514). Philadelphia: Lippincott Raven Publishers.

Hester, J.T., and J. Falkel. 1984. Isokinetic evaluation of tibial rotation: Assessment of a stabilization technique. *J Orthop Sports Phys Ther* 6(1): 46-51.

Hewett, T.E. 2000. Neuromuscular and hormonal factors associated with knee injuries in female athletes: Strategies for Intervention. *Sports Med* 29(5): 313-327.

Hewett, T.E., K.R. Ford, and G.D. Myer. 2006. Anterior cruciate ligament injuries in female athletes: Part 2, A meta-analysis of neuromuscular interventions aimed at injury prevention. *Am J Sports Med* 34: 1-9.

Hewett, T.E., T.N. Lindenfeld, J.V. Riccobene, and F.R. Noyes. 1999. The effect of neuromuscular training on the incidence of knee injury in female athletes. A prospective study. *Am J Sports Med* 27(6): 699-706.

Hewett, T.E., G.D. Myer, et al. 2005a. Biomechanical measures of neuromuscular control and valgus loading of the knee predict ACL injury risk in female athletes. *Am J Sports Med* 33(4):492-501.

Hewett, T.E., G.D. Myer, and K.R. Ford. 2004. Decrease in neuromuscular control about the knee with maturation in female athletes. *J Bone Joint Surg* 86A: 1601-1608.

Hewett, T.E., G.D. Myer, and K.R. Ford. 2005d. Reducing knee and anterior cruciate ligament injuries among female athletes: A systematic review of neuromuscular training interventions. *J Knee Surg* 18: 82-88.

Hewett, T.E., G.D. Myer, K.R. Ford, R.S. Heidt Jr., A.J. Colosimo, S.G. McLean, A.J. van den Bogert, M.V. Paterno, and P. Succop. 2005b. Biomechanical measures of neuromuscular control and valgus loading of the knee predict anterior cruciate ligament injury risk in female athletes: A prospective study. *Am J Sports Med* 33(4): 492-501.

Hewett, T.E., M.V. Paterno, and G.D. Myer. 2002. Strategies for enhancing proprioception and neuromuscular control of the knee. *Clin Orthop* 402: 76-94.

Hewett, T.E., A.L. Stroupe, T.A. Nance, and F.R. Noyes. 1996. Plyometric training in female athletes. Decreased impact forces and increased hamstring torques. *Am J Sports Med* 24(6): 765-773.

Hewett, T.E., B.T. Zazulak, G.D. Myer, and K.R. Ford. 2005c. A review of electromyographic activation levels, timing differences, and increased anterior cruciate ligament injury incidence in female athletes. *Br J Sports Med* 39: 347-350.

Hewson, G.F., R.A. Mendini, and J.B. Wang. 1986. Prophylactic knee bracing in college football. *Am J Sports Med* 14: 262-266.

Hirokawa, S., M. Solomonow, Z. Luo, and R. D'Ambrosia. 1991. Muscular co-contraction and control of knee stability. *J Electromyog Kinesiol* 1(3): 199-208.

Hirschman, H.P., D. Daniel, and K. Miyasaka. 1990. The fate of unoperated knee ligament injuries. In: D. Daniel (Ed.), *Knee ligaments: Structure, function, injury and repair* (pp. 481-503). New York: Raven Press.

Ho, K.K.Y., and A.J. Weissberger. 1992. Impact of short-term estrogen administration on growth hormone secretion and action: Distinct route-dependent effects on connective and bone tissue metabolism. *J Bone Min Res* 7: 821-827.

Hodges, P.W., and C.A. Richardson. 1997. Contraction of the abdominal muscles associated with movement of the lower limb. *Phys Ther* 77(2):132-142; discussion 142-144.

Holm, I., M.A. Fosdahl, A. Friis, M.A. Risberg, G. Myklebust, and H. Steen. 2004. Effects of neuromuscular training on proprioception, balance, muscle strength, and lower limb function in female team handball players. *Clin J Sport Med* 14: 88-94.

Horton, M.G., and T.L. Hall. 1989. Quadriceps femoris angle: Normal values and relationship with gender and selected skeletal measures. *Phys Ther* 69: 897-901.

Hosokawa, M., M. Ishii, K. Inoue, C.S. Yao, and T. Takeda. 1981. Estrogen induces different responses in dermal and lung fibroblasts: Special reference to collagen. *Conn Tissue Res* 9: 115-120.

Houglum, P.A. 2005. *Therapeutic exercise for musculoskeletal injury*. Champaign: Human Kinetics.

Hruska, R. 1998. Pelvic stability influences lower extremity kinematics. *Biomechanics* 6: 23-29.

Hsieh, H.-H., and P.S. Walker. 1976. Stabilizing mechanisms of the loaded and unloaded knee joint. *J Bone Joint Surg Am* 58-A(1): 87-93.

Hsu, R.W., S. Himeno, M.B. Coventry, and E.Y. Chao. 1990. Normal axial alignment of the lower extremity and load-bearing distribution at the knee. *Clin Orthop Rel Res* 255: 215-227.

Hurd, W.J., T.L. Chmielewski, and L. Snyder-Mackler. 2006. Perturbation-enhanced neuromuscular training alters muscle activity in female athletes. *Knee Surg Sports Traumatol Arthrosc* Jan. 14(1): 60-9. Epub 2005 Jun 4.

Huston, L.J., M.L.V.H. Greenfield, and E.M. Wojtys. 2000. Anterior cruciate ligament injuries in the female athlete: Potential risk factors. *Clin Orthop Rel Res* 372: 50-63.

Huston, L.J., B. Vibert, and E.M. Wojtys. 2001. Gender differences in knee angle when landing from a drop-jump. *Am J Knee Surg* 14: 215-219.

Huston, L.J., and E.M. Wojtys. 1996. Neuromuscular performance characteristics in elite female athletes. *Am J Sports Med* 24(4): 427-436.

Hutchinson, M.R., and M.L. Ireland. 1995. Knee injuries in female athletes. *Sports Med* 19(4): 288-302.

Hutchinson, M.R., R.I. Williams, and M.L. Ireland. Knee injuries. 2002. In: M.L. Ireland and A. Nattiv (Eds.), *The female athlete* (pp. 387-419). Philadelphia: Saunders.

Ilahi, O.A., and H.W. Kohl. 1998. Lower extremity morphology and alignment and risk of overuse injury. *Clin J Sports Med* 8: 38-42.

Imran, A., and J.J. O'Connor. 1997. Theoretical estimates of cruciate ligament forces: Effects of tibial surface geometry and ligament orientations. *Proc Inst Mech Eng* [H] 211(6): 425-439.

Indelicato, P.A. 1983. Nonoperative treatment of complete tears of the medial collateral ligament of the knee. *J Bone Joint Surg* 65A: 323-329.

Indelicato, P.A., and E.S. Bittar. 1985. A perspective of lesions associated with anterior ligament insufficiency of the knee. *Clin Orthop Relat Res* Sept. (198):77-80

Ireland, M.L. 1999. Anterior cruciate ligament injury in female athletes: Epidemiology. *J Athl Train* 34(2): 150-154.

Ireland, M.L. 2002. The female ACL: Why is it more prone to injury? *Orthop Clin North Am* 33: 637-651.

Ireland, M.L. 2005. The female athlete: Entitled to compete, predetermined to tear her anterior cruciate ligament? Invited commentary. *Curr Sports Med Rep* 4: 57-60.

Ireland, M.L., B.T. Ballantyne, K. Little, and I.S. McClay. 2001. A radiographic analysis of the relationship between the size and shape of the intercondylar notch and anterior cruciate ligament injury. *Knee Surg, Sports Traumatol, Arthrosc* 9: 200-205.

Ireland, M.L., M. Gaudette, and S. Crook. 1997. ACL injuries in the female athlete. *J Sport Rehab* 6: 97-110.

Ireland, M.L., J.D. Wilson, B.T. Ballantyne, and I.M. Davis. 2003. Hip strength in females with and without patellofemoral pain. *J Orthop Sports Phys Ther* 33(Nov, 11): 671-676.

Irmischer, B.S., C. Harris, R.P. Pfeifer, M.A. DeBeliso, K.J. Adams, and K.G. Shea. 2004. Effects of a knee ligament injury prevention exercise program on impact forces in women. *J Strength Cond Res* 18: 703-707.

Israel, R., D.R. Mishell, S.C. Stone, I.H. Thorneycroft, and D.L. Moyer. 1972. Single luteal phase serum progesterone assay as an indicator of ovulation. *Am J Obstr Gynecol* 112(8): 1043-1046.

Jackson, D.W., E.S. Grood, B.T. Cohn, S.P. Arnoczky, T.M. Simon, and J.F. Cummings. 1991. The effect of in situ freezing on the anterior cruciate ligament. An experimental study in goats. *J Bone Joint Surg* 73A: 201-213.

Jansson, A., T. Saartok, S. Werner, and P. Renstrom. 2004. General joint laxity in 1845 Swedish school children of different ages: Age- and gender-specific distributions. *Acta Paediatrica* 93(9): 1202-1206.

Järvinen, M., A. Natri, S. Laurila, et al. 1994. Mechanisms of anterior cruciate ligament ruptures in skiing. *Knee Surg, Sports Traumatol, Arthrosc* 2: 224-228.

Jiang, C., K. Yip, and T. Liu. 1994. Posterior slope angle of the medial tibial plateau. *J Formas Med Assoc* 93: 509-512.

Johannson, H., P. Sjolander, and P. Sojka. 1990. Activity in receptor afferents from the anterior cruciate ligament evokes reflex events on fusimotor neurons. *Neurosci Res* 8: 54-59.

Johansson, H., P. Sjolander, and P. Sojka. 1991. A sensory role for the cruciate ligaments. *Clin Orthop* 268: 161-178.

Johnson, R.J. 1988. Prevention of cruciate ligament injuries. In: J.A. Feagin Jr.(Ed.), *The crucial ligaments* (pp. 349-356). New York: Churchill Livingstone.

Johnson, R.J. 2001. The ACL injury in female skiers. In: L.Y. Griffin (Ed.), *Prevention of noncontact ACL injuries* (pp. 107-111). Rosemont, IL: American Academy of Orthopaedic Surgeons.

Johnson, R.J., B.D. Beynnon, C.E. Nichols, et al. 1992. The treatment of injuries of the anterior cruciate ligament. *J Bone Joint Surg* 74A: 140-148.

Johnson, R.J., and C.F. Ettlinger. 1982. Alpine ski injuries: Changes through the years. *Clin Sports Med* 1: 181-197.

Johnson, R.J., C.F. Ettlinger, and J.E. Shealy. 1989. Skier injury trends. In: R.J. Johnson, C.D. Mote Jr., and M-H Binet (Eds.), *Skiing trauma and safety* (pp. 25-31). Seventh International Symposium. ASTM STP 1022. Philadelphia: American Society for Testing and Materials.

Johnson, R.J., C.F. Ettlinger, and J.E. Shealy. 1993. Skier injury trends: 1972 to 1990. In: R.J. Johnson, C.D. Mote Jr., and J. Zelcer (Eds.), *Skiing trauma and safety* (pp. 11-22). Ninth International Symposium. ASTM STP 1182. Philadelphia: American Society for Testing and Materials.

Johnson, R.J., C.F. Ettlinger, and J.E. Shealy. 1997. Skier injury trends: 1972 to 1994. In: R.J. Johnson, C.D. Mote Jr., and A. Ekeland (Eds.), *Skiing trauma and safety* (pp. 37-48). Eleventh International Symposium. ASTM STP 1289. Philadelphia: American Society for Testing and Materials.

Johnson, R.J., C.F. Ettlinger, and J.E. Shealy. 2003. Lower extremity injuries involving traditional alpine skis versus short skis with non-release bindings. In: R.J. Johnson, M. Lamont, and J.E. Shealy (Eds.), *Skiing trauma and safety* (Vol. 14, pp. 105-112). ASTM STP 1440. West Conshohocken, PA: American Society for Testing and Materials.

Johnson, R.J., C.F. Ettlinger, and J.E. Shealy. 2004. Skier injury trends. A 30-year investigation. *Knee Surg, Sports Traumatol, Arthrosc* 12: 170-177.

Johnson, R.J., and M.H. Pope. 1978. Functional anatomy of the meniscus. In: *American Academy of Orthopaedic Surgeons: Symposium on reconstruction of the knee* (p. 3). St. Louis: Mosby.

Johnson, R.J., and M.H. Pope. 1991. Epidemiology and prevention of skiing injuries. *Ann Chir Gynaecol* 80: 110-115.

Johnson, R.J., M.H. Pope, and C.F. Ettlinger. 1974. Ski injuries and equipment function. *J Sports Med* 2: 299-307.

Johnson, R.J., J.E. Shealy, and C.F. Ettlinger. 2005. Injury trends and risk factors involving ACL injuries in alpine skiing. Presented at the Sixteenth International Symposium on Ski Trauma and Skiing Safety, Arai Mountain, Niigata, Japan, April 17-23.

Johnston, R.B., M.E. Howard, P.W. Cawley, and G.M. Losse. 1998. Effect of lower extremity muscular fatigue on motor control performance. *Med Sci Sports Exerc* 30(12): 1703-1707.

Joseph, B. 1998. Treatment of internal rotation gait due to gluteus medius and minimus overactivity in cerebral palsy: Anatomical rationale of a new surgical procedure and preliminary results in twelve hips. *Clin Anat* 11: 22-28.

Junge, A., D. Rosch, L. Peterson, T. Graf-Baumann, and J. Dvorak. 2002. Prevention of soccer injuries: A prospective intervention study in youth amateur players. *Am J Sports Med* 30: 652-659.

Kahn, C.R. 1994. Picking a research problem. The critical decision. *New Engl J Med* 330: 1530-1533.

Kain, C.C., J.A. McCarthy, S. Arms, M.H. Pope, J.R. Steadman, P.R. Manske, and R.A. Shively. 1988. An in vivo analysis of the effect of transcutaneous electrical stimulation of the quadriceps and hamstrings on anterior cruciate ligament deformation. *Am J Sports Med* 16: 147-152.

Kannus, P., and R.J. Johnson. 1991. Downhill skiing injuries: Trends to watch for this season. *J Musculoskel Med* 8: 12-32.

Karageanes, S.J., K. Blackburn, and Z.A. Vangelos. 2000. The association of the menstrual cycle with the laxity of the anterior cruciate ligament in adolescent female athletes. *Clin J Sports Med* 10(3): 162-168.

Karter, A.J., M.R. Stevens, W.H. Herman, S. Ettner, D.G. Marrero, M.M. Safford, M.M. Engelgau, J.D. Curb, and A.F. Brown. 2003. Out-of-pocket costs and diabetes preventive services: The Translating Research Into Action for Diabetes (TRIAD) study. *Diab Care* 26(8): 2294-2299.

Kendall, F.P., and E.K. McCreary. 1983. *Muscles: Testing and function.* Baltimore: Williams & Wilkins.

Kennedy, J.C., I.J. Alexander, and K.C. Hayes. 1982. Nerve supply of the human knee and its functional importance. *Am J Sports Med* 10: 329-335.

Kernozek, T.W., and N.L. Greer. 1993. Quadriceps angle and rearfoot motion: Relationships in walking. *Arch Phys Med Rehab* 74(4): 407-410.

Kernozek, T.W., M.R. Torry, H. Van Hoof, H. Cowley, and S. Tanner. 2005. Gender differences in frontal and sagittal plane biomechanics during drop landings. *Med Sci Sports Exerc* 37: 1003-1012.

Kibler, W.B., T.J. Chandler, L. Cabell, and R. Shapiro. 2001. Gender differences in muscle activation around the hip, knee, and ankle in cutting maneuvers. *Clin Biomech* 16: 945.

Kim, A.W., A.M. Rosen, et al. 1995. Selective muscle activation following electrical stimulation of the collateral ligaments of the human knee joint. *Arch Phys Med Rehab* 76(8): 750-757.

Kineane, J.E. 1914, April 14-15. National Association of Industrial Accident Boards and Commissions first meeting, Lansing, MI.

Kirkendall, D.T., and L.H. Calabrese. 1983. Physiological aspects of dance. *Clin Sports Med* 2(3): 525-537.

Kirkendall, D.T., and W.E. Garrett Jr. 2000. The anterior cruciate ligament enigma. Injury mechanisms and prevention. *Clin Orthop* 372: 64-68.

Kissick, W.L. 1994. *Medicine's dilemmas: Infinite need versus finite resources.* New Haven: Yale University Press.

Kjaer, M., and B. Larsson. 1992. Physiological profile and incidence of injuries among elite figure skaters. *J Sports Sci* 10: 29-36.

Kocher, M.S., W.I. Sterett, K.K. Briggs, D. Zurakowski, and J.R. Steadman. 2003. Effect of functional bracing on subsequent knee injury in ACL-deficient professional skiers. *J Knee Surg* 16(2): 87-92.

Koutedakis, Y., A. Agrawal, and N.C.C. Sharp. 1998. Isokinetic characteristics of knee flexors and extensors in male dancers, Olympic oarsmen, Olympic bobsleighers and non-athletes. *J Dance Med Sci* 2(2): 63-67.

Koutedakis Y., M. Khalouha, P.J. Pacy, et al. 1997. Thigh peak torques and lower-body injuries in dancers. *J Dance Med Sci* 1(1): 12-15.

Kozaci, L.D. 1997. Degradation of type II collagen, but not proteoglycan, correlates with matrix metalloproteinase activity in cartilage explant cultures. *Arthritis Rheum* 40: 164-174.

Kraemer, W.J., N.D. Duncan, and J.S. Volek. 1998. Resistance training and elite athletes: Adaptations and program considerations. *J Orthop Sports Phys Ther* 28: 110-119.

Kraemer, W.J., K. Hakkinen, N.T. Triplett-Mcbride, A.C. Fry, L.P. Koziris, N.A. Ratamess, J.E. Bauer, J.S. Volek, T. McConnell, R.U. Newton, S.E. Gordon, D. Cummings, J. Hauth, F. Pullo, J.M. Lynch, S.J. Fleck, S.A. Mazzetti, and H.G. Knuttgen. 2003. Physiological changes with periodized resistance training in women tennis players. [Erratum appears in *Med Sci Sports Exerc* 35(May, 5): 889, 2003.] *Med Sci Sports Exerc* 35: 157-168.

Krane, S.M. 1996. Different collagenase gene products have different roles in degradation of type I collagen. *J Biol Chem* 271: 28509-28515.

Krivickas, L.S. 1997. Anatomical factors associated with overuse sports injuries. *Sports Med* 24(2): 132-146.

Krosshaug, T., and R. Bahr. 2005. A model-based image-matching technique for three-dimensional reconstruction of human motion from uncalibrated video sequences. *J Biomech* 38: 919-929.

Kujala, U.M., J. Kettunen, H. Paananen, T. Aalto, M.C. Battie, O. Impivaara, T. Videman, and S. Sarna. 1995. Knee osteoarthritis in former runners, soccer players, weight lifters, and shooters. *Arthritis Rheum* 38: 539-546.

Kujala, U.M., S. Sarna, J. Kaprio, and M. Koskenvuo. 1996. Hospital care in later life among world class athletes. *JAMA* 276: 216-220.

Kulas, A.S., T.C. Windley, et al. In press. Effects of abdominal postures on lower extremity energetics during single leg landings. *J Sport Rehab.*

Kumagai, M., S. Naoto, et al. 1997. Functional evaluation of hip abductor muscles with use of magnetic resonance imaging. *J Bone Joint Surg* 15: 888-893.

Kurosawa, H., T. Fukubayashi, and H. Nakajima. 1980. Load-bearing mode of the knee: Physical behaviour of the knee joint with and without menisci. *Clin Orthop* 149: 283-290.

Kvist, J. 2004. Rehabilitation following anterior cruciate ligament injury: Current recommendations for sports participation. *Sports Med* 34(4): 269-280.

LaFortune, M.A., P.R. Cavanagh, H.J. Sommer, and A. Kalenak. 1994. Foot inversion-eversion and knee kinematics during walking. *J Orthop Res* 12(3): 412-420.

Lahm, A., C. Erggelet, M. Steinwachs, et al. 1998. Articular and osseous lesions in recent ligament tears: Arthroscopic changes compared with magnetic resonance imaging findings. *Arthroscopy* 14: 597-604.

Lam, C.K., W.Y. Leung, W.C. Wu, and J. Lam. 1997. Orthopaedic ice-skating injuries in a regional hospital in Hong Kong. *Hong Kong Med J* 3(2): 131-134.

Lambson, R.B., B.S. Barnhill, and R.W. Higgins. 1996. Football cleat design and its effect on anterior cruciate ligament injuries: A three-year prospective study. *Am J Sports Med* 24: 155-159.

Lamontagne M., D.L. Benoit, D.K. Ramsey, A. Caraffa, G. Cerulli. 2005. What can we learn from in vivo biomechanical investigation of lower extremity? In: *Proceedings of XXIII International Symposium of Biomechanics in Sports,* pp. 49-56.

Landgren, B.M., A.L. Unden, and E. Deczfalusy. 1980. Hormonal profile of the cycle in 68 normal menstruating women. *Acta Endocrinol* 94: 89-98.

LaPrade, R.F., and Q.M. Burnett. 1994. Femoral intercondylar notch stenosis and correlation to anterior cruciate ligament injuries. *Am J Sports Med* 22(2): 198-302.

Larsen, P.R., H.M. Kronenberg, S. Melmed, and K.S. Polonsky. 2003. *Williams textbook of endocrinology.* Philadelphia: Saunders.

Larsson, L.G., J. Baum, and G.S. Mudholkar. 1987. Hypermobility: Features and differential incidence between the sexes. *Arthritis Rheum* 30: 1426-1430.

Lauder, T.D., S.P. Baker, G.S. Smith, and A.E. Lincoln. 2000. Sports and physical training injury hospitalizations in the army. *Am J Prev Med* 18 (Suppl.): 118-128.

Lee, H.J., W.R. Holcomb, et al. 2004. Hamstring to quadriceps strength ratios: An analysis and strength training study. *J Athl Train* 39(2): S-29.

Leetun, D.T., M.L. Ireland, et al. 2004. Core stability measures as risk factors for lower extremity injury in athletes. *Med Sci Sports Exerc* 36(6): 926-934.

Lehnhard, R.A., H.R. Lehnhard, R. Young, et al. 1996. Monitoring injuries on a college soccer team: The effect of strength training. *J Strength Cond Res* 10: 115-119.

Lenton, E.A., G.F. Lawrence, R.A. Coleman, and I.D. Cooke. 1983. Individual variation in gonadotropin and steroid concentrations and in the lengths of the follicular and luteal phases in women with regular menstrual cycles. *Clin Reprod Fertil* 2: 143-150.

Lephart, S.M., J.P. Abt, et al. 2002a. Neuromuscular contributions to anterior cruciate ligament injuries in females. *Curr Opin Rheumatol* 14: 168-173.

Lephart, S.M., J.P. Abt, C.M. Ferris, T.C. Sell, T. Nagai, J.B. Myers, and J.J. Irrgang. 2005. Neuromuscular and biomechanical characteristic changes in high school athletes: A plyometric versus basic resistance program. *Br J Sports Med* 39: 932-938.

Lephart, S.M., C.M. Ferris, B.L. Riemann, J.B. Myers, and F.H. Fu. 2001. Gender differences in neuromuscular patterns and landing strategies. *Clin Biomech* 16: 941-959.

Lephart, S.M., C.M. Ferris, B.L. Riemann, J.B. Myers, and F.H. Fu. 2002b. Gender differences in strength and lower extremity kinematics during landing. *Clin Orthop Rel Res* 401: 162-169.

Lephart, S.M., F.H. Fu, P.A. Borsa, et al. 1995. Proprioception of the knee and shoulder joint in normal, athletic, capsuloligamentous pathological, and post-reconstruction individuals. *Orthop Trans* 18: 1157.

Lephart, S.M., M.S. Kicher, F.H. Fu, et al. 1992. Proprioception following anterior cruciate ligament reconstruction. *J Sport Rehab* 1: 188-196.

Levy, A.S., M.J. Wetzler, M. Lewars, and W. Laughlin. 1997. Knee injuries in women collegiate rugby players. *Am J Sports Med* 25(3): 360-362.

Levy, I.M., D.A. Torzilli, and R.F. Warren. 1982. The effect of medial meniscectomy on anterior-posterior motion of the knee. *J Bone Joint Surg* 64A: 883-888.

Lewandrowksi, K-U, J. Muller, and G. Schollmeier. 1997. Concomitant meniscal and articular cartilage lesions in the femorotibial joint. *Am J Sports Med* 25: 486-494.

Li, G., L.E. DeFrate, H.E. Rubash, and T.J. Gill. 2005. In vivo kinematics of the ACL during weight-bearing knee flexion. *J Orthop Res* 23: 340-344.

Li, G., T.W. Rudy, M. Sakane, A. Kanamori, C.B. Ma, and S.L.Y. Woo. 1999. The importance of quadriceps and hamstring muscle loading on knee kinematics and in-situ forces in the ACL. *J Biomech* 32(4): 395-400.

Li, G., S. Zayontz, E. Most, L.E. DeFrate, J.F. Suggs, and H.E. Rubash. 2004. In situ forces of the anterior and posterior cruciate ligaments in high knee flexion: An in vitro investigation. *J Orthop Res* 22: 293-297.

Lindenfeld, T.N., D.J. Schmitt, M.P. Hendy, et al. 1994. Incidence of injury in indoor soccer. *Am J Sports Med* 22(May-June, 3): 364-371.

Lindsay, D.M., M.E. Maitland, et al. 1992. Comparison of isokinetic internal and external hip rotation torques using different testing positions. *J Orthop Sports Phys Ther* 16(1): 43-50.

Liu, S.H., R.A. Al-Shaikh, V. Panossian, and G.M. Finerman. 1996. Primary immunolocalization of estrogen and progesterone target cells in the human anterior cruciate ligament. *Orthop Res Soc* 14: 526-533.

Liu, S.H., R.A. Al-Shaikh, V. Panossian, G.A. Finerman, and J.M. Lane. 1997. Estrogen affects the cellular metabolism of the anterior cruciate ligament. *Am J Sports Med* 25(5): 704-709.

Lloyd, D.G. 2001. Rationale for training programs to reduce anterior cruciate ligament injuries in Australian football. *J Orthop Sports Phys Ther* 31(11): 645-54; discussion 661.

Lloyd, D.G., and T.S. Buchanan. 1996. A model of load sharing between muscles and soft tissues at the human knee during static tasks. *J Biomech Eng* 118(3): 367-376.

Lloyd, D.G., and T.S. Buchanan. 2001. Strategies of muscular support of varus and valgus isometric loads at the human knee. *J Biomech* 34: 1257-1267.

Lofvenberg, R., J. Karrholm, G. Sundelin, and O. Ahlgren. 1995. Prolonged reaction time in patients with chronic lateral instability of the ankle. *Am J Sports Med* 23(4): 414-417.

Lohmander, L.S. 1994. Temporal patterns of stromelysis-1, tissue inhibitor, and proteoglycan fragments in human knee joint fluid after injury to the cruciate ligament or meniscus. *J Orthop Res* 12: 12-18.

Lohmander, L.S., A. Ostenberg, M. Englund, and H. Roos. 2004. High prevalence of knee osteoarthritis, pain, and functional limitations in female soccer players twelve years after anterior cruciate ligament injury. *Arthritis Rheum* 8(10): 3145-3152.

Lombardo, S., P.M. Sethi, and C. Starkey. 2005. Intercondylar notch stenosis is not a risk factor for anterior cruciate ligament tears in professional male basketball players: An 11-year prospective study. *Am J Sports Med* 33(1): 29-34.

London, R.S., A. Chapdelaine, D. Upmalis, W. Olson, and J. Smith. 1992. Comparative contraceptive efficacy and mechanism of action of the norgestimate-containing triphasic oral contraceptive. *Acta Obstr Gynecol Scand* 71: 9-14.

Loudon, J.K. 2000. Measurement of knee-joint-position sense in women with genu recurvatum. *J Sport Rehab* 9: 15-25.

Loudon, J.K., W. Jenkins, and K.L. Loudon. 1996. The relationship between static posture and ACL injury in female athletes. *J Orthop Sports Phys Ther* 24(2): 91-97.

Louie, J., and C. Mote. 1987. Contribution of the musculature to rotary laxity and torsional stiffness at the knee. *J Biomech* 20: 281-300.

Lucca, J.A., and S.J. Recchiuti. 1983. Effect of electromyographic biofeedback on an isometric strengthening program. *Phys Ther* 63: 200-203.

Lund-Hanssen, H., J. Gannon, L. Engebretsen, K.J. Holen, S. Anda, and L. Vatten. 1994. Intercondylar notch width and the risk for anterior cruciate ligament rupture. *Acta Orthop Scand* 65(5): 529-532.

Lund-Hanssen, H., J. Gannon, L. Engebretsen, K.J. Holen, and S. Hammer. 1996. Isokinetic muscle performance in healthy female handball players with a unilateral anterior cruciate ligament reconstruction. *Scand J Med Sci Sports* 6: 172-175.

Lynch, M.A., and C.E. Henning. 1994. Osteoarthritis in the ACL-deficient knee. In: J. Feagin (Ed.), *The crucial ligaments* (pp. 385-391). New York: Churchill Livingstone.

Lynch, M.A., C.E. Henning, and K.R. Glick Jr. 1983. Knee joint surface changes. *Clin Orthop* 172: 148-153.

MacDonald, P.B., D. Hedden, O. Pacin, et al. 1996. Proprioception in anterior cruciate ligament-deficient and reconstructed knees. *Am J Sports Med* 24: 774-778.

MacWilliams, B.A., D.R. Wilson, J.D. DesJardins, J. Romero, and E.Y. Chao. 1999. Hamstrings co-contraction reduces internal rotation, anterior translation, and anterior cruciate ligament load in weight-bearing flexion. *J Orthop Res* 17: 817-822.

Maitland, M.E., S.V. Ajemian, and E. Suter. 1999. Quadriceps femoris and hamstring muscle function in a person with an unstable knee. *Phys Ther* 79: 66-75.

Malinzak, R.A., S.M. Colby, D.T. Kirkendall, B. Yu, and W.E. Garrett. 2001. A comparison of knee joint motion patterns between men and women in selected athletic tasks. *Clin Biomech* 16: 438-445.

Malone, T.R., W.T. Hardaker, W.E. Garrett, et al. 1993. Relationship of gender to anterior cruciate ligament injuries in intercollegiate basketball players. *J South Orthop Assoc* 2: 36-39.

Mandelbaum, B. 2002. ACL prevention strategies in the female athlete and soccer: Implementation of a neuromuscular training program to determine its efficacy on the incidence of ACL injury. Abstract presented at the AOSSM 2002 Specialty Day, Dallas, TX.

Mandelbaum, B.R., H.J. Silvers, D.S. Watanabe, J.F. Knarr, S.D. Thomas, L.Y. Griffin, D.T. Kirkendall, and W. Garrett Jr. 2005. Effectiveness of a neuromuscular and proprioceptive training program in preventing anterior cruciate ligament injuries in female athletes: 2-year follow-up. *Am J Sports Med* 33(7): 1003-1010.

Mankin, H.J. 1982. Current concepts review: The response of articular cartilage to mechanical injury. *J Bone Joint Surg* 64A: 4560-4566.

Mankin, H.J., and K.D. Brandt. 1992. Biochemistry and metabolism of cartilage in osteoarthritis. In R Moskowitz (Ed.), *Osteoarthritis: Diagnosis and medical/surgical management* (2nd ed., pp. 109-154). Philadelphia: Saunders.

Mankin, H.J., V.C. Mow, and J.A. Buckwalter. 1994. Form and function of articular cartilage. In: S.R. Simon (Ed.), *Orthopaedic basic science* (pp. 1-144). Rosemont, IL: American Academy of Orthopaedic Surgeons.

Markolf, K.L., D.M. Burchfield, M.M. Shapiro, M.F. Shepard, G.A.M. Finerman, and J.L. Slauterbeck. 1995. Combined knee loading states that generate high anterior cruciate ligament forces. *J Orthop Res* 13: 930-935.

Markolf, K.L., A. Graff-Radford, and H.C. Amstutz. 1978. In vivo knee stability: A quantitative assessment using an instrumented clinical testing apparatus. *J Bone Joint Surg Am* 60-A(5): 664-674.

Markolf, K.L., J.S. Mensch, and H.C. Amstutz. 1976. Stiffness and laxity of the knee: The contributions of the supporting structures. *J Bone Joint Surg Am* 58-A(5): 583-595.

Markolf, K.L., J.R. Slauterbeck, K.L. Armstrong, M.S. Shapiro, and G.A. Finerman. 1997. A biomechanical study of replacement of the posterior cruciate ligament with a graft. Part II: Forces in the graft compared with forces in the intact ligament. *J Bone Joint Surg* 79A: 381-386.

Marks, P.H., M. Cameron, and W. Regan. 1998. Fracture of the fabella: a case of posterolateral knee pain. *Orthopedics* 21(6): 713-714.

Marks, P.H., J.A. Goldenberg, W.C. Vezina, et al. 1992. Subchondral bone infractions in acute ligamentous knee injuries demonstrated on bone scintigraphy and magnetic resonance imaging. *J Nuclear Med* 33: 516-520.

Maroudas, A., J. Mizrahi, E.P. Katz, et al. 1986. Physiochemical properties and functional behaviour of normal and osteoarthritic human cartilage. In: K. Kvettner (Ed.), *Articular cartilage biochemistry* (3rd ed.). New York: Raven Press.

Marshall, J.L., and R.J. Johnson. 1977. Mechanisms of the most common ski injuries. *Phys Sports* 5(12): 49-54.

Martin, D.F. 1994. Pathomechanics of knee osteoarthritis. *Med Sci Sports Exerc* 26: 1429-1434.

Martineau, P.A., F. Al-Jassir, E. Lenczner, M.L. Burman. 2004. Effect of oral contraceptive pill on ligamentous laxity. *Clin J Sports Med* 14: 281-286.

Mascal, C.L., R. Landel, et al. 2003. Management of patellofemoral pain targeting hip, pelvis, and trunk muscle function: 2 case reports. *J Orthop Sports Phys Ther* 33: 647-660.

Matrisian, L.M. 1994. Matrix metalloproteinase gene expression. *Ann NY Acad Sci* 732: 42-50.

McClay, I., and K. Manal. 1997. Coupling parameters in runners with normal and excessive pronation. *J Appl Biomech* 13: 109-125.

McClay-Davis, I., and M.L. Ireland. 2001. ACL research retreat: The gender bias April 6-7, 2001. *Clin Biomech* 16: 937-939.

McClay-Davis, I., and M.L. Ireland. 2003. ACL research retreat II: The gender bias. *J Orthop Sports Phys Ther* 35(8): A1-A30.

McConkey, J.P. 1986. Anterior cruciate ligament rupture in skiing: A new mechanism of injury. *Am J Sports Med* 14(2): 160-164.

McDaniel, W.J., and T.B. Dameron. 1980. Untreated ruptures of the anterior cruciate ligament. A follow-up study. *J Bone Joint Surg* 62A: 696-705.

McDevitt, C.A., and R.J. Webber. 1989. The ultrastructure and biochemistry of meniscal cartilage. *Clin Orthop* 252: 8-18.

McDevitt, E.R., D.C. Taylor, M.D. Miller, J.P. Gerber, G. Ziemke, D. Hinkin, J.M. Uhorchak, R.A. Arciero, and P.S. Pierre. 2004. Functional bracing after anterior cruciate ligament reconstruction: A prospective, randomized, multicenter study. *Am J Sports Med* 32(8): 1887-1892.

McGrail, M.P.J., S.P. Tsai, and E.J. Bernacki. 1995. A comprehensive initiative to manage the incidence and cost of occupational injury and illness. Report of an outcomes analysis. *J Occup Environ Med* 37(11): 1263-1268.

McLean, S.G., X. Huang, et al. 2004. Sagittal plane biomechanics cannot injure the ACL during sidestep cutting. *Clin Biomech* 19: 828-838.

McLean, S.G., X. Huang, and A.J. van den Bogert. 2005. Association between lower extremity posture at contact and peak knee valgus moment during sidestepping: Implications for ACL injury. *Clin Biomech* 20: 863-870.

McLean, S.G., R.J. Neal, P.T. Myers, and M.R. Walters. 1999. Knee joint kinematics during the sidestep cutting maneuver: Potential for injury in women. *Med Sci Sports Exerc* 31(7): 959-968.

McNair, P.J., and R.N. Marshall. 1994. Landing characteristics in subjects with normal and anterior cruciate ligament deficient knee joints. *Arch Phys Med Rehab* 75: 584-589.

McNair, P.J., R.N. Marshall, and J.A. Matheson. 1990. Important features associated with acute anterior cruciate ligament injury. *NZ Med J* 103: 537-539.

McNair, P.J., H. Prapavessis, and K. Callender. 2000. Decreasing landing forces: Effects of instruction. *Br J Sports Med* 34: 293-296.

McNitt-Gray, J.L. 1993. Kinetics of the lower extremities during drop landings from three heights. *J Biomech* 26: 1037-1046.

Meeuwisse, W.H. 1994. Assessing causation in sport injury. *Clin J Sports Med* 4: 166-170.

Meeuwisse, W.H., B.E. Hagel, N.G. Mohtadi, et al. 2000. The distribution of injuries in men's Canada West university football. A 5-year analysis. *Am J Sports Med* 28: 516-523.

Meeuwisse, W.H., R. Sellmer, and B.E. Hagel. 2003. Rates and risks of injury during intercollegiate basketball. *Am J Sports Med* 31(3): 379-385.

Meikle, M.C. 1994. Immunolocalization of matrix metalloproteinases and TIMP-1 (tissue inhibitor of metalloproteinase) in human gingival tissues from periodontitis patients. *J Periodontal Res* 29: 118-126.

Merchant, A.C. 1965. Hip abductor muscle force: An experimental study of the influence of hip position with particular reference to rotation. *J Bone Joint Surg Am* 47: 462-476.

Messina, D.F., W.C. Farney, and J.C. DeLee. 1999. The incidence of injury in Texas high school basketball: A prospective study among male and female athletes. *Am J Sports Med* 27(3): 294-299.

Meyers, M.C., and B.S. Barnhill. 2004. Incidence, causes, and severity of high school football injuries on FieldTurf versus natural grass: A 5-year prospective study. *Am J Sports Med* 32(7): 1626-1638.

Micheli, L.J., J.D. Metzl, J. Di Canzio, and D. Zurakowski. 1999. Anterior cruciate ligament reconstructive surgery in adolescent soccer and basketball players. *Clin J Sports Med* 9(3): 138-141.

Miller, K.E., D.F. Sabo, M.P. Farrell, G.M. Barnes, and M.J. Melnick. 1999. Sports, sexual behavior, contraceptive use, and pregnancy among female and male high school students: Testing cultural resource theory. *Sociol Sport J* 16(4): 366-387.

Millett, P.J., T.L. Wickiewicz, and R.F. Warren. 2001. Motion loss after ligament injuries to the knee. Part I: Causes. *Am J Sports Med* 29: 664-675.

Mink, J.H., and A.L. Deutsch. 1989. Occult cartilage and bone injuries of the knee: Detection, classification, and assessment with MR imaging. *Radiology* 170: 823-829.

Miyasaka, K.C., D.M. Daniel, M.L. Stone, and P. Hirshman. 1991. The incidence of knee ligament injuries in the general population. *Am J Knee Surg* 4: 3-8.

Mizrahi, J., and Z. Susak. 1982a. Analysis of parameters affecting impact force attenuation during landing in human vertical freefall. *Eng Med* 11: 141-147.

Mizrahi, J., and Z. Susak. 1982b. In-vivo elastic and damping response of the human leg to impact forces. *J Biomed Eng* 104: 63-65.

Mizuta, H., M. Shiraishi, K. Kubota, K. Kai, and K. Takagi. 1992. A stabilometric technique for evaluation of functional instability in anterior cruciate ligament-deficient knee. *Clin J Sports Med* 2(4): 235-239.

Mjolsnes, R., A. Arnason, et al. 2004. A 10-week randomized trial comparing eccentric vs. concentric hamstring strength training in well-trained soccer players. *Scand J Med Sci Sports* 14: 311-317.

Moore, K.L. 1992. *Clinically oriented anatomy.* Baltimore: Williams & Wilkins.

More, R.C., B.T. Karras, R. Neiman, D. Fritschy, S.L. Woo, and D.M. Daniel. 1993. Hamstrings—an anterior cruciate ligament protagonist. An in vitro study. *Am J Sports Med* 21: 231-237.

Moreland, J.D., M.A. Thomson, and A.R. Fuoco. 1998. Electromyographic biofeedback to improve lower extremity function after stroke: A meta-analysis. *Arch Phys Med Rehab* 79: 134-140.

Moul, J.L. 1998. Differences in selected predictors of anterior cruciate ligament tears between male and female NCAA division I collegiate basketball players. *J Athl Train* 33: 118-121.

Mulder, S. 2002. In-line skating. *Accid Anal Prev* 34(1): 65-70.

Murphy, D.F., D.A.J. Connolly, and B.D. Beynnon. 2003. Risk factors for lower extremity injury: A review of the literature. *Br J Sports Med* 37: 13-29.

Myer, G.D., K.R. Ford, J.L. Brent, T.E. Hewett. 2006b. The Effects of Plyometric versus Dynamic Balance Training on Power, Balance and Landing Force in Female Athletes. *J Strength Cond Res* 20(2):345-53.

Myer, G.D., K.R. Ford, J.G. Divine, et al. 2004. Specialized dynamic neuromuscular training can be utilized to induce neuromuscular spurt in female athletes. *Med Sci Sports Exerc* 36(5): 343-344.

Myer, G.D., K.R. Ford, and T.E. Hewett. 2004a. Methodological approaches and rationale for training to prevent anterior cruciate ligament injuries in female athletes. *Scand J Med Sci Sports* 14(5): 275-285.

Myer, G.D., K.R. Ford, and T.E. Hewett. 2004b. Rationale and clinical techniques for anterior cruciate ligament injury prevention among female athletes. *J Athl Train* 39: 352-364.

Myer, G.D., K.R. Ford, and T.E. Hewett. 2005b. The effects of gender on quadriceps muscle activation strategies during a maneuver that mimics a high ACL injury risk position. *J Electromyog Kinesiol* 15: 181-189.

Myer, G.D., K.R. Ford, S.G. McLean, and T.E. Hewett. 2006a. The effects of plyometric versus dynamic stabilization and balance training on lower extremity biomechanics. *Am J Sports Med* 34: 1-11.

Myer, G.D., K.R. Ford, J.P. Palumbo, and T.E. Hewett. 2005a. Neuromuscular training improves performance and lower-extremity biomechanics in female athletes. *J Strength Cond Res* 19: 51-60.

Myklebust, G., and Bahr R. 2005. Return to play guidelines after anterior cruciate ligament surgery. *Br J Sports Med* Mar 39(3):127-31.

Myklebust, G., L. Engebretsen, I.H. Braekken, A. Skjolberg, O.E. Olsen, and R. Bahr. 2003. Prevention of anterior cruciate ligament injuries in female team handball players: A prospective intervention study over three seasons. *Clin J Sports Med* 13: 71-78.

Myklebust, G., S. Maehlum, L. Engebretsen, T. Strand, and E. Solheim. 1997. Registration of cruciate ligament injuries in Norwegian top level team handball. *Scand J Med Sci Sports* 7(5): 289-292.

Myklebust, G., S. Maehlum, I. Holm, and R. Bahr. 1998. A prospective cohort study of cruciate ligament injuries in elite Norwegian team handball. *Scand J Med Sci Sports* 8: 149-153.

Najibi, S., and J.P. Albright. 2005. The use of knee braces, part 1: Prophylactic knee braces in contact sports. *Am J Sports Med* 33(4): 602-611.

Nakajima, H., M. Kondo, H. Kurosawa, and T. Fukubayashi. 1979. Insufficiency of the anterior cruciate ligament. Review of our 118 cases. *Arch Orthop Trauma Surg* 95: 233-240.

Nashner, L.M. 1977. Fixed patterns of rapid postural responses among leg muscles during stance. *Exp Brain Res* 30(1): 13-24.

Nathan, C., and M. Sporn. 1991. Cytokines in context. *J Cell Biol* 113: 9811-9816.

National Coalition for Women and Girls in Education. 2002. *Title IX at 30: Report card on gender equity.* Washington, DC. Available at www.ncwge.org. June

National Collegiate Athletic Association. 2002. *NCAA injury surveillance system summary.* Indianapolis: NCAA.

National Collegiate Athletic Association. 2004. *1981-82–2003-04 Sports sponsorship and participation report.* Prepared by Corey Bray, Associate Director of Research, National Collegiate Athletic Association. Indianapolis: NCAA.

National Federation of State High School Associations (NFHS). 2005. *2004-2005 High school athletics participation survey.* National Federation of State High School Associations: Indianapolis.

Naylor, A.H., D. Gardner, and L. Zaichowsky. 2001. Drug use patterns among high school athletes and nonathletes. *Adolescence* 36(144): 627-639.

Neilson, A.B., and J. Yde. 1991. Epidemiology of acute knee injuries: A prospective hospital investigation. *J Trauma* 31: 1644-1648.

Neitfeld, J.J., B. Wilbrink, M. Helle, et al. 1990. Interleukin-I induced interleukin-6 is required for the inhibition of proteoglycan synthesis by interleukin-i in human cartilage. *Arthritis Rheum* 33: 1695-1701.

Neptune, R.R., I.C. Wright, et al. 1999. Muscle coordination and function during cutting movements. *Med Sci Sports Exerc* 31(2): 294-302.

Nestour, E.L., J. Marraoui, N. Lahlou, M. Roger, D.D. Ziegler, and P. Bouchard. 1993. Role of estradiol in the rise in follicle-stimulating hormone levels during the luteal-follicular transition. *J Clin Endocrinol Metabol* 77: 439-442.

Neumann, D.A. 1989. Biomechanical analysis of selected principles of hip joint protection. *Arthritis Care Res* 2(4): 146-155.

Newton, R.U., W.J. Kraemer, and K. Hakkinen. 1999. Effects of ballistic training on preseason preparation of elite volleyball players. *Med Sci Sports Exerc* 31: 323-330.

Nguyen, D. 2001. In-line skating injuries in children: A 10-year review. *J Pediatr Orthop* 21(5): 613-618.

Nicholas, J.A. 1970. Injuries to knee ligaments: Relationship to looseness and tightness in football players. *JAMA* 212: 2236-2239.

Nichols, A., L. Yu, J. Garrick, and R. Requa. 1998. Anterior cruciate ligament injury in two international figure skaters. Mechanism of injury. Third Congress on the Sports Medicine and Sports Science of Skating, Philadelphia, January.

Nigg, B. 1985. Biomechanics. Load analysis and sports injuries in the lower extremities. *Sports Med* 2: 367-379.

Nilsson, C., J. Leanderson, A. Wykman, and L.E. Strender. 2001. The injury panorama in a Swedish professional ballet company. *Knee Surg, Sports Traumatol, Arthrosc* 9: 242-246.

Norkin, C.C., and P.K. Levangie. 1992. *Joint structure and function: A comprehensive analysis.* (pp. 312-313). Philadelphia: F.A. Davis Company.

Noyes, F.R., R.W. Basset, E.S. Grood, et al. 1980. Arthroscopy in acute traumatic hemarthrosis of the knee: Incidence of anterior cruciate tears and other injuries. *J Bone Joint Surg* 62A: 687-695.

Noyes, F.R., D.S. Matthews, P.A. Mooar, and E.S. Grood. 1983. The symptomatic anterior cruciate-deficient knee, part II: The results of rehabilitation, activity modification, and counseling on functional disability. *J Bone Joint Surg Am* 65: 163-174.

Nunley, R.M., D. Wright, J.B. Renner, B. Yu, and W.E. Garrett. 2003. Gender comparison of patellar tendon tibial shaft angle with weight bearing. *Res Sports Med* 11: 173-185.

Nyland, J.A., D.N. Caborn, et al. 1997. Fatigue after eccentric quadriceps femoris work produces earlier gastrocnemius and delayed quadriceps femoris activation during crossover cutting among normal athletic women. *Knee Surg, Sports Traumatol, Arthrosc* 5(3): 162-167.

Nyland, J., S. Kuzemchek, M. Parks, and D.N. Caborn. 2004. Femoral anteversion influences vastus medialis and gluteus medius EMG amplitude:composite hip abductor EMG amplitude ratios during isometric combined hip abduction-external rotation. *J Electromyog Kinesiol* 14(2): 255-261.

Oates, K.M., D.P. Van Eenenaam, K. Briggs, K. Homa, and W.I. Sterett. 1999. Comparative injury rates of uninjured, anterior cruciate ligament-deficient, and reconstructed knees in a skiing population. *Am J Sports Med* 27(5): 606-610.

Oliphant, J.G., and J.P. Drawbert. 1996. Gender differences in anterior cruciate ligament injury rates in Wisconsin intercollegiate basketball. *J Athl Train* 31(3): 245-247.

Olmstead, T.G., H.W. Wevers, et al. 1986. Effect of musculature activity on valgus/varus laxity and stiffness of the knee. *J Biomech* 19(8): 565-577.

Olsen, O-E, G. Myklebust, L. Engebretsen, and R. Bahr. 2004. Injury mechanisms for anterior cruciate ligament injuries in team handball. *Am J Sports Med* 32(4): 1002-1012.

Olsen, O.E., G. Myklebust, L. Engebretsen, I. Holme, and R. Bahr. 2003. Relationship between floor type and risk of ACL injury in team handball. *Scand J Med Sci Sports* 13(5): 299-304.

Olsen, O.E., G. Myklebust, L. Engebretsen, I. Holme, and R. Bahr. 2005. Exercises to prevent lower limb injuries in youth sports: Cluster randomised controlled trial. *Br Med J* doi:10.1136/bmj.38330.632801.8F (published February 7, 2005).

Onate, J.A., S.W. Guskiewicz, W.E. Marshall, and W.E. Garrett. 2003. Jump-landing knee flexion angle differences between gender. *Med Sci Sports Exerc* 35 Suppl. 1: S306.

Onate, J.A., K.M. Guskiewicz, S.W. Marshall, C. Giuliani, B. Yu, and W.E. Garrett. 2005. Instruction of jump-landing technique using videotape feedback: Altering lower extremity motion patterns. *Am J Sports Med* 33: 831-842.

Orchard, J.W., and J.W. Powell. 2003. Risk of knee and ankle sprains under various weather conditions in American football. *Med Sci Sports Exerc* 35(7): 1118-1123.

Orchard, J., H. Seward, J. McGivern, and S. Hood. 1999. Rainfall, evaporation and the risk of non-contact anterior cruciate ligament injury in the Australian Football League. *Med J Aust* 170(7): 304-306.

Orchard, J., H. Seward, J. McGivern, and S. Hood. 2001. Intrinsic and extrinsic risk factors for anterior cruciate ligament injury in Australian footballers. *Am J Sports Med* 29(2): 196-200.

Otis, C.L., B. Drinkwater, M. Johnson, A. Loucks, and J.H. Wilmore. 1997. ACSM position stand on the female athlete triad. *Med Sci Sports Exerc* 29(5): i-ix.

Padua, D.A., C.R. Carcia, B.L. Arnold, and K.P. Granata. 2005. Gender differences in leg stiffness and stiffness recruitment strategy during two-legged hopping. *J Mot Behav* Mar 37(2):111-25.

Padua, D.A., C.R. Carcia, S.E. Wilson, and K.P. Granata. 2002. Altered lower extremity stiffness and stiffness recruitment strategies between males and females during hopping. *Med Sci Sports Exerc* 32(5): S.

Padua, D.A., M. Distefano, A.M. VanDoren, W.E. Prentice, J.T. Blackburn, and S.G. Karas. 2005. Gender Differences in Trunk Kinematics and Muscle Activation During Cutting in Division I Soccer Athletes. 2005 American Orthopaedic Society for Sports Medicine Annual Meeting, Keystone, CO.

Padua, D.A., S.W. Marshall, A.I. Beutler, M. DeMaio, J.A. Onate, B. Yu, K.M. Guskiewicz, and W.E. Garrett. 2004. Sex comparison of jump landing kinematics and technique. *Med Sci Sports Exerc* 36 Suppl.: S348.

Paletta, G.A. Jr., D.S. Levine, S.J. O'Brien, et al. 1992. Patterns of meniscal injury associated with acute anterior cruciate ligament injuries in skiers. *Am J Sports Med* 20: 542-547.

Pandy, M.G., and K.B. Shelburne. 1997. Dependence of cruciate-loading on muscle forces and external load. *J Biomech* 30: 1015-1024.

Pasciak, M., T.M. Stoll, and F. Hefti. 1996. Relation of femoral to tibial torsion in children measured by ultrasound. *J Pediatr Orthop* 5(4): 268-272.

Paterno, M.V., G.D. Myer, K.R. Ford, and T.E. Hewett. 2004. Neuromuscular training improves single-leg stability in young female athletes. *J Orthop Sports Phys Ther* 34(6): 305-316.

Pattee, G.A., J.M. Fox, W. Del Pizzo, et al. 1989. Four to ten year follow-up of unreconstructed anterior cruciate ligament tears. *Am J Sports Med* 17(3): 430-435.

Paul, J.J., K.P. Spindler, J.T. Andrish, R.D. Parker, M. Secic, and J.A. Bergfeld. 2003. Jumping versus nonjumping anterior cruciate ligament injuries: A comparison of pathology. *Clin J Sports Med* 13: 1-5.

Paulos, L.E. 1992. Revision ACL surgery. Why Failures Occur Symposium. American Orthopaedic Society for Sports Medicine Eighteenth Annual Meeting, San Diego, July.

Paulus, D., A. Saint-Remy, and M. Jeanjean. 2000. Oral contraception and cardiovascular risk factors among adolescents. *Contraception* 62: 113-116.

Pearl, A.J. 1993. *The athletic female* (pp. 302-303). Champaign, IL: Human Kinetics.

Pelletier, J.P., P.J. Roughley, J.H. DiBattista, et al. 1991. Are cytokines involved in osteoarthritis pathophysiology? *Semin Arthritis Rheum* 20 (Suppl. 2) 12-25.

Petersen, W., C. Braun, W. Bock, K. Schmidt, A. Weimann, W. Drescher, E. Eiling, R. Stange, T. Fuchs, J. Hedderich, and T. Zantop. 2005. A controlled prospective case control study of a prevention training program in female team handball players: The German experience. *Arch Orthop Trauma Surg* 125(9): 614-621.

Pfeiffer, R.P., K. Shea, S. Grandstrand, and D. Roberts. 2004. Effects of a knee ligament injury prevention (KLIP) exercise program on impact forces in women. Prsented at AOSSM Specialty Day, San Francisco, CA.

Pinals, R.S. 1996. Mechanisms of joint destruction, pain and disability in osteoarthritis. *Drugs* 52 Suppl. 3: 14-20.

Pokorny, M.J., T.D. Smith, S.A. Calus, and E.A. Dennison. 2000. Self-reported oral contraceptive use and peripheral joint laxity. *J Orthop Sports Phys Ther* 30:683-692.

Pollard, C.D., I. Davis McClay, and J. Hamill. 2004. Influence of gender on hip and knee mechanics during a randomly cued cutting maneuver. *Clin Biomech* 19: 1022-1031.

Pollard, C.D., B.C. Heiderscheit, R.E. van Emmerik, and J. Hamill. 2005. Gender differences in lower extremity coupling variability during an unanticipated cutting maneuver. *J Appl Biomech* 21: 143-152.

Pope, R.P. 2002. Rubber matting on an obstacle course causes anterior cruciate ligament ruptures and its removal eliminates them. *Mil Med* 167(4): 355-358.

Powers, C.M. 2003. The influence of altered lower-extremity kinematics on patellofemoral joint dysfunction: A theoretical perspective. *J Orthop Sports Phys Ther* 33: 639-646.

Powers, C.M., S.M. Sigward, S. Ota, et al. 2004. The influence of an ACL injury training program on knee mechanics during a side-step cutting maneuver. *J Athl Train* 39: S27.

Prapavessis, H., and P.J. McNair. 1999. Effects of instruction in jumping technique and experience jumping on ground reaction forces. *J Orthop Sports Phys Ther* 29: 352-356.

Prapavessis, H., P.J. McNair, K. Anderson, and M. Hohepa. 2003. Decreasing landing forces in children: The effect of instructions. *J Orthop Sports Phys Ther* 33: 204-207.

Prasad, R., S. Vettivel, B. Isaac, L. Jeyaseelan, and G. Chandi. 1996. Angle of torsion of the femur and its correlates. *Clin Anat* 9(2): 109-117.

Quatman, C.E., K.R. Ford, G.D. Myer, and T.E. Hewett. 2006. Maturation leads to gender differences in landing force and vertical jump performance: A longitudinal study. *Am J Sports Med* May 34(5): 806-813

Quinn, A., V. Lun, J. McCall, and T. Overend. 2003. Injuries in short track speed skating. *Am J Sports Med* 31(4): 507-510.

Quirk, R. 1983. Ballet injuries: The Australian experience. *Clin Sports Med* 2: 507-514.

Rabe, T., D.C. Nitsche, and B. Runnebaum. 1997. The effects of monophasic and triphasic oral contraceptives on ovarian function and endometrial thickness. *Eur J Contracept Reprod Health Care* 2: 39-51.

Rajabi, M.R. 1991. Immunochemical and immunohistochemical evidence of estrogen-mediated collagenolysis as a mechanism of cervical dilatation in the guinea pig at parturition. *Endocrinology* 128: 371-378.

Ramesh, R., O. VonArx, T. Azzopardi, and P.J. Schranz. 2005. The risk of anterior cruciate ligament rupture with generalised joint laxity. *J Bone Joint Surg Br* 87-B: 800-803.

Ramseier, E.W., and R. Odermatt. 1993. "Warm-up!" Prevention of skiing accidents. A preventive campaign by the Swiss Accident Insurance Organization. *Z Unfallchir Versicherungsmed* 86(3): 194-199.

Reinbolt, J.A., J.F. Schutte, B.J. Fregly, B.I. Koh, R.T. Haftka, A.D. George, and K.H. Mitchell. 2005. Determination of patient-specific multi-joint kinematic models through two-level optimization. *J Biomech* 38: 621-626.

Renstrom, P., S.W. Arms, T.S. Stanwyck, R.J. Johnson, and M.H. Pope. 1986. Strain within the anterior cruciate ligament during hamstring and quadriceps activity. *Am J Sports Med* 14(1): 83-87.

Renstrom, P., and R.J. Johnson. 1990. Anatomy and biomechanics of the menisci. *Clin Sports Med* 9: 523-538.

Rizzo, M., S.B. Holler, and F.H. Bassett. 2001. Comparison of males' and females' ratios of anterior-cruciate-ligament width to femoral-intercondylar-notch width: A cadaveric study. *Am J Orthop* 30(8): 660-664.

Roberts, D., G. Andersson, and T. Friden. 2004. Knee joint proprioception in ACL-deficient knees is related to cartilage injury, laxity and age. *Acta Orthop Scand* 75(1): 78-83.

Romani, W., J. Patrie, L.A. Curl, and J.A. Flaws. 2003. The correlations between estradiol, estrone, estriol, progesterone, and sex hormone-binding globulin and anterior cruciate ligament stiffness in healthy, active females. *J Wom Health* 12(3): 287-297.

Roos, E.M. 2005. Joint injury causes knee osteoarthritis in young adults. *Curr Opin Rheumatol* 17: 195-200.

Roos, H. 1998. Are there long-term sequelae from soccer? *Clin Sports Med* 17: 819-831.

Roos, H., T. Adalberth, L. Dahlberg, et al. 1995. Osteoarthritis of the knee after injury to the anterior cruciate ligament or meniscus: The influence of time and age. *Osteo Cartilage* 3: 261-267.

Rosen, M.A., D.W. Jackson, and P.E. Berger. 1991. Occult osseous lesions documented by magnetic resonance imaging associated with anterior cruciate ligament ruptures. *Arthroscopy* 7: 45-51.

Rosene, J.M., and T.D. Fogarty. 1999. Anterior tibial translation in collegiate athletes with normal anterior cruciate ligament integrity. *J Athl Train* 34(2): 93-98.

Rossi, M.J., J.H. Lubowitz, and D. Guttmann. 2003. The skier's knee. *J Arthrosc Rel Surg* 19(1): 75-84.

Rossmanith, W.G., B. Schenkel, and R. Benz. 1994. Role of androgens in the regulation of the human menstrual cycle. *Gynecol Endocrinol* 8: 151-159.

Rothenberger, L.A., J.I. Chang, and T.A. Cable. 1988. Prevalence and types of injuries in aerobic dancers. *Am J Sports Med* 16(4): 403-407.

Rovere, G.D., L.X. Webb, A.G. Gristina, and J.M. Vogel. 1983. Musculoskeletal injuries in theatrical dance students. *Am J Sports Med* 11(4): 195-198.

Rozzi, S.L., S.M. Lephart, W.S. Gear, and F.H. Fu. 1999. Knee joint laxity and neuromuscular characteristics of male and female soccer and basketball players. *Am J Sports Med* 27(3): 312-319.

Ruiz, A.L., M. Kelly, and R.W. Nutton. 2002. Arthroscopic ACL reconstruction: A 5-9 year follow-up. *Knee* 9(3): 197-200.

Ryder, S.H., R.J. Johnson, B.D. Beynnon, and C.F. Ettlinger. 1997. Prevention of ACL injuries. *J Sport Rehab* 6: 80-96.

Saklatuala, J. 1989. Tumour necrosis factor-alpha stimulates resorption and inhibits synthesis of proteoglycan in cartilage. *Nature* 322: 547-549.

Salamonsen, L.A., and D.E. Woolley. 1996. Matrix metalloproteinases in normal menstruation. *Hum Reprod* 11 Suppl. 2: 124-133.

Salci, Y., B.B. Kentel, C. Heycan, S. Akin, and F. Korkusuz. 2004. Comparison of landing maneuvers between male and female college volleyball players. *Clin Biomech* 19: 622-628.

Sarna, S., T. Sahi, M. Koskenvuo, and J. Kaprio. 1993. Increased life expectancy of world class male athletes. *Med Sci Sports Exerc* 25: 237-244.

Satku, K., V.P. Kumar, and S.S. Ngoi. 1986. Anterior cruciate ligament injuries. To counsel or to operate. *J Bone Joint Surg* 68B: 458-461.

Sbriccoli, P., M. Solomonow, B.H. Zhou, Y. Lu, and R. Sellards. 2005. Neuromuscular response to cyclic loading of the anterior cruciate ligament. *Am J Sports Med* 33: 543-551.

Scarvell, J.M., P.N. Smith, K.M. Refshauge, H. Galloway, and K. Woods. 2005. Comparison of kinematics in the healthy and ACL injured knee using MRI. *J Biomech* 38: 255-262.

Schauberger, C.W., B.L. Rooney, L. Goldsmith, D. Shenton, P.D. Silva, and A. Schaper. 1996. Peripheral joint laxity increases in pregnancy but does not correlate with serum relaxin levels. *Am J Obstr Gynecol* 174(2): 667-671.

Schmitz, R.J., B.L. Riemann, et al. 2002. Gluteus medius activity during isometric closed chain hip rotation. *J Sport Rehab* 11: 179-188.

Schneikert, J. 1996. Androgen receptor-ets protein interaction is a novel mechanism for steroid hormone-mediated down-modulation of matrix metalloproteinase expression. *J Biol Chem* 271: 23907-23913.

Schot, P., J.S. Dufek, and B.T. Bates. 1991. Individual joint contributions to shock absorption during vertical drop landings. Presented at the American Society of Biomechanics annual meeting. Tempe, AZ.

Schultz, R.A., D.C. Miller, C.S. Kerr, and L. Micheli. 1984. Mechanoreceptors in human cruciate ligaments. *J Bone Joint Surg Am* 66-A(7): 1072-1076.

Schutte, M.J., E.J. Dabezies, M.L. Zimney, et al. 1987. Neural anatomy of the human anterior cruciate ligament. *J Bone Joint Surg* 69A: 243-247.

Sciore, P., C.G. Frank, and D.A. Hart. 1998. Identification of sex hormone receptors in human and rabbit ligaments of the knee by reverse transcription-polymerase chain reaction: Evidence that receptors are present in tissue from both male and female subjects. *J Orthop Res* 16: 604-610.

Sciore, P., S. Smith, C.B. Frank, and D.A. Hart. 1997. Detection of receptors for estrogen and progesterone in human ligaments and rabbit ligaments and tendons by RT-PCR. 43rd Annual Meeting of the Orthopaedic Research Society, San Francisco.

Seckinger, P., K. Williamson, and J.F. Balavoine. 1987. A urine inhibitor of interleukin-i activity affects both interleukin-ia and ib but not tumour necrosis factor-a. *J Immunol* 139: 1541-1545.

Self, B.P., and D. Paine. 2001. Ankle biomechanics during four landing techniques. *Med Sci Sports Exerc* 33: 1338-1344.

Sell, T., C.M. Ferris, et al. 2004. Predictors of anterior tibia shear force during a vertical stop-jump. *J Orthop Sports Phys Ther* 34(1-PL 14).

Sell, T.C., C.M. Ferris, J.P. Abt, Y-S Tsai, J.B. Myers, F.H. Fu, and S.M. Lephart. 2006. The effect of direction and reaction on the neuromuscular and biomechanical characteristics of the knee during tasks that simulate the noncontact anterior cruciate ligament injury mechanism. *Am J Sports Med* 34(1): 43-54.

Seneviratne, A., E. Attia, R.J. Williams, S.A. Rodeo, and J.A. Hannafin. 2004. The effect of estrogen on ovine anterior cruciate ligament fibroblasts. *Am J Sports Med* 32(7): 1613-1618.

Seward, H., T. Wrigley, G. Waddington, and N. Lacey. 1999. A comparative study of balance board and jump landing training on Australian footballers. Presented at the Fifth IOC World Congress on Sport Sciences, Sydney, NSW, Oct. 31-Nov. 5.

Shangold, M., and G. Mirkin. 1988. *Women and exercise.* Philadelphia: Davis.

Sharma, L. 2004. The role of proprioceptive deficits, ligamentous laxity, and malalignment in development and progression of knee osteoarthritis. *J Rheumatol* 31: 87-92.

Sharma, L., K.W. Hayes, D.T. Felson, T.S. Buchanan, G. Kirwan-Mellis, C. Lou, Y.C. Pai, and D.D. Dunlop. 1999a. Does laxity alter the relationship between strength and physical function in knee osteoarthritis? *Arthritis Rheum* 42(1): 25-32.

Sharma, L., C. Lou, D.T. Felson, D.D. Dunlop, G. Kirwan-Mellis, K.W. Hayes, D. Weinrach, and T.S. Buchanan. 1999b. Laxity in healthy and osteoarthritic knees. *Arthritis Rheum* 42(5): 861-870.

Sharma, L., and Y.C. Pai. 1997. Impaired proprioception and osteoarthritis. *Curr Opin Rheumatol* 9: 253-258.

Shea, K.G., R. Pfeiffer, J.H. Wang, M. Curtin, and P.J. Apel. 2004. Anterior cruciate ligament injury in pediatric and adolescent soccer players: An analysis of insurance data. *J Pediatr Orthop* 24(6): 623-628.

Shealy, J.E. 1985. Overall analysis of NSAA/ASTM data on skiing injuries for 1978 through 1981. In: R.J. Johnson and C.D. Mote Jr. (Eds.), *Skiing trauma and safety* (pp. 302-313). Fifth International Symposium. ASTM STP 860. Philadelphia: American Society for Testing and Materials.

Shealy, J.E. 1993. Comparison of downhill ski injury patterns: 1978-81 vs 1988-90. In: R.J. Johnson, C.D. Mote Jr., and J. Zelcer (Eds.), *Skiing trauma and safety* (pp. 23-32). Ninth International Symposium. ASTM STP 1182. Philadelphia: American Society for Testing and Materials.

Shealy, J.E., C.F. Ettlinger, and R.J. Johnson. 2003. What do we know about ski injury research that relates binding function to knee and lower leg injuries? In: R.J. Johnson, M. Lamont, and J.E. Shealy (Eds.), *Skiing trauma and safety* (Vol. 14, pp. 36-52). ASTM STP 1440. West Conshohocken, PA: American Society for Testing and Materials.

Shelbourne, K.D., T.J. Davis, and T.E. Klootwyk. 1998. The relationship between intercondylar notch width of the femur and the incidence of anterior cruciate ligament tears: A prospective study. *Am J Sports Med* 26: 402-408.

Shelbourne, K.D., T.E. Klootwyk, J.H. Wilckens, and M.S. De Carlo. 1995. Ligament stability two to six years after anterior cruciate ligament reconstruction with autogenous patellar tendon graft and participation in accelerated rehabilitation program. *Am J Sports Med* 23(5): 575-579.

Shelbourne, K.D., and P.A. Nitz. 1991. The O'Donoghue triad revisited. Combined knee injuries involving anterior cruciate and medial collateral ligament tears. *Am J Sports Med* 19: 474-477.

Shepard, M.K., and Y.D. Senturia. 1977. Comparison of serum progesterone and endometrial biopsy for confirmation of ovulation and evaluation of luteal function. *Fertil Steril* 28(5): 541-548.

Sherman, M.F., R.F. Warren, J.L. Marshall, et al. 1998. A clinical and radiographical analysis of 127 anterior cruciate insufficient knees. *Clin Orthop* 227: 229-237.

Shikata, J., H. Sanda, T. Yamamuro, and T. Takeda. 1979. Experimental studies of the elastic fiber of the capsular ligament: Influence of aging and sex hormones on the hip joint capsule of rats. *Conn Tissue Res* 7: 21-27.

Shimokochi, Y., R.J. Schmitz, S.Y. Lee, T.C. Windley, and S.J. Shultz. 2005. Plantar flexor to dorsiflexor isokinetic eccentric strength ratio and ankle eversion predict tibial internal rotation during a single-leg landing. *J Athl Train* 40(2): S-33.

Shultz, S.J., C.R. Carcia, and D.H. Perrin. 2004a. Knee joint laxity affects muscle activation patterns in the healthy knee. *J Electromyog Kinesiol* 14: 475-483.

Shultz, S.J., B.G. Gansneder, T.C. Sander, S.E. Kirk, and D.H. Perrin. 2006a. Absolute hormone levels predict the magnitude of change in knee laxity across the menstrual cycle. *J Orthop Res.*24:124-131.

Shultz, S.J., P.A. Houglum, and D.H. Perrin. 2005a. *Examination of musculoskeletal injuries.* Champaign: Human Kinetics.

Shultz, S.J., S.E. Kirk, T.C. Sander, and D.H. Perrin. 2005b. Sex differences in knee laxity change across the female menstrual cycle. *J Sports Med Phys Fit* 45:594-603.

Shultz, S.J., and D.H. Perrin. 1999a. The role of dynamic hamstring activation in preventing knee ligament injury. *Athl Ther Today* 4: 49-53.

Shultz, S.J., and D.H. Perrin. 1999b. Using surface electromyography to assess sex differences in neuromuscular response characteristics. *J Athl Train* 34: 165-176.

Shultz, S.J., D.H. Perrin, et al. 2000. Assessment of neuromuscular response characteristics at the knee following a functional perturbation. *J Electromyog Kinesiol* 10(3): 159-170.

Shultz, S.J., D.H. Perrin, J.M. Adams, B.L. Arnold, B.M. Gansneder, and K.P. Granata. 2001. Neuromuscular response characteristics in men and women after knee perturbation in a single-leg weight-bearing stance. *J Athl Train* 36(1): 37-43.

Shultz, S.J., D.H. Perrin, B.M. Gansneder, K.P. Granata, J.M. Adams, and B.L. Arnold. 1999c. Effect of lower extremity limb alignment on muscular activation patterns. *Med Sci Sports Exerc* 31:S284.

Shultz, S.J., T.C. Sander, S.E. Kirk, M. Johnson, and D.H. Perrin. 2004b. Relationship between sex hormones and anterior knee laxity across the menstrual cycle. *Med Sci Sports Exerc* 36(7): 1165-1174.

Shultz, S.J., Y. Shimokochi, A. Nguyen, J.P. Ambegaonkar, R.J. Schmitz, B.D. Beynnon, and D.H. Perrin. 2006b. Non-weight bearing anterior knee laxity is related to anterior tibial translation during transition from non-weight bearing to weight bearing. *J Orthop Res.* 24:516-523.

Sigward, S.M., and C.M. Powers. 2006. The influence of gender on knee kinematics, kinetics and muscle activation patterns during side-step cutting. *Clin Biomech* 21: 41-48.

Silvers, H.J., and B.R. Mandelbaum. 2001. Preseason conditioning to prevent soccer injuries in young women. *Clin J Sports Med* 11: 206.

Simon, W.H., S. Freidenberg, and S. Richardson. 1973. Joint congruence: A correlation of joint congruence and thickness of articular cartilage in dogs. *J Bone Joint Surg* 55A: 1614.

Sitler, M., J. Ryan, W. Hopkinson, J. Wheller, J. Santomier, R. Kolb, and D. Polley. 1990. The efficacy of a prophylactic knee brace to reduce knee injuries in football. A prospective randomized study at West Point. *Am J Sports Med* 18(3): 310-315.

Slauterbeck, J., C. Clevenger, W. Lundberg, and D.M. Burchfield. 1999. Estrogen level alters the failure load of the rabbit anterior cruciate ligament. *J Orthop Res* 17: 405-408.

Slauterbeck, J.R., S.F. Fuzie, M.P. Smith, R.J. Clark, K. Xu, D.W. Starch, and D.M. Hardy. 2002. The menstrual cycle, sex hormones, and anterior cruciate ligament injury. *J Athl Train* 37: 275-278.

Slauterbeck, J.R., and D.M. Hardy. 2001. Sex hormones and knee ligament injuries in female athletes. *Am J Med Sci* 322(4): 196-199.

Slauterbeck, J.R., J.R. Hickox, K.T. Xu, and D.M. Hardy. 2004a. Expression of remodeling genes in human anterior cruciate ligament varies by gender. *J Orthop Res Trans* 29: 1304.

Slauterbeck, J.R., K. Pankratz, K.T. Xu, S.C. Bozeman, and D.M. Hardy. 2004b. Canine ovariohysterectomy and orchiectomy increases the prevalence of ACL injury. *Clin Orthop Rel Res* 429: 301-305.

Slemenda, C.W. 1992. The epidemiology of osteoarthritis of the knee. *Curr Opin Rheumatol* 4: 546-551.

Smidt, J.G. 1973. Biomechanical analyses of knee flexion and extension. *J Biomech* 6: 79-82.

Smillie, J.S. 1971. *Injuries of the knee joint* (4th ed., p. 68). Edinburgh: Churchill Livingstone.

Smith, A.D., and R. Ludington. 1989. Injuries in elite pair skaters and ice dancers. *Am J Sports Med* 17: 482-488.

Smith, A.D., and L.J. Micheli. 1982. Injuries in competitive figure skaters. *Physician Sportsmed* 19: 36-47.

Smith, B.A., G.A. Livesay, and S.L.Y. Woo. 1993. Biology and biomechanics of the anterior cruciate ligament. *Clin Sports Med* 12(4): 637-670.

Smith, K.D., L.J. Rodriguez, R.K. Tcholakian, and E. Steinberger. 1979. The relation between plasma testosterone levels and the lengths of phases of the menstrual cycle. *Fertil Steril* 32(4): 403-407.

Snellman, K., J. Parkkari, P. Kannus, J. Leppala, I. Vuori, and M. Jarvinen. 2001. Sports injuries in floorball: A prospective one-year follow-up study. *Int J Sports Med* 22(7): 531-536.

Sobel, E., S. Levitz, M. Caselli, Z. Brentnall, and M.Q. Tran. 1999. Natural history of the rearfoot angle: Preliminary values in 150 children. *Foot Ankle Int* 20(2): 119-125.

Soderman, K., H. Alfredson, T. Pietila, et al. 2001. Risk factors for leg injuries in female soccer players: A prospective investigation during one out-door season. *Knee Surg, Sports Traumatol, Arthrosc* 9: 313-321.

Soderman, K., S. Werner, T. Pietila, B. Engstrom, and H. Alfredson. 2000. Balance board training: Prevention of traumatic injuries of the lower extremities in female soccer players? A Prospective Randomized Intervention Study. *Knee Surg, Sports Traumatol, Arthrosc* 8: 356-363.

Sojka, P., H. Johansson, P. Sjolander, R. Lorentson, and M. Djupsjobacka. 1989. Fusimotor neurons can be reflexively influenced by activity in receptor afferents from the posterior cruciate ligament. *Brain Res* 483: 177-183.

Solomon, R.L., and L.J. Micheli. 1986. Technique as a consideration in modern dance injuries. *Physician Sportsmed* 14(8): 83-92.

Solomon, R., L.J. Micheli, J. Solomon, et al. 1995. The "cost" of injuries in a professional ballet company: Anatomy of a season. *Med Probl Perform Art* 10(1): 3-10.

Solomonow, M., R. Baratta, and R. D'Ambrosia. 1989. The role of the hamstrings in the rehabilitation of the anterior cruciate ligament-deficient knee in athletes. *Sports Med* 7: 42-48.

Solomonow, M., R. Baratta, B.H. Shou, H. Shoji, W. Bose, C. Beck, and R. D'Ambrosia. 1987. The synergistic action of the anterior cruciate ligament and thigh muscles in maintaining joint stability. *Am J Sports Med* 15(3): 207-213.

Solomonow, M., and M. Krogsgaard. 2001. Sensorimotor control of knee stability. A review. *Scand J Med Sci Sports* 11(2): 64-80.

Sommerlath, K. 1989. The importance of the meniscus in unstable knees: A comparative study. *Am J Sports Med* 17: 773-777.

Sommerlath, K., and J. Gillquist. 1987. Knee function after meniscus repair and total meniscectomy. A 7-year follow-up study. *Arthroscopy* 3: 166-169.

Souryal, T.O., and T.R. Freeman. 1993. Intercondylar notch size and anterior cruciate ligament injuries in athletes. *Am J Sports Med* 21(4): 535-539.

Souryal, T.O., H.A. Moore, and J.P. Evans. 1988. Bilaterality in anterior cruciate ligament injuries. *Am J Sports Med* 16(5): 449-454.

Speer, K.P., C.E. Spritzer, F.H. Bassett III, J.A. Feagin Jr., and W.E. Garrett Jr. 1992. Osseous injury associated with acute tears of the anterior cruciate ligament. *Am J Sports Med* 20: 382-389.

Speer, K.P., R.F. Warren, T.L. Wickiewicz, L. Horowitz, and L. Henderson. 1995. Observations on the injury mechanism of anterior cruciate ligament tears in skiers. *Am J Sports Med* 23(1): 77-81.

Spindler, K.P., J.P. Schlis, J.A. Bergfeld, J.T. Andrish, G.G Weiker, T.E. Anderson, D.W. Piriano, B.J. Richmond, and S.V. Medendorf. 1993. Prospective study of osseous, articular, and meniscal lesions in recent anterior cruciate ligament tears by magnetic resonance imaging and arthroscopy. *Am J Sports Med* 21(4): 551-557.

Stacoff, A., X. Kaelin, and E. Stuessi. 1988. The impact in landing after a volleyball block. In: A.P. Hollander, P.A. Huijing, and G.J. van Ingen Schenau (Eds.), *Biomechanics XI-B* (pp. 694-700). Amsterdam: Free University Press.

Staeubli, H.U., O. Adam, W. Becker, and R. Burgkart. 1999. Anterior cruciate ligament and intercondylar notch in the coronal oblique plane: Anatomy complemented by magnetic resonance imaging in cruciate ligament-intact knees. *Arthroscopy* 15(4): 349-359.

Staheli, L.T., M. Corbett, C. Wyss, and H. King. 1985. Lower extremity rotational problems in children. Normal values to guide management. *J Bone Joint Surg Br* 67A(1): 39-47.

Stauffer, R.N., E.Y. Chao, and A.N. Gyory. 1997. Biomechanical gait analysis of the diseased knee joint. *Clin Orthop* 126: 246-255.

Steele, J.R. 1986. A kinetic and kinematic analysis of a cruciate ligament rupture in netball. *Abstracts of the XXII FIMS World Congress of Sports Medicine,* Brisbane, Queensland, September 20-28, p. 262.

Steele, J.R., and J.M.M. Brown. 1999. Effects of chronic anterior cruciate ligament deficiency on muscle activation patterns during an abrupt deceleration task. *Clin Biomech* 14: 247-257.

Steele, J.R., and P.D. Milburn. 1987a. Ground reaction forces in netball. *J Hum Mvmnt Stud* 13: 399-410.

Steele, J.R., and P.D. Milburn. 1987b. A kinematic analysis of netball landing techniques. *Aust J Sci Med Sport* 19: 23-27.

Stevenson, H., J. Webster, R. Johnson, and B. Beynnon. 1998. Gender differences in knee injury epidemiology among competitive alpine ski racers. *Iowa Orthop J* 18: 64-66.

Strand, T., R. Tvedte, L. Engebretsen, and A. Tegnander. 1990. [Anterior cruciate ligament injuries in handball playing. Mechanisms and incidence of injuries]. *Tidsskr Nor Laegeforen* 110: 2222-2225.

Strickland, S.M., T.W. Belknap, S.A. Turner, T.M. Wright, and J.A. Hannafin. 2003. Lack of hormonal influences on mechanical properties of sheep knee ligaments. *Am J Sports Med* 31(2): 210-215.

Tan, V., R.M. Seldes, and A. Daluiski. 2001. In-line skating injuries. *Sports Med* 31(9): 691-699.

Tang, W.M., Y.H. Zhu, and K.Y. Chiu. 2000. Axial alignment of the lower extremity in Chinese adults. *J Bone Joint Surg Am* 82-A(11): 1603-1608.

Teitz, C.C. 2002. Dance. In: M.L. Ireland and A. Nattiv (Eds.), *The female athlete* (pp. 611-618). Philadelphia: Saunders.

Teitz, C.C., B.K. Hermanson, R.A. Kronmal, and P.H. Diehr. 1987. Evaluation of the use of braces to prevent injury to the knee in collegiate football players. *J Bone Joint Surg* 69(A): 2-9.

Teitz, C.J. 2001. Video analysis of ACL injuries. In: L.Y. Griffin (Ed.), *Prevention of noncontact injuries* (pp. 87-92). Rosemont, IL: American Academy of Orthopedic Surgeons.

Thompson, H.W., and P.A. McKinley. 1995. Landing from a jump: The role of vision when landing from known and unknown heights. *Neuroreport* 6(3): 581-584.

Thompson, W.O., and F.H. Fu. 1993. The meniscus in the cruciate-deficient knee. *Clin Sports Med* 12: 771-796.

Tillman, M.D., K.R. Smith, J.A. Bauer, J.H. Cauraugh, A.B. Falsetti, and J.L. Pattishall. 2002. Differences in three intercondylar notch geometry indices between males and females: A cadaver study. *Knee* 9: 41-46.

Tis, L.L., D.H. Perrin, et al. 1991. Isokinetic strength of the trunk and hip in female runners. *Isok Exerc Sci* 1: 22-25.

Torzilli, P.A., X. Deng, and R.F. Warren. 1994. The effect of joint-compressive load and quadriceps muscle force on knee motion in the intact and anterior cruciate ligament-sectioned knee. *Am J Sports Med* 22(1): 105-112.

Traina, S.M., and D.F. Bromberg. 1997. ACL injury patterns in women. *Orthopedics* 20(6): 545-549.

Trimble, M.H., M.D. Bishop, B.D. Buckley, L.C. Fields, and G.D. Rozea. 2002. The relationship between clinical measurements of lower extremity posture and tibial translation. *Clin Biomech* 17: 286-290.

Tropp, H., J. Ekstrand, and J. Gillquist. 1984. Stabilometry in functional instability of the ankle and its value in predicting injury. *Med Sci Sports Exerc* 16: 64-66.

Tropp, H., and P. Odenrick. 1988. Postural control in single-limb stance. *J Orthop Res* 6: 833-839.

Tulchinsky, D., C.J. Hobel, E. Yeager, and J.R. Marshall. 1972. Plasma estrone, estradiol, estriol, progesterone, and 17-hydroxyprogesterone in human pregnancy. *Am J Obstr Gynecol* 112(8): 1095-1100.

Tyler, T., and M.P. McHugh. 2001. Neuromuscular rehabilitation of a female Olympic ice hockey player following anterior cruciate ligament reconstruction. *J Orthop Sports Phys Ther* 31(10): 577-587.

Uhorchak, J.M., C.R. Scoville, G.N. Williams, R.A. Arciero, P. St. Pierre, and D.C. Taylor. 2003. Risk factors associated with non-contact injury of the anterior cruciate ligament: A prospective four-year evaluation of 859 West Point cadets. *Am J Sports Med* 31(6): 831-842.

United States Department of Health and Human Services. 1996. *Physical activity and health: A report of the Surgeon General.* Atlanta: U.S. Department of Health and Human Services, Centers for Disease Control and Prevention.

United States Department of Health and Human Services. 2004, August. Guide to Medicare's preventive services. Accessed at www.medicare.gov/publications/pubs/pdf/10110.pdf> on September 8, 2005.

United States Department of Justice, Civil Rights Division. Title IX legal manual. 2001, January 11. www.usdoj.gov/crt/cor/coord/ixlegal.pdf>.

Urabe, Y., R. Kobayashi, S. Sumida, K. Tanaka, N. Yoshida, G.A. Nishiwaki, E. Tsutsumi, and M. Ochi. 2005. Electromyographic analysis of the knee during jump landing in male and female athletes. *Knee* 12: 129-134.

van Eijden, T.M.G.J., W. De Boer, and W.A. Weijs. 1985. The orientation of the distal part of the quadriceps femoris muscle as a function of the knee flexion-extension angle. *J Biomech* 18: 803-809.

Van Lunen, B.L., J. Roberts, D. Branch, and E.A. Dowling. 2003. Association of menstrual cycle hormone changes with anterior cruciate ligament laxity measurements. *J Athl Train* 38(4): 298-303.

van Mechelen, W., H. Hlobil, and H.C. Kemper. 1992. Incidence, severity, aetiology and prevention of sports injuries. A review of concepts. *Sports Med* 14: 82-99.

Vellet, A.D., P.H. Marks, P.J. Fowler, et al. 1991. Occult post-traumatic osteochondral lesions of the knee: Prevalence, classification, and short term sequelae evaluated with MR imaging. *Radiology* 178: 271-276.

Vermont Safety Research. 1996. ACL Awareness '96: Parts 1 & 2. Video. Vermont Safety Research, P. O. Box 85, Underhill Ctr., VT 05490, 1994, 1995.

Viola, R.W., J.R. Steadman, S.D. Mair, K.K. Briggs, and W.I. Sterett. 1999. Anterior cruciate ligament injury incidence among male and female professional alpine skiers. *Am J Sports Med* 27(6): 792-795.

Wahl, L.W. 1977. Effect of hormones on collagen metabolism and collagenase activity in the pubic symphysis ligament of the guinea pig. *Endocrinology* 100: 571-579.

Wallace, G.G., P.C. Innis, J.R. Steele, D. Zhou, and G.M. Spinks. 2003. *Feedback device having electrically conductive fabric.* WO 03/014684; PCT/AU02/1074; AU 2002313397.

Warme, W.J., J.A. Feagin Jr., P. King, et al. 1995. Ski injury statistics, 1982 to 1993, Jackson Hole Ski Resort. *Am J Sports Med* 23: 597-600.

Warren, R.F., and J. Marshall. 1978. Injuries of the anterior cruciate and medial collateral ligaments of the knee. *Clin Orthop* 136: 191-197.

Washington, E.L. 1978. Musculoskeletal injuries in theatrical dancers: Site, frequency, and severity. *Am J Sports Med* 6: 75-98.

Wedderkopp, N.K.M., R. Holm, and K. Froberg. 2003. Comparison of two intervention programmes in young female players in European handball, with and without ankle disc. *Scand J Med Sci* 13: 371-375.

Wedderkopp, N., M. Kaltoft, B. Lundgaard, et al. 1999. Prevention of injuries in young female players in European team handball. A prospective intervention study. *Scand J Med Sci Sports* 9(1): 41-47.

Wentorf, F.A., K. Sudoh, C. Moses, E.A. Arendt, and C. Carlson. In press. The effects of estrogen on material and mechanical properties of the intra- and extra-articular knee structures. *Am J Sports Med.*

Westacott, C.I., and M. Sharif. 1996. Cytokines in osteoarthritis: Mediators or markers of joint destruction? *Semin Arthritis Rheum* 25: 254-272.

Westblad, P., L.T. Fellander, and C. Johansson. 1995. Eccentric and concentric knee extensor muscle performance in professional ballet dances. *Clin J Sports Med* 5: 48-52.

White, K.K., S.S. Lee, A. Cutuk, A.R. Hargens, and R.A. Pedowitz. 2003. EMG power spectra of intercollegiate athletes and anterior cruciate ligament injury risk in females. *Med Sci Sports Exerc* 35: 371-376.

Wiegratz, I., E. Kutschera, J.-H. Lee, C. Moore, U. Mellinger, U.H. Winkler, and H. Kuhl. 2003. Effect of four different oral contraceptives on various sex hormones and serum-binding globulins. *Contraception* 67: 25-32.

Wild, M.J., P.S. Rudland, and D.J. Black. 1991. Metabolism of the oral contraceptive steroids ethinyl estradiol and norgestimate by normal (HUMA7) and malignant (MCF-7 and ZR-75-1) human breast cells in culture. *J Ster Biochem Mol Biol* 39(4A): 535-543.

Wilk, K.E., R.F. Escamilla, et al. 1996. A comparison of tibiofemoral joint forces and electromyographic activity during open and closed kinetic chain exercises. *Am J Sports Med* 24(4): 518-527.

Wilkerson, G.B., M.A. Colston, et al. 2004. Neuromuscular changes in female collegiate athletes resulting from a plyometric jump-training program. *J Athl Train* 39(1): 17-23.

Williamson, D.M., and I.M.R. Lowden. 1986. Ice skating injuries. *Injury* 17: 205-207.

Winter, E.M., and F.B. Brookes. 1991. Electromechanical response times and muscle elasticity in men and women. *Eur J Appl Physiol Occup Physiol* 63(2): 124-128.

Wirtz, P.D. 1982. High school basketball knee ligament injuries. *J Iowa Med Soc* 72(3):105-106.

Wojtys, E.M. 2000. Letter to the editor (author's response). *Am J Sports Med* 28(1): 131.

Wojtys, E.M., J.A. Ashton-Miller, and L.J. Huston. 2002. A gender-related difference in the contribution of the knee musculature to sagittal-plane shear stiffness in subjects with similar knee laxity. *J Bone Joint Surg* 84-A: 10-16.

Wojtys, E.M., and L.J. Huston. 1994. Neuromuscular performance in normal and anterior cruciate ligament-deficient lower extremities. *Am J Sports Med* 22(1): 89-104.

Wojtys, E.M., L.J. Huston, et al. 1996. Neuromuscular adaptations in isokinetic, isotonic, and agility training programs. *Am J Sports Med* 24(2): 187-192.

Wojtys, E.M., L. Huston, M.D. Boynton, K.P. Spindler, and T.N. Lindenfeld. 2002. The effect of menstrual cycle on anterior cruciate ligament in women as determined by hormone levels. *Am J Sports Med* 30(2): 182-188.

Wojtys, E.M., L.J. Huston, T.N. Lindenfeld, T.E. Hewett, and M.L. Greenfield. 1998. Association between the menstrual cycle and anterior cruciate ligament injuries in female athletes. *Am J Sports Med* 26(5): 614-619.

Wojtys, E.M., L.J. Huston, H.J. Schock, J.P. Boylan, and J.A. Ashton-Miller. 2003. Gender differences in the muscular protection of the knee in torsion in size-matched athletes. *J Bone Joint Surg* 85A: 782-789.

Woo, S.L., K.N. An, and S.P. Arnoczky. 1994. Anatomy, biology and biomechanics of tendon, ligament and meniscus. In: S.R. Simon (Ed.), *Orthopaedic basic science* (pp. 45-88). Rosemont, IL: American Academy of Orthopaedic Surgeons.

Wood, D.J. 1987. Design and evaluation of a back injury prevention program within a geriatric hospital. *Spine* 12(2): 77-82.

Woodford-Rogers, B., L. Cyphert, and C.R. Denegar. 1994. Risk factors for anterior cruciate ligament injury in high school and college athletes. *J Athl Train* 29(4): 343-346.

Woodland, L.H., and R.S. Francis. 1992. Parameters and comparisons of the quadriceps angle of college-aged men and women in the supine and standing positions. *Am J Sports Med* 20(2): 208-211.

Woods, G.M., and D.R. Chapman. 1984. Repairable posterior meniscocapsular disruption in anterior cruciate ligament injuries. *Am J Sports Med* 12: 381-385.

Wreje, U., J. Brynhildsen, H. Aberg, B. Bystrom, M. Hammar, and B. VonSchoultz. 2000. Collagen metabolism markers as a reflection of bone and soft tissue turnover during the menstrual cycle and oral contraceptive use. *Contraception* 61: 265-270.

Yasuda, K., A.R. Erickson, R.J. Johnson, et al. 1992. Dynamic strain behavior in the medial collateral and anterior cruciate ligaments during lateral impact loading. *Trans Orthop Res Soc* 17: 127.

Young, L.R. 1981. Skier fall modes and injury patterns. In: W. Hauser, J. Karlsson, and M. Magi (Eds.), *Ski trauma and skiing safety IV, proceedings of the fourth conference* (pp. 217-226). Munich: TUEV.

Yu, B., J.D. Chappell, and W.E. Garrett. 2006a. Authors' response to letter to the editor. *Am J Sports Med.*

Yu, B., D.T. Kirkendall, T.N. Taft, and W.E. Garrett. 2002. Lower extremity motor control-related and other risk factors for noncontact anterior cruciate ligament injuries. In: J.H. Beaty (Ed.), *Instructional course lectures* (51, pp. 315-324). Rosemont, IL: American Academy of Orthopaedic Surgeons.

Yu, B., C.F. Lin, and W.E. Garrett. 2006b. Lower extremity biomechanics during the landing of a stop-jump task. *Clin Biomech* Mar 21(3): 297-305.

Yu, B., S.B. McClure, J.A. Onate, K.M. Guskiewicz, D.T. Kirkendall, and W.E. Garrett. 2005. Age and gender effects on lower extremity kinematics of youth soccer players in a stop-jump task. *Am J Sports Med* 33: 1356-1364.

Yu, L., and A.D. Smith. 2002. Figure skating. In M.L. Ireland and A. Nattiv (Eds.), *The female athlete* (pp. 651-660). Philadelphia: Saunders.

Yu, W.D., J.D. Hatch, V. Panossian, G.A. Finerman, and S.H. Liu. 1997. Effects of estrogen on cellular growth and collagen synthesis of the human anterior cruciate ligament: An explanation for female athletic injury. Presented at the 43rd Annual Meeting of the Orthopaedic Research Society. San Francisco, CA.

Yu, W.D., S.H. Liu, J.D. Hatch, V. Panossian, and G.A. Finerman. 1999. Effect of estrogen on cellular metabolism of the human anterior cruciate ligament. *Clin Orthop Rel Res* 366: 229-238.

Yu, W.D., V. Panossian, J.D. Hatch, S.H. Liu, and G.A. Finerman. 2001. Combined effects of estrogen and progesterone on the anterior cruciate ligament. *Clin Orthop Rel Res* 383: 268-281.

Zavatsky, A.B., and H.J.K. Wright. 2001. Injury initiation and progression in the anterior cruciate ligament. *Clin Biomech* 16: 47-53.

Zazulak, B.T., P.L. Ponce, S.J. Straub, M.J. Medvecky, L.A. Avedisian, and T.E. Hewett. 2005. The effect of gender on hip muscle activity during landing. *J Orthop Sports Phys Ther* 35(5): 292-299.

Zazulak, B.T., T.E. Hewett, N.P. Reeves, B. Goldberg, and J. Cholewicki. Forthcoming. The effects of core proprioception on knee injury: A prospective biomechanical-epidemiological study. *Am J Sports Med*.

Zazulak, B.T., T.E. Hewett, N.P. Reeves, B. Goldberg, and J. Cholewicki. Forthcoming. Factors related to core stability predict knee ligament injury. *Am J Sports Med*.

Zeller, B.L., J.L. McCrory, W.B. Kibler, and T.L. Uhl. 2003. Differences in kinematics and electromyographic activity between men and women during the single leg squat. *Am J Sports Med* 31(3): 449-456.

Zhang, S.N., B.T. Bates, and J.S. Dufek. 2000. Contributions of lower extremity joints to energy dissipation during landings. *Med Sci Sports Exerc* 32: 812-819.

Zimney, M.L. 1988. Mechanoreceptors in articular tissues. *Am J Anat* 182: 16-32.

Zimney, M.L., M. Schutte, and E. Dabezies. 1986. Mechanoreceptors in the human anterior cruciate ligament. *Anat Record* 214: 204-209.

Index

Note: Page numbers followed by an italicized *f* or *t* refer to the figure or table on that page, respectively.

About the AOSSM

The **American Orthopaedic Society for Sports Medicine (AOSSM)** is a national organization of orthopaedic surgeons specializing in sports medicine, including national and international sports medicine leaders. The AOSSM works closely with many other sports medicine specialists and clinicians, including family physicians, emergency physicians, pediatricians, athletic trainers, and physical therapists, to improve the identification, prevention, treatment, and rehabilitation of sports injuries.

Formed in 1972 primarily as a forum for education and research, AOSSM has increased its membership from its modest initial membership of fewer than 100 to over 2,000. There are 67 Accreditation Council for Graduate Medical Education approved fellowships in orthopaedic sports medicine in the United States and Canada.

Members must demonstrate continuing active research and educational activities in the field of sports medicine. Such activities may include service as a team physician at any level of competition; educating persons involved with the health of athletes; service to local, regional, national, and international competitions; and the presentation of scientific research papers at sports medicine meetings. The unifying interest of the membership is their concern with the effects of exercise and the monitoring of its impact on active individuals of all ages, abilities, and levels of fitness.